† HOUSE OF PAIN †

† HOUSE OF PAIN †

NJ Travis

LOTUS WELLBEING, INC. PUBLICATIONS

LOTUS WELLBEING, INC. PUBLICATIONS

House of Pain
NJ Travis

Copyright © 2013 by Nancy Jean Travis
All Rights Reserved

Cover Art: Vincent Stephens
Cover Design: NJ Travis
Copyediting: Jessica Winston, RYT

Web: www.houseofpainthebook.com

ISBN 978-0-61577-845-7 (paperback)

First Edition

For Rocky, Flea and all the Lost Boys

"The best use of a physician's knowledge is to teach patients how to heal themselves." ~ Dr. David Simon

NJ Travis

PREFACE

Dear Reader, kindly be advised that this is a kinky tale about fast boys, rough sex, hard drugs, Tantric yoga and human consciousness. My aim is to inspire you to get all your koshas on the same page, to create union, yoga.

Bad language, explicit sex and gratuitous violence were inevitable ingredients in order for me to exorcise the sickness which inspired me to write this, the sickness which blinds us from enlightenment and causes us to suffer unnecessary bondage to Maya, the illusion of concrete reality.

May all Beings be freed from suffering. May all Beings be at peace.

Om Namah Shivaya
Om Trayambakam Yajamahe

NJ Travis, PYT, RYT-500
Point Richmond, California
January 2013

NJ Travis

✝ HOUSE OF PAIN ✝

Part One: HERE AND NOW

*"How can you hear the Buddha singing
when that dog between your legs
keeps doing circus tricks?"* ~ Hafiz

Part One

HERE AND NOW

†

S&M

It's flat again and flat is nothing but trouble. There'll be blood before the night is over. When Mother Ocean struts her stuff and the Point is breaking head high the boys are too busy to raise hell.

The truth is all the troublemakers seem to disappear into thin air when the surf gets big, probably hiding under the bed. But on days like this there'll be a bit of random mayhem, just because. A full moon with the ocean as flat as a baby girl is a lethal combo.

DJ will be in ecstasy. He never starts stuff, but he comes out of his shell when there's a fight or a reef cut or even a good black eye. There's something dark about my little soul brother, but I'm trying to enlighten him and light him up.

Me, I don't care much for mayhem and bloodshed. I prefer things a lot more methodical. Disciplined. Intentional. Power is the manifestation of intention, desire and control. I like the way it tastes.

Today the ocean is behaving like a girl trying to suck up all my attention unless I've got something better to do and believe me, honey, I don't. My specialty is just being here and now. I've got all the time in the world and I'm absolutely killing it with relish.

The Point Guard doesn't require my services today apparently so my plan is to get my friends off the street tonight. I'm thinking about an early night with Darrell and DJ and some nice bourbon. Then I'll hit the gym tomorrow to stay strong. Maybe. Nothing is ever sealed with a kiss in hot wax as far as I'm concerned.

No one is even slowing down to look for sets let alone park it's so flat. But DJ and Nick are bobbing like corks in the bed of seaweed on the outside reef. Nick's out there because she's half woman half fish and DJ because he follows her around like a bloodthirsty predator. He's too young to know he's just flogging his own heart.

She pretends not to notice him or maybe he doesn't even register on her radar. Like all the boys, he's just background noise. She doesn't think twice about running over any of them, even me, if we get in her way on a wave.

Which is why I call her Nick, because of the damage she does. Her real name is Nancy, but Nick suits her like a wet t-shirt. She's put more dings in the crew's boards than all of the reef and rocks combined. She stings.

Nick never drops in or snakes anyone, takes off deep and follows perfect wave etiquette. You know she has the right of way if she hits you. You bought it: no excuses, returns or refunds. No apologies accepted. All those gym dues she's paid are money in the bank.

The beach is quiet and at it's beautiful best, but most of it is still under water from the full moon high tide. The ocean sucks and hisses like a snake against the rocks and sand. Long boas of seaweed are getting tangled up in the rocks and stranded at the tide line.

My toes are screaming with pleasure as they hug the wet sand. Everything starts in the toes and blows through the top of the head. It's the way humans are wired. Enlightenment starts at your feet. If you can dig that, you can get the chakras.

Which is exactly why I fucking hate shoes! I can almost not be fucked going to the gym because of shoes. But I put up with it because I can destroy myself pretty quickly with the right weights. With yoga at least you get bare feet as a requirement.

I work a couple nights a week teaching yoga. If I fill the room my cut is about $250 or $300 a night and baby I can fill a room. I make more money than a stripper without even breathing hard, in my bare feet. If I had to work a job where I needed shoes, I'd be a very poor man.

I reach down to rescue one of the seaweed boas from its worldly entanglement and wrap it once around my neck for good looks. I wish Nick would paddle in so I can hassle her with a seaweed boa strip tease.

My jeans are soaked and dirty and I'm ecstatic for no reason at all, the best kind of happiness. You can't buy this. It's better than money. I put a hand up to shade my eyes, watching DJ watching Nicky watching Mother Ocean for a sign of life. I'm tempted to just swim out and harass them, because I can and because I love them both, more than air, more than water.

No shoes, no shirt, no brain, no pain. It's irresistible and I dive in with just my jeans and my boa. The water is friggin' frigid 52F as usual so I know I've only got 15 minutes or so before hypothermia sets in. The bone deep pain of the cold water and the ice cream headache feels like a punch in the face and I like it.

There's nothing like pain to remind me I'm alive and kicking. Pain is my favorite teacher. I'm screaming now and laughing as I swim out the hundred yards to the reef. Everything is beginning to go in slow motion and I see Nick turn around and start to laugh at me. DJ smirks. Three's a crowd.

I get that. But he knows I can have any girl I want at the Point if I could be fucked trying. But I've got too much of nothing to do. I don't make time, I take time and I kill it without mercy.

"DJ!" I scream. "Dracula, she's not your type. B positive. Plus she's soooo cold blooded. Come in and drink some bourbon with me and Darrell tonight."

I'm running out of breath, but manage to choke out a few more words. "It's a good night to lock the doors."

Already I feel the numbness in my feet. With hypothermia, first the feeling goes, then your mind starts shutting down. But the most amusing part is when your motor skills disappear. You think about moving your hands but your hands laugh at you. I like the chill but I'm not excited about drowning today.

Nick snarls, "Hello, baby, how's my sweet S&M today?" She usually calls me Sim for short, but now drawls out the longer version "ess-an-em", just playing me up. I don't care what she calls me. It sounds sexy the way she spits it through her teeth.

DJ's mouth drops in famishment. I never fail to be amused by his insatiable hunger. He's just that much younger than I am, seven years younger, that I can laugh at it. I remember it well. Ignorance and craving are the principle causes of pain and suffering in the world. So said Buddha. And DJ knows better because I'm his teacher.

Nick plays me and teases me because she knows I can't be fucked with her. She can rip my heart out of my chest and serve it as an hors d'oeuvre, but she ignores DJ because he's a puppy. She doesn't want to hurt anyone.

"Yeah, bourbon. How about some Tantra with that?" he laughs. I see her cock her head just for a second, listening, then she pretends she didn't hear any of it. But I can read her mind. What could a little shit like DJ possibly know about Tantra?

"See you on the inside, Sim," he says. He gives a long lost look at Nicky and paddles for the beach. I grab the rail of her longboard and splash her a little but she ignores it.

"Shit, Nick!" I beg. "Paddle me in, I'm losing the plot here." My teeth are already chattering and my voice is cracking up an octave. She gives me a pure pity smile and scoots up to the front of her 9'2" so she can haul me up on the back like a dead fish out of the fricking freezing ocean.

I'm lying behind her, my chest between her thighs, my head pillowed on her ass and I'm so numb I don't feel a thing but sweet ecstasy. Then she paddles me into the beach with deep powerful strokes. Her gym dues are paying interest. I can always count on Nick.

DJ is waiting on the beach with a scowl. She kisses me on the mouth just to string him out before she climbs up the cliff with her board. From the sidewalk at the top she yells down,

"Behave yourselves, boys."

"Fuck you, Nick!" I yell back up with my most beautiful drop dead gorgeous lady killer smile. I know how good I look standing here dripping wet in my jeans and bare chest with my green seaweed boa. And she laughs at me because she knows I know and she can't touch me. I own her.

DJ shakes his head hard like he's shaking off a bad dream and looks lovingly back over the flat Pacific and groans, "Nick."

"Not today, buddy." I thump him across his heart hard enough to hurt. "Not likely tomorrow either, honey. Bourbon at my place. Four o'clock sharp. Bring Darrell."

"Sure," he says. "I'll bring some food, too."

"Nothing too bloody, Dracula. Some fish would be good."

It's a brilliant full moon plan. I've got a lemon tree on my deck to tie the fish and bourbon together like a knot. My zucchini is on the vine dying to be eaten, just begging for olive oil, sea salt and cracked pepper. Add a little brown rice and it's a balanced diet.

DJ scratches up the cliff after Nick and I start walking home down the beach, dragging my frozen feet in the hot sand. I pass a girl standing ankle deep on the tide line. I might have seen her a million times, or else a million like her. She doesn't surf. She's as white as a ghost, but I guess she has a right to walk on the beach. I would normally run a stake through her heart by ignoring her but I'm feeling a touch manic today. I'm having fun.

With all the USDA Prime beef I've got on display right now—tan, wet, half-naked—she'd probably turn to stone if she looked me in the eye. God help her if she checks out my construction. I'm betting she's too shy to look.

I'm not smiling so much as purely smirking at her as I walk by playing with my seaweed boa. I can't be fucked talking to her, even saying hi, but I'm tempted to give her a rude wolf whistle. Instead, I settle for a low growl.

She shocks me when she turns her head and looks me up and down and winks. Who the hell does she think she is winking at me? But it's money in the bank. Any girl if I wanted. Then I just ignore her and watch my feet kicking sprays of sand as I walk away. I'm so cool I'm cold. I'm freezing.

Two crack heads in black mugger knit hats, black hoodies and shoes for God's sake are coming down the deck stairs. Shoes! On my beach! Gang banger dealers from across town I'm guessing. I don't know them. They must be new, so they've got to be taught here and now.

I wish Darrell were here to back me up, but it's just me. I take a good look so I can ID them later for Sean. Then I give them the Point Guard dirt stare to let them know they don't belong here.

They look away from me but as they walk by one says "S&M?"

I'm surprised and a little shocked by that, Nicky's pet name for me. I stop and say, "Yeah. What?" I'm ready to take them here and now.

"Thought so, asshole," says his partner as he pulls a gun from his hoodie and fires. One. Two. The pain is bigger than my wildest dreams. My stomach explodes through my back, and the beach reaches up to kiss me.

They're laughing and bolting for the stairs and I hear her scream. I'm far underneath the sea, swimming into her arms as she cries. Then she's whispering in my ear, stay with me, stay with me, stay with me.

I open my eyes for an eternity and see such pain and fear in her eyes it scares me. She's bloody, covered with blood. Is she bleeding? I'm starting to get confused. I want to say goodbye but I've never even said hello. All I can manage to say before I go is "Hold me, honey." I'm so completely fucked.

†

SEAN

Nicky is leaning through the window of the squad car, her smiling eyes dancing like the Milky Way. She makes my day every time.

"Officer Sean, you should arrest me today. I feel so good it has to be illegal," she laughs. She shifts from one foot to the other so her hips are swinging from side to side as she's bending over. I have the best office in the world, beachfront patrol.

DJ is leaning helplessly against the rail at the edge of the cliff like a wild animal caught in the headlights. She's ignoring him, but he can't leave and he can't stop admiring her rear view. It's pretty funny but he's not laughing. He's probably not even breathing.

I get out of the patrol car and walk around to her side. She has to stand tall to continue getting in my face and I think DJ starts breathing again. I smile at him and put my hand on my heart in sympathy. "Hey, Sean," is all he manages.

Something catches Nick's eye on the beach below and I turn to see Sim strutting like a god past a local girl. The girl turns to look but he doesn't miss a step.

"Mr. Untouchable," Nick sneers. "She's another notch for his belt."

"You should talk, girl," I say. "How many hearts have you strung out today?"

"Just S&M and DJ – and now you, Sean. Nobody else was out today. It's dead." She gives me a fake frown and her nose crinkles. I notice a little bit of the dark tan peeling off the end of it. One side of her mouth twitches into a smirk and she gives me the ten-mile dirt stare that all the boys work so hard to perfect, the 'stink eye'. She's got it nailed like a closed coffin and she's putting that fish hook right through my heart, hanging me up to dry. But I'm bulletproof. Sim taught me.

"Not as dead as I'd like," I say as I pick out the two crackers in black death beanies going down the stairs. I've been watching them for a while hanging on the street before going down to the beach. Obviously, they're not the beach type.

I've got them sussed as dealers and I know Sim will give me their details. We're on the same mission, environmental cleanup, keeping drugs off the beach. We started the Point Guard years ago as an alliance between the local crew and the police to keep the beach safe and clean. So I wait for him.

I watch them walk past Sim. There are words and he stops and turns back. Then one of them fires two shots point blank into him. Nick's mouth drops open in shock and DJ turns around confused.

I don't have that kind of time. I grab the radio, press the call button and shove it at Nick. "Ambulance." And then I scramble straight down the cliff face and run.

The girl already has her arms around him and she's talking to him, talking and talking, and she's covered with his blood. Sim is out cold and there's so much blood I can't even try to stop it.

His stomach is wide open and his back is a horror. I scoop him up in my arms and carry him up the stairs. It feels like he weighs nothing.

By the time I get back to the car I can hear the siren. He's still breathing but he looks like a bad horror movie. His skin is cold and wet and his face is blue. His heart is beating so slow I wonder if it will stop. Maybe it's a good thing he's so cold. Hypothermia has shut his metabolism down so much it might save his life.

Nick has her face buried on DJ's neck and they're both speechless. There's too much blood even for Dracula Junior. He's horrified and it doesn't even seem to register that he's got his goddess in his arms.

The medics get Sim in and out so fast my head spins. "Steven Mack," I tell them. "Dr. Mack's little brother. I'll call him. I'll follow you. Thanks, guys."

Then the adrenalin starts running out and I have to lean on the car for my breath.

The girl is still kneeling down on the beach, rooted to the spot. I have to talk to her but I haven't got that kind of time now. I grab DJ and give him a hard shake, but he's so far out of it he can't help me. I give him my cell phone and tell him to get in the car.

Nick is made out of everlasting steel. I can count on her. I give her my card and tell her to have the girl call me. "Get her home, Nick. I'll send another car to pick you up, okay? Call me."

Then I hit the siren and the lights and chase after the ambulance with DJ in the back.

I used to drive Darrell and Sim around in the back when they were kids just to get them off the street. Sim always insisted on being handcuffed so he could pretend he was under arrest. Darrell just wanted to go along for the ride, usually begging me in vain to turn on the siren.

Dr. Mack was putting in long hours at the hospital and little brother Steven, was running wild and free. Unstoppable. No parents, no school, no worries, no control.

All those years of babysitting Mack's brother and his friends paid off in spades. As Sim goes, so goes the neighborhood. There's not one of the Point Guard crew who doesn't love the police like family, especially the lost boys who don't have any.

My heart sinks as I think of Sim as a teenager in handcuffs howling at the moon in the back of the police cruiser fifteen years ago. He never got into serious trouble. He was a good kid. Crazy, reckless, scrappy, absolutely maniacal, but he was always solid. Even now the only hell he raises is with the Point Guard, running the dealers off the beach. I'd like to see him grow old.

I tell DJ to call Mack. I hate it that I know the hospital phone number by heart. Then I get on the radio and ask dispatch to send another car to pick up the girls.

I'm concentrating hard on traffic but in the back of my head I want to pull the car over and throw up. Then DJ gets a flash of enlightenment in the back seat and groans, "There goes the neighborhood."

†

MACK

My day screeches to a stop when I take the call. It's a kid I don't know and he's stammering. I can hear a siren on the line and someone in the background telling him what to say.

"Tell him to meet us at Emergency". But instead the kid says, "Dr. Mack, I think he's dead. Sim. He looks dead." Then the other voice yells, "Damn it, DJ. He's not dead."

The kid says, "We're going to the hospital. Officer Sean wants you to meet us there. Someone shot him." I hear him ask, "What should I say?" And then he stammers some more and hangs up.

I can hear the sirens coming closer. It never lets up at the hospital. I haven't seen my brother in months and I don't want to see him like this.

Jain comes up behind me as I wait by the Emergency entrance and puts a hand on my shoulder. "My shift, Mack. I've got him."

I've never been so happy to see him even though he looks like shit. Both of us are old before our time, only eight years older than Steven, but we look middle-aged. I'm useless with this. I'm a neurologist. But Jain is one of the best trauma surgeons around so I'm grateful he's here.

"I'm sorry," he says. "I can use all the help I can get from what the medics said. If you want to assist – " His words trail off. I don't want to do it but I can't do anything else. I'm here now.

Outside the doors the lot is blazing with flashing lights and then there's a chilling silence as the sirens suddenly stop. The doors slide open and a small parade rushes in with the gurney, two medics, Sean and a young guy bringing up the rear. Steven is laid out with a blood bag and oxygen. His face is gun metal blue.

Jain directs them to OR 1 but I stay behind and shake Sean's hand. "Fuck," I say Steven's favorite word. "He's blue. I've never even seen a corpse that color. Did he drown? I though he was shot." It makes no sense to me.

"Shot twice. We got lucky, Mack. If he were alone on the beach he'd be dead. I was nearby and we got him in fast."

"But he *looks* dead."

"More luck. He was swimming in the ocean without a wetsuit. He's frozen. Hypothermic. Thaw him out slowly, okay?" He's trying to joke but he looks sick.

"Was he in a fight?" I ask.

The kid with him looks up at me when I say that, shocked, startled or excited, I'm not sure which. He could be Steven's much younger brother. He has the same black hair and steel blue eyes. The same tough stare and hard set mouth. Dark bronze tan and tiny silver handcuffs on a chain around his neck, just like Steven. He worries me.

"No, Mack. It's a gang hit. He's high profile. Let me work on it. I've got a witness, a girl. You guys just fix him and I'll be back. I'm praying hard, Mack. And look. No word to anyone. This stays out of the paper for now. His life depends on it."

He sees me staring at the kid and introduces me. "Mack, this is DJ, the teacher's pet. DJ meet Dr. Mack, Sim's brother. Your teacher's teacher."

With that, DJ unleashes an angelic smile on me as if he is truly happy to meet me. Then he hugs me hard and says, "Help him, Doc. Fix him."

Sean pulls him off me and says, "Let's go, DJ. See you soon, Mack."

DJ smiles at me again and points his fist to the ground, thumb and pinkie extended out in a brotherly shaka mudra, just like I've seen Steven do. The "I'm-too-cool-to-lift-my-arm-but-I-love-you-bro" shaka.

Then they're gone, without the lights and siren. I call the shift nurse and tell her to cancel everything for me. Everything. Everyone. I tell her I'm sick and have to take some personal leave. Then I scrub up and head for OR 1.

†

NICK

This could get me evicted. Escorted home in a police car with a bloody girl on my arm – geez, this ought to ruin my rep with the neighbors!

I get her inside, show her to the shower and give her some of my clean clothes, jeans, a tank top and a beautiful pink kimono to wrap herself in. She's shaking but I get her name and call Sean while she's cleaning up. He's on his way here. "I'm coming, Nick," he says. I would normally play him up on that but I don't much feel like it now.

S&M is in surgery. He's alive. I pick up the empty barbell from the living room floor and start curling it idly. All my blood rushes into my arms and I feel the relief as my heart warms and falls into a steady rhythmic pulse. I count the reps in Spanish for more distraction.

Uno. Dos. Tres. I count to Ocho. The shots are still echoing in my head. Uno. Dos. Uno. Dos. I set the bar down against the wall and get two Belgian ales from the fridge. Uno. Dos.

Brandy comes in with wet hair, looking lost and I hand her a bottle of beer. I don't care too much for alcohol but it does the job and she looks like she needs a drink.

She sits in the stuffed chair and takes a thoughtful swig from the bottle. "Who is he?" she asks.

"Steven Alexander Mack, our local 'walks-on-water' god. We call him Sim. Its a little twist on his initials." Cause he's a little twisted, but I keep that to myself. More like S&M than SAM.

Surfer, soul mate, Tantric yogi, bodybuilder, den mother, police informant, heartbreaker, psychoneurotic scientist, seriously freaky free spirit with a sweet heart, I wonder how much of that is left in him now. How much of S&M is going to be left at the end of the day?

I can read her mind. "Yeah, he's still alive. But I'll bet all the tea in China he wishes he were dead right now. He doesn't like hospitals and he doesn't like needles."

She takes another long drink. "I saw him come out of the water with you. Your boyfriend?"

That's hysterical. I wonder how much I should tell her. Just enough to warn her off I think. She saw him come out of the water with me, but I've seen him come without me just sitting there with his shirt off. Yeah, he's my boyfriend but he's the kinkiest ever. We don't do straight sex.

"He's not wired that way, honey. He may look like God's gift to women, but he's a very kinky boy. The kind you don't take home to mother," I can't help but bare my teeth in a big grin at her.

"Gay?" she asks.

"Gay? No way. Oh, God, he's not even straight! He gets turned on looking at his own reflection. He's celibate but he's a real player. He likes to pull the wings off little angels like you for fun."

And he likes to get physical with little devils like me, I muse, but it's none of her business what S&M likes to do.

I try to give her a sweet friendly smile but realize I'm out of practice.

I'll bet he's never been properly kissed before, not like I can kiss. I think he could be had, but it would be like sleeping with my brother so I'm not going there. Two can play this game and I learned it directly from him.

Uno. Dos. Sean knocks twice and I invite him in. DJ is right behind him looking around the room with morbid curiosity. It makes me nervous because none of the boys know where I live. I liked it that way. I can't be fucked with them coming around. I just hope he doesn't start stalking me now.

"What's *he* doing here?" I hiss sweetly.

"I'm babysitting, Nick. Another lost boy. You want him?"

"Hell, no, Sean. Darrell can look after him."

Brandy looks like a ghost with her pale skin wrapped in my pink kimono. And she looks like she's seen a ghost as she stares at DJ, the spitting image of S&M when he was seven years younger.

I shake my finger in her face. "Oh, no! No. No. No. That's a very bad idea, Brandy. He's more dangerous than Sim. DJ doesn't know any better."

DJ frowns at me and I hand him my full beer. "Peace, baby," I say. "And forget you even know where I live, okay?"

He smiles and winks at me. I'm fucked. Maybe I can get police protection.

"Well, here you go, Sean," I sigh. "Her name's Brandy Petersen. She saw everything. She's a nursing student and she's missing training right now. But she got extra credit in acute trauma this afternoon. She's all yours."

Sean sits in a chair near her and starts going over the scene, what she saw, what she did, what she heard. It's sickening to hear it all again so I go get beer bottle numero tres for myself.

Brandy holds her empty bottle out to me when I come back and begs, "More?" so I give it to her. DJ holds his out too so I go back for cervezas numero cuatro y cinco.

I haven't even had a sip yet and I'm almost out. I thank God Sean's on duty and not drinking. There's not enough alcohol on the planet to ease my heart.

When I return, Sean is asking her if Sim said anything. I snort. She looks up at me and asks him "When?"

"Did he say who they were? Any info? Anything?"

"Before they came, he was just walking down the beach. He had this long piece of seaweed around his neck and he was twirling one of the ends like a stripper with a boa. I swear he looked like a porn star and he almost gave me a heart attack when he growled at me. He was so sexy I winked at him, but he didn't say anything."

Cold day in hell, I think.

"After they shot him, when I was holding him, he just said 'hold me' before he passed out. That's it. 'Hold me, honey,' I think."

Oh, wow! She got some traction with him! I make a mental note that it takes a few bullets to sweeten him up. Maybe I should have hit him harder. There's one beer left in the fridge and I'll be damned if anyone but me drinks it. God, I love him.

†

DJ

"My House is full of pain and it's driving me insane
If the House were my skin, I'd invite it in,
but the House is my mind and its making me blind.
The House is my heart being torn apart.
The House is my soul losing control.
The House is full of Pain. Again. Again. Again."

Darrell gives me a drop dead stare. "Those aren't even the words, DJ," he complains. I've been banging my fists in time to the beat on the tabletop. And so I stop.

"They are *my* words. The original song sucked." I say. But I've been thinking that pain is coming into the house from every direction. I am the House, so why am I letting it in?

Sim taught me yoga and the koshas, how to protect myself on different levels: physical, emotional, mental, psychological, spiritual: how to heal and how to use pain as a teacher.

He said the first Noble Truth of Buddha is that the world is pain and suffering. The second Truth is that the cause of pain is ignorance and attachment. And the third Truth is that suffering is optional if you understand the cause.

The fourth Truth is the path to remove pain by understanding, thought, speech, action, livelihood, effort, mindfulness and concentration. He made me memorize all eight remedies to remove pain until I could recite them by heart.

The way he teaches yoga, he always throws that stuff in because he says Buddha was one of the greatest yogis. Sim says pain is the most brilliant teacher on the planet. Number one, it makes you stronger. Number two, it teaches you not to do stupid stuff.

He hasn't taught me the chakras yet because he says Tantra is a little too sexy for me. I'm waiting patiently for that part. I've been nosing through the textbooks at his house but I can't say I get it.

After we left the hospital, Sean took the time to pick up Darrell and drop us at Sim's beach house. He told us to stay indoors and wait to hear from him. I couldn't remember how to get back to Nick's if I wanted to, I'm that lost. I would like to be sleeping at the foot of her bed, just watching over her.

We got a call a few hours ago from Sean saying he's still in surgery. Stay put. If Sim is alive, he's an attempted murder witness and a target. If he dies, you're all murder witnesses. It's messy. Even with me and Nick, we didn't see much but how would they know?

We're keeping a vigil with all the candles in the house lit and we're drinking Sim's bourbon with lemon, but there's not going to be a barbeque tonight because we've lost our taste for anything else.

I put my shot glass down for another pour of bourbon. It's so much cooler than beer and so much warmer. The moon is rising and putting a beautiful silver trail across the water. Sim would approve. He'd just sit here and absorb it and tell us to shut up, breathe and drink, so I do.

I met his brother today. He looks old enough to be his father, but I liked him right off. I wonder if he understands Sim. Then I wonder how much of what Sim knows he taught him.

If Sim were here, he'd tell me. But it's just me and Darrell. Darrell didn't get to see the horror show today but he's pacing me shot for shot. He's Sim's wingman and he's supposed to be in charge now but he's not talking.

"Darrell, it's been ten hours. Call the hospital, okay?"

"No news is good news, but okay." He dials 411 then punches the number in. "Hey, I'm checking on a friend. He's been in surgery all day. Steven Mack.Yeah. How is he? No? Well maybe he's under a different name. Sam? How about Sim? Yeah, Mack is the last name for sure.

"How about S&M?" he winces as he says it, because no one calls him that but us. It's personal. Then he shakes his head at me and listens for a minute. "Come on. Are you sure this is Memorial Hospital?" Then he hangs up.

"What? Is he okay?"

"He's not there. She said Dr. Mack works there but he's on indefinite sick leave. They don't have a patient by any of those names. He's fucking disappeared."

"Call the cops," I say. I'm nervous and start banging on the table again. He calls Capitola station and asks for Sean, then hangs up and smiles.

"It's got to be police protection. They won't tell me where Sean is either. I'll bet he's guarding Sim at the hospital."

"Then call Nick," I demand.

"It's 2am, DJ. Do you think I'd call her even if I had the number? Uh, don't tell me you've got it."

I raise an eyebrow but he calls my bluff. I'm a little drunk and she would have already hung up on me if I had her number.

"Yeah. Didn't think so. Go to sleep. You've got the futon, Dracula. I've got the bed. Sweet dreams."

He staggers into Sim's bedroom, but I don't move. I sit in lotus and put my fingers together in the mudra for wisdom, as Sim taught me. There's a long highway across the sky ahead of the full moon before its gone and a lot of bourbon left to get me there.

I start to wonder who invented bourbon and where did the moon come from and why the surf breaks on a low tide and dies on a high tide. I *know* why. It's physics. But who designed it? Where would I be without the moon?

I wonder how drunk I am. I can't tell without standing up and I'm not going to push my luck any more today.

I inhale through the left nostril and exhale through the right. Inhale through the right and exhale through the left. Again. Again. Again. 99 times counting backwards. I've got a lot of time to kill and I have no mercy on it.

†

DJ

Sim was teaching me yoga one day in the ocean. He said don't bother coming to his class, the physical practice is over-rated. The real practice can be learned sitting still.

I told him I'm happy to learn the physical part if that could help with my sex life and he laughed so hard he almost choked.

"DJ, you're such a baby. You haven't got a clue about sex if you think it's physical. What if I could teach you how to have a hundred orgasms without taking your pants off?"

"I don't mind taking my pants off," I say, especially for a hundred orgasms.

"Of course you don't, baby. But you've got to learn to walk before you run. I can teach you Tantric sex. Or maybe Nick will teach you. But first you have to learn how you're wired. You've got to get the Big Picture."

Now he's got me seriously interested, if Nick knows this stuff, too. Sim is a great teacher but Nick is hot. I want Nick to teach me!

"I'm listening," I say. I'm just about breathless listening.

"Every part of your awareness, every part of sex, every thing you do happens on many different levels. The deeper it goes, the further it takes you."

"What do you mean levels?"

"You've got five koshas, five "coats" or layers of consciousness. Like the layers of an onion, but not they're not physical. All of them are connected and all working together to help you evolve and grow."

"It sounds complicated."

"Well it isn't. It's ridiculously simple." He holds up his hand, five fingers and counts them off. "One: body. Two: energy. Three: mind. Four: experience. Five: spirit."

Then he holds up his first finger.

"One. Your body is on the outside. Annamaya Kosha. That's Sanskrit for the Body made of Food. Bones, muscles, blood, nerves, joints, all the things Western doctors love to cut up and replace.

"But it's not a real body. Maya means an illusionary layer and kosha means something like a coat. You might think the food layer is the physical "you" but its just dead meat without the other layers.

"Two. Pranamaya Kosha. Prana is the energy flowing to all your cells. It's the psycho-neuro system that informs your body's intelligence. Again, it's an illusionary layer because it's useless without the outer and the inner layers. It connects the mind and body. Got it?"

"Yeah, okay, but that doesn't sound too simple."

"Stay with me, buddy, I'm going to make this as clear as sunshine. You are an incredibly complicated being, but it's easy enough to understand.

"Three. The mental layer, Manomaya Kosha. You know this one because most people live in their mind and don't even notice their body or their energy. Your ego hangs out at that level. And trust me, your ego isn't real either. You just keep making it up as you go."

"Four. The experiential layer, a higher consciousness based on your wisdom and your understanding of the world around you. Vijnanamaya Kosha. At that level you detach from your ego and feel your connection to others.

"That's a pretty important layer for good sex," he smiles. "Trust me on that. The fourth layer connects your mind to your soul.

"Five. The layer made of bliss, Anandamaya kosha. This is your deepest core and it's said to contain happiness inside your heart and soul. It's your natural state. You're born with bliss.

"Remember, they are only illusions of separate bodies, like layers of clothing. But they all work in harmony unless you get scattered. The meaning of yoga is union, getting all your layers on the same page.

"But that's really just the blue print for the House. Do you want to know how it's actually built?"

"Sure," I say. I'm still a little confused by all the Sanskrit. I don't understand how it ties together.

"Remember the time you hit the reef and did a face plant on your board?"

"Yeah, I got a seriously bloody nose from that," I smile at the thought. I don't mind blood much.

"Hurt much?" he asks.

"Not really."

"Why do you think it didn't hurt?"

"Cause I was frozen?" I guess.

"Nah. Because it's only physical. It's only skin deep and then it's over."

"Let me show you how it works. Pain is a brilliant teacher."

He untied a leather thong coiled around his left wrist.

"Pull your sleeve up."

I folded the wetsuit arm up a few inches.

"Give me your arm." I could see where this was going.

He whacked me as hard as he could with the wet leather across my forearm, snapping it back so it stung like hell but didn't leave a mark. Then I didn't feel a thing.

"Where's the pain now? Where did it go?" he asked with a grin.

"No pain. Just a memory."

"Right. It's just a sting and then it disappears into thin air. It's just a physical sensation. I didn't hurt you."

"Now, say I did some actual physical damage, say I broke your nose – which I'm not going to do by the way. But say I did it by accident. The pain will go into the next level, the energetic system, because pain is a messenger. It's sending information and instructions to start the healing process. You need it.

"It might take a few days or weeks to heal. But it could go even deeper into the third mental level if you start thinking 'S&M is a real bastard because he broke my nose', even though it was an accident.

"Then it could go even deeper into your experience layer if you let it. Maybe you start to believe I used to be your friend but you can't trust me anymore.

"It keeps radiating inwards if you let it go further. And it can go the other way, outward sometimes. Like mental problems becoming physical, a nervous breakdown or something."

"How about the fifth level?"

"That's your core, your soul. If it gets that deep, you've got some serious pain. You really own it. Now you've lost your teacher and your soul brother because you let it go too far. Your karma is screwed.

"All I did was whack you on the wrist and it didn't hurt. Like I said, that is the simplest kind of pain there is.

"It didn't even register on a mental level because I'm your teacher and you trust me. It didn't get emotional because we're blood brothers. It stopped as soon as it started. It was just temporary."

"Okay, I think I'm getting it."

"Let's see if you do. What if some stranger came up and whacked you with a leather strap like that for no reason?"

"Fucking last thing he would see is my fist on automatic pilot!" I feel angry just talking about it.

"Yeah? Even though it didn't really hurt you or do any damage, you just jumped right past your nervous system and went all mental and emotional on him cause you don't know him. Now it's war, baby. You lost control."

I frown. "So what are you saying? Turn the other cheek?" That didn't sound right. Sim never backs down. He wouldn't be in the hospital now if he did.

"No. What I'm saying is be aware of where the pain is coming from. That knowledge of yourself gives you control. Is it just in your mind? I would just laugh at the guy because he didn't hurt me. He can't touch me that easily. You've got to pick your fights."

"Okay. I got it. But what if you broke my nose because you really meant to hurt me?"

"Then we wouldn't even be having this conversation. It would be Game On and we'd both lose, inside and out."

A nice set was building on the horizon so I took the first wave and left the bigger second wave for Sim. He'd do the same for me. Later on the beach, I asked him how he knows that stuff. Who was *his* teacher?

"Its just yoga, baby. You watch it and it looks like it's physical, but when you practice it you notice the layers, how the prana starts to flow, how it gets into your mind and calms you down. Then you start to feel all tuned up and connected as all the layers unite to create bliss. It works the same way as sex. It's how you're wired. You can get a lot of mileage out of that if you understand it."

He stopped for a few minutes and stared at the ocean. I waited to see if he was going to get into any of the sexy stuff yet. If you could use the koshas to keep pain out, maybe you could use them to let sex in. I wanted to hear more but he just gave a happy sigh.

"My brother Mack was my first teacher, then I studied as much as I could on my own. But now, I'm teaching Nick how to be my teacher. She can really deliver a message to any kosha I ask her for. Body, mind, heart, soul, she really kills me.

"But only because I let her take control. I like to play, so I let her in." He grinned and bit his lip, then spit it back out with a mantra, "Vam!"

†

S&M

I can hear them whispering, but I can't wake up. I can open my eyes but I'm not here in my body. There is fog outside the window and it's impossible to tell if its morning or afternoon. There is fog inside the room too and fog in my head.

It's impossible to tell where the room ends and where my body begins. I can't feel it. There's Mack sitting in a chair and his buddy Dr. Jain is playing with needles. Jain says, "Okay, he's not really cognizant but I don't want him awake yet. I'm going to put him back down for a while." He says, "Rest." Then he turns all my headlights off.

I wake up in the middle of the night and Mack is still parked in the same chair. He's watching me. Sean is in his police uniform in another chair drinking coffee. My whole body is numb. I can't find any of my fingers or toes. I haven't talked to Mack in months and I'd like to say hello but I can't find my words.

He comes over to the bed and checks the IVs. Is that my arm or his? He says, "Good to see you, Steven," as he sticks another needle in some one's arm. What the fuck, I think? He smiles and asks how is the pain on a scale of 1 to 10. None I want to say, but I can just shake my head no.

"It's the strongest narcotic known to man," he laughs. "Go back to sleep, buddy."

A warm flood of opiates washes away my consciousness in a tidal wave, and I think that I'm already dead. I can never be the same person again no matter what happens. It's the set wave of impermanence and enlightenment. I'm not real. I never was. It's all a karmic illusion. I'm so completely fucked.

The third time is the charm. There's soft daylight, and I think its morning because Mack is sleeping in the chair. I can find my hands this time at the end of my arms. One of the arms has got tubes taped to it and there's another tube to my nose.

I like the oxygen but I don't want the needles, so I pull them both out. There's some blood but there's no pain at all. There's no such thing as pain now. Right away a little alarm starts going off beeping.

Mack wakes up and then jumps up and says, "What are you doing? You need this." He rings for a nurse and a young guy comes and takes a look at the drips dripping and the blood bleeding. He starts hooking me up again as Jain comes in.

"Nah," I say. I still can't talk. I don't want that shit in me. I am more stoned than 20 junkies.

Jain says, "Look, Steven. You're not thinking straight. You have no idea what's going on. You'll be really sorry without this."

Then he whispers with Mack and the nurse comes back with leather restraining cuffs. Pretty kinky for a hospital I think. What's up with that? The nurse puts the cuffs around my biceps and straps them to the bed rails. Now I can move my hands but I can't reach the IVs.

Jain gets another needle and inserts it into the IV before hooking it back to the drip. He says, "Sorry, buddy. You're down for the count. Take it easy. We've got you."

He gives me enough of it that I quit caring about any of it. The cuffs make me feel kind of safe, like I can't fall out of bed if I wanted to. I'm much happier now that I'm tied down.

†

S&M

Mack has been sitting there forever. He never leaves. Jain comes and goes but Mack is parked permanently in the chair except for occasional pacing and bathroom breaks.

I'm starting to like the drugs. There's a push button on the drip that I can control every 10 minutes and I'm entertaining myself with a boost of the warm rush. There's nothing else to do.

Mack says we've been here for eight days now. There's no visitors allowed except Sean and another cop. I want to get out. I can't eat. Jain told me he reconstructed my stomach so I'm on liquids. I don't mind fasting; it's not a problem. Food is optional. I run on an alternative energy source, but I can't seem to remember how that works.

There's damage to my ribs and nice sized exit wounds in the middle of my back. Mack says I look like Frankenstein pieced together but that Jain did a damn good job sewing me up. "You still look beautiful, brother," he assures me. "Just a little bit messy."

I can't tell how bad it is because I can't feel it; they won't let me feel anything.

Dr. Jain comes in later to keep Mack company while he eats his hospital dinner. I think I can speak now but I don't care; I've got nothing to say to anyone anymore. I'm just playing around with the control button on the narcotics drip. I've got a method now and I can tell when 10 minutes is up without looking at the clock.

"You ought to go home, Mack," he says. "You know I've got him."

"I'll go home when he does, Jain. I want to take him with me."

"I don't think so. He's going to need intensive care for a long time."

"I can do that. I can handle anything but surgery at home. I'll get a nurse to help me if I have to. I'm not going back to work until he's better. I want to get him out of here. He's going crazy. I'm going crazy, too."

"I don't know. You need security."

"Way up there, it's not likely anyone will know we're on the mountain. It's pretty private. I've got an idea. Sean's also been guarding the girl, the witness. He can guard both of them at my house. She's a nurse almost. I can use her. And I know you'll come over to check on us. What about it?"

I haven't been speaking to either of them all week, but I change my mind now and croak, "Hey. Get me the hell out of here!"

†

NICK

Brandy and I have been holed up at my place all week. We've got a cop watching us and Sean comes by every day to tell us how S&M is doing.

"Same as usual, Nick. Pretty fucked up, stoned on meds and mad at the world. No visitors allowed."

I don't miss the beach. It's been flat and after what I saw last time I'm a little cautious about going back there till we get the all clear. Brandy is trying to study for her exams next month but she's missing classes. Sean says it's not safe for her to go back yet.

Today is different. Sean calls and said he's bringing someone who wants to talk with Brandy. When they come in I offer them some tea. Sean introduces the stranger as Dr. Jain, S&M's surgeon. He's a big gorgeous blond bodybuilder. I know I've seen him at the gym before. A bit older, but really heartstopping handsome. I could have some fun with him, but he's more interested in talking to Brandy.

"I'm a friend of Dr. Mack," he says. "We went to med school together. I'm here to talk to you about Steven, because Mack won't leave the hospital room. But he wants your help."

"How's he doing?" I interrupt. Talk to *me*! I'm his friend not her!

"The same, I guess. Pissed, a little difficult to deal with. It's just going to take some time and patience, but we've got him under control."

"Under control? S&M?" I raise my eyebrows at Sean. "I'll *bet* he's pissed!"

Sean doesn't want to elaborate, so I look to Dr. Jain. "What's up with that?"

"He just wants to get out and off the drugs, but we can't do that yet, he's not ready. But Mack wants to get him out of the hospital and take him home. Which is why I'm here. We made a deal with him."

"You're negotiating control with S&M?" I laugh. "I wish I was there. He can be a lot of fun."

Jain turns red. "I'm not sure what you call fun. We had to restrain him to keep him from pulling all the IVs out."

"Oh, very interesting! Then its Game On," I say. "He knows that one."

Every one in the room falls silent. Sean gives me a glare and I give him a dirtier look back. Then we both wink. I know he knows S&M likes handcuffs. It's Sean's fault for playing cops with him.

Sean says, "I'm not sure if it pisses him off or turns him on or both. The cuffs. I think he's bored enough to make the best of it. He's playing with the IV drip controls to see how high he can get."

"The cuffs just mean he trusts you enough to let you drive," I say. "It means he feels safe with you." I know my boy much better than this doctor.

Jain is speechless for a minute and swigs the tea like it was bourbon.

"That may be so if he agreed to it but he's not feeling very safe in there. He trusts his brother Mack and he trusts me because I've know him since he was twelve, but I can tell you he doesn't trust anything about the hospital or medicine in general. We don't see eye to eye on what he needs to heal."

"So what's the deal you made?" I ask. I want to know how far he's managed to manipulate everyone if he's that stoned.

"Um," he stammers. "We're going to let him go home with Dr. Mack. Mack wants to set up an ICU in his home and bring in a nurse to help. Sean agrees it will be safer to guard Steven there than the hospital. And Steven has agreed to co-operate with us if we get him out of there."

"And you're here why?" I ask.

"They need a nurse. We're guarding Brandy anyway. We can kill two birds at once," Sean says.

"Not really," Jain says with a smirk. "We can kill half a dozen. Brandy's missing school and I'm offering to tutor her and make sure she her passes her exams. She'll get the opportunity to work in private practice doing real IVs, wound care and, not least of all, dealing with a patient. Mack gets to start the private clinic he wants so he can get out of the hospital. And the patient, the wild boy, apparently gets to control everybody in his wake. How many birds is that?"

Now I'm the one who's speechless. S&M is doing just fine. Game On.

†

MAC

We got everything we needed to set up shop within a day. And even a little more than we bargained for. Brandy accepted Jain's invitation without thinking twice, but asked if we would bring her roommate Sunny up to help. I need all the help I can get, so I agreed. They can share the guest room.

With one doctor and one nurse handling intensive care 24/7, the shifts would be long. But with an extra nurse, we could break it up into four-hour shifts, two a piece a day. More time for sleep, and she'd have a classmate to help her study.

I had no trouble getting a hospital bed delivered. I ordered the optional restraints. A deal is a deal, but Steven is Steven. I leased an oxy-pulsometer, racks, drips, and a concentrator. I already had a lot of medical supplies left from when I was taking care of my wife including a wheel chair. It brought back some hard memories, but it got me busy again.

Between Jain and myself we signed out enough controlled substances to knock all of us into next month, each of us signing off on the other's order. We had the ambulance deliver some blood when they brought Steven home. I didn't think he'd need much more after he'd practically drained the blood bank during surgery. Anyway, I'm his type in case of emergency.

Jain rode up the mountain in the ambulance to make sure there was no trauma from getting moved and Steven made it in one piece, very stoned and very happy to see me again.

The medics tucked him in bed without any drama, restraints or IVs. We're all still in the bargaining stage and he's had enough dope to last a couple hours before it starts to wear off.

There's a nice view of the backyard and the pool from the ICU. He hasn't been up here in a long time. It's too far from the beach, nestled in the coastal mountains, very quiet and secluded. I've always dreamed of turning it into a retreat center or a wellness clinic and now I'm trying to turn lemons into lemonade.

"When's happy hour start?" he smiles.

"You're there permanently, buddy," I say. "But I think Jain and I deserve a drink now. Jain? I'll get it. Watch him like a hawk, okay? Keep him out of the pool." I wink at my brother.

When I come back with bourbon and ice, Jain is setting up his chart, taking his pulse, temperature, blood pressure, hooking up the oxypulse.

"Your O2 levels are borderline, Steven," he says. "84% saturation resting is not good. I want you over 90. Are you okay with some oxygen?" He's negotiating patiently. Steven nods, fine, so he hooks up the concentrator.

"How about your pain level, from 1 to 10?"

"None. Can you give me some? I'll take 10."

Jain laughs at him.

"No, I'm serious, Doc. I can't feel anything except fuzzy. Anything would be better than nothing."

"It's coming, buddy." Jain says grimly. "We've got some pain on order. Let's see how long you last without your meds."

We promised to switch him to something lighter, maybe orals, if he stays stable. We've got bucket loads of Norco, morphine and bags of fentanyl which is 100 times stronger than that. We can even go stronger with the surgical stuff if he needs that.

He hasn't got a clue how much damage he's got. Jain told me there are still shrapnel fragments next to his spine but at some point he just had to stop digging and close him up. Besides the bullet holes and the organ damage, it's hard to tell how much nerve and concussive damage was done. It was point blank with a big caliber gun and meant to kill.

For now we just want to let some of the organs and nerves start healing and get the inflammation and swelling down. We've had a long discussion about what could happen if we hit him with traumatic shock and withdrawals at the same time.

It's hard to say which one will make him scream bloody murder first, but its most likely going to be a combination. It's a fine line to walk and we don't want to go too far too fast. Which is why we asked Sean not to bring the nurses up until tomorrow. We don't want to scare them off with arm cuffs and negotiations.

It's nice that he's talking to us again. I need his feedback if we're going to do this.

"How do you want to do this, little brother? What can we do here that you didn't have at the hospital?"

"Give me some latitude," he begs. "I can't heal with nothing but drugs and surgery. There's a big difference between sickness care and wellness care. You know that. Why else did you want to leave the hospital?"

"At this point, we're not talking sickness and wellness, we're talking about life and death. It could kill you if we take you off everything.

"But I understand what you're saying. What can we do to help you heal better? I know we can't do that part for you but how can we help? You can't do yoga."

"Sure I can. I can't do the physical asana but I can do Tantra: meditation, nidra, mantra, all the subtle stuff. I just need to get my mind clear enough."

"Okay, we can work with you on that. Besides taking you off drugs what else can we do to clear your mind?"

"Start with Ayurveda, just help me get back in synch. The last week was all florescent lights and unconsciousness. What time is it now?"

"3pm." I answer.

"Not Daylight Savings. Put the clocks on sun time, real time. So it's only 2pm?"

"Right. Agreed. We'll change the clocks."

"Soooo," he yawns a little. He's wearing down. "Two o'clock. It's Vata time. Vata is air and movement. It's a good time to make some plans and changes. Discussions. Let's talk. You know this stuff, basic stuff, Mack. You taught me a long time ago. Perfect Health 101."

"Yeah, 2-6 is Vata, 6-10 is Kapha and 10-2 is Pitta," I explain to Jain because they don't get teach Ayurveda in med school or at the gym.

"It's Greek to me," Jain says, sipping the bourbon. "What's it mean?"

"Ayurveda means the wisdom of living. It's the sister science of yoga, encompassing herbalism, diet, lifestyle, color, aromatherapy, and sound. It also includes massage and detoxification.

"Steven's into it; I actually taught him. It's the most complete system of holistic medicine on the planet, the study of being in tune with nature, the sun, the seasons, and our Circadian rhythms. There are certain times of day when we're quiet, active or burning up."

"So that's why he wants the clocks turned back?"

"The sun doesn't observe Daylight Savings," Steven says. "The sun rises and sets according to the seasons and it's always straight up at noon."

"And medical science agrees with him," I add. "All the Vata elements — movement, transition, most of our bodily functional changes — happen from 2-6 a.m. Bone marrow gets rebuilt, hormones are released, organs are replenished, which is why we should be sleeping then."

"Is that why we night shift guys are getting old so fast?" Jain laughs.

"It's also why it's the most critical time for patients; it's a rough time with all the changes going on. Most of our waking activity goes on from 2 to 6 pm. It's a volatile time; it's happy hour. So you want to do this, Steven, work with an Ayurvedic schedule?"

Speaking of changes, I look at him and he's gone somewhere else with a studious frown on his face.

"Mack, I could use a shot," he whispers.

"Morphine?"

"No. Bourbon. I'm feeling it."

"No bourbon for you, brother. We're not trained to do pain management with alcohol. We can clean your wounds with it if you like, though."

Jain looks concerned. "How's the pain, Steven? On a scale from 1 to 10?"

But he's gotten back on point, ignoring him. "10 to 2 is Pitta time. Fire and digestion. The best time to eat is noon. 10 to 2 at night is a good time to fast."

"It's all based on common sense and observation," I tell Jain. "Simple stuff."

Jain is watching Steven's face closely as he rambles on.

"6 to 10 is Kapha time. Sunrise. Sunset. Quiet. Surf. Sex. Meditation."

He's fading fast. His eyes are a little wild and he's staring at Jain. "8," he says. "Maybe 9."

"Do you want to stop there?" Jain asks. "I can fix it. Let's see if we can dial it down."

He just stares.

"No drips," Jain says. "Just let me use a needle. A little bit."

"Yes. A little bit."

"I'm not going to knock you out, just get you stable. Keep talking to me."

He uses the fentanyl so he only hits him with a tiny bit and it works in seconds.

"We'll get it dialed," he says. "We've got you, buddy".

"What the hell?" Steven says. "I'm missing some parts."

"What do you feel?" I ask.

"Everything between my waist and my heart is missing. My third chakra is totally fucked."

Jain looks at me confused.

"Stomach, ribs, mid back," I explain. "He's talking about the mid central nervous system. The third chakra is all about power and control. That's got to be messing with him pretty hard."

"There's no pain there?"

"There's pain everywhere else. But it's just deadness there. It's like a river with a damn dam across it."

"Yeah, you've got some shrapnel in your back, buddy. It's just temporary."

"All this shit is," he whines. I've never heard him sound so hopeless. "All this shit is temporary! The whole bleeding world is just a dance. Its on and off, like the lights. I'm so totally fucked."

"Yeah, you're fucked, brother. But keep dancing."

†

MACK

I offer Jain the guest room, but who are we kidding? We're staying up all night between the kitchen and the den, drinking coffee and checking on Steven. Jain gives him a hit every four hours to keep him stable.

Steven sleeps pretty well for most of the night so Jain and I stay up talking about the plan. The more we talk, the better I like it.

I'll put one of the nurses on Kapha shifts and one on Pitta. I'll take the Vata shifts because they're the most volatile. Also, that's the best time for them to study, from 2 to 6 in the afternoon.

Jain can teach them a couple afternoons a week and I can do hands on training with them during my shift. None of us works longer than 4 hours at a time and we all get 8 consecutive hours rest.

It's beautiful and Jain gets the hang of it quickly. Then he starts applying it to the drug therapy. We'll keep him stable with the fentanyl during the volatile Vata hours and try using Norco during the quieter Kapha times. We can play 10 to 2 by ear depending on how he's going, maybe morphine or maybe take him off meds for a few hours.

He's pretty sure he's got the minimum med levels dialed in now and writes out the calculations for the nurses and me. Drips or needle, whichever he prefers, on a four hour dose. At dawn, we give him a couple Norco tabs with some watered down juice.

Sean arrives around 8am with the girls in his patrol car. There's been another police car across the road watching us all night. He waves him off and the car pulls away. All's quiet on the mountain except a few birds celebrating Kapha hours.

The girls are pretty young but I'm grateful. We can teach them exactly what we want, not just rote hospital procedure. I show them all to my office, then give Sean a cup of coffee and take him to see Steven.

"Can I leave you two alone?" He looks rested and a little stoned but he nods, so I go back to the office.

"Thank you, ladies. We're going to be quick. I'll be working with you and teaching you what we need. Dr. Jain will be training you for exams from 2 to 6, but not today cause we've been up all night.

"You're going to get the best training of your life. Jain's time is priceless. You're also going to learn a lot you won't get in nursing school, alternative therapies. But right now, I'm hammered and need some rest.

"I need one of you to take over the shift from 10-2 today and tonight 10-2 again. And the other one comes on from 6-10 tonight and again tomorrow morning 6-10. Who wants the late shift?"

I don't know why I bothered to ask. Sunny is full of fire, red sun bleached hair and green eyes, a Pitta poster child. Brandy is quiet and shy with sweet brown eyes, a Kapha girl.

Sunny says she'll take the late shift. Of course. I say, "Done deal. Brandy's got 6 to 10. You've got time to get settled in your room. Top of the stairs on the left.

"Let me know if you need anything and come back down at 10. I'll introduce you to Damien then. I mean Steven. Just kidding."

Brandy laughs and says, "I know him. Sim. I um - - met him and his friend, Nick."

"You helped save his life. That's why you're here, Brandy."

I see Jain out and go back to the den. Sean is laughing at something Steven said.

"Mack, I can't get used to seeing my anti-drug crusader this stoned. It's amusing," he laughs. "Scary even."

"Yeah. Scary," I say and pull just enough fentanyl into the needle to maintain him at a perfect 4. Before the nurses' shifts start today, I'm going to dial him down to a 2.

†

S&M

I woke myself up screaming last night from all the nightmares the dope is giving me. I think it shook Mack up a bit, but his answer to everything is just to hit me again with another shot. This is not the way I want to play this hand.

I'm not the worrying kind of guy, but now I've got two doctors and two nurses and they all know how to inject. I swear I never want to learn how to use a needle. Even if they get me strung out on this stuff I won't know how to shoot it if I wanted it.

I was dreaming of an old witch but what she was up to in my nightmare has been erased from my memory. What's really haunting me now is the ghost girl. I know her. Dr. Jain brought the two nurses in yesterday and showed them how to set up the drips and how to do the math so they're don't give me an overdose.

I like Jain. I like him very much. He's been my brother's best friend as long as I can remember and I trust him very much. But when he walked in with those two girls my heart stopped. The red haired girl looked a little on the mean side, but the ghost girl I remember had blood all over her arms and so much fear in her eyes it scared me.

I mean she doesn't have any blood on her now, but it's etched in my mind, a far away memory of death that's walked back into the room. I growled at her and then she was covered with blood. Two guys in black called my name and the whole ocean was destroyed.

Mack takes care of me from 2 'til 6. He organized the shifts on Ayurveda time like I asked him. The Kapha girl, the ghost girl, comes on at 6.

To tell the truth, I'm fucking scared. "Don't leave me with her, Mack," I beg.

He laughs at me. He's been up all night but he's easily amused. "You're scared of a girl? You? The sex god of Pleasure Point? That's pretty entertaining."

"I'm not scared," I lie. "I just don't want her touching me or looking at me or talking to me." And that part is true. It's just too damn intimate. She can hurt me real bad and I've got all the pain I can handle now.

At six sharp she taps on the door and comes in the room. She's not just smiling, she's being very familiar like she already knows me. Didn't she wink at me on the beach?

"Mack," I say in a tone that my brother knows all too well, my non-negotiable hard limit tone, "I don't want her near me."

And he gives me his best big-brother condescending tone of voice, "Buddy, she helped save your life. I think you'll be safe with her for four hours.

"Brandy, I'll stay with him while you get some tea. He's a little nicer once he's had some. No sugar. This is as sweet as he gets."

As she heads back out the door, he calls after her, "And honey, do yourself a favor and don't talk to him or touch him or look at him unless you have to. I'm serious. He has some real issues."

†

SEAN

I'm doing the security graveyard shift at the Mack house, six pm to six am. It's a long day, but it's a nice assignment watching over people I know and like. It gets me off the street during the day and from what I know, that's not a good place to be at the moment.

I escorted the nurses up here yesterday and I'm happy to be out of the hospital environment. Both ladies are beautiful and the house is quiet except for Sim's occasional nightmares.

I hang out in the kitchen when I'm not sitting with Sim, drink coffee and talk to the nurses when they take breaks. Mack works from 2 to 6 am and then the girls get to sleep.

Tonight is our second night and Brandy comes into the kitchen to unwind a little after Sunny relieves her. She's looking a little tired and sad so I try to make small talk and cheer her up. She's been under police guard for nearly two weeks.

"Feel safer here, Brandy?" I ask. I felt safe guarding Sim at the hospital, but very insecure when I was guarding her at Nick's beach house. It was getting violent down there.

"Safe, yes, but I'm not feeling welcome. He doesn't like me. Dr. Mack asked me not to talk to him."

"Geez, Brandy, I'm really sorry you feel like that. He's a very compassionate guy actually. I've known him fifteen years or so. What's wrong?"

"I don't know. I like him. I want to help him. Dr. Mack said he has issues. Nick said he's mean to women. But Sunny is doing just fine. She talks to him, no problem."

"What do *you* think?" Sometimes the most important thing we do is just shut up and listen.

"I don't know, Sean. I want to be a good nurse. I can't figure it out. I was there when he was shot, just like you. I tried to help him just like you. I can't figure it out."

Sunny comes in for some tea and I ask how he is. She said fine, sleeping off and on, definitely on a lot of meds. I ask if he's on different doses for their shifts and she says, yes, a much stronger drug at night.

"That could be part of it, Brandy," I offer. "Talk to Mack about it."

When we're alone again, I put my foot in my mouth, but she seems so depressed that I just go for it. "Look, Brandy, if you'd like to get out the house and go for a bite sometime, I'm off during the day. If you need someone to talk to, I mean."

I'm sorry I said it right away because she blushes and says no without even giving it a thought. "Sorry, Sean, I'm not free."

"No offense meant, Brandy. I meant as your friend and a friend of the Macks. You've been under house restriction for nearly two weeks."

Mack walks in for coffee and sits down with us. It's getting on towards 11.

"What's eating Sim?" I ask. "Brandy's feeling a little shut out."

"Maybe we should have a talk in my office before you go to sleep, Brandy. I have some ideas."

And with that they leave me to mull over my coffee alone.

†

BRANDY

Dr. Mack's study is very formal but comforting and inviting, as if a lot of love and work has gone on in here and more than a little is still in the room. The chairs and sofas are old worn leather, soft and distressed with use.

There are very few personal effects in the room except books, both texts and journals. But there's a small bar on one of the bookshelves with cut crystal glasses and decanters.

"You're off for the night, Brandy. Do you drink?" he offers as he pours himself one. "I still have three hours to sober up before my shift. Steven is putting my sobriety to the test."

I shake my head no.

"So let's see if I've got this right. Steven isn't talking to you, won't look at you, and doesn't want you to touch him. At first I thought he was afraid because you reminded him of what happened, but he doesn't scare that easily.

"I've been thinking about it a bit. It's not that he's got an ego problem, because he doesn't. He just has very high standards and self-esteem. When you first met him, or saw him – because he doesn't talk to strange women – he was probably in the best shape of his life.

"But you saw him get crushed. I think he's embarrassed to have you see him like this. He's really just a simple guy at heart, not as complicated as you might think."

He takes a drink and waits to see my reaction. He has my full attention.

"And you, I don't know you, but I'm a great judge of character. You really seem to care about taking care of him, doing a good job, am I right?"

I nod.

"Do you like him?"

I can't answer him.

"Stupid question, I guess. A beautiful free-spirited man who's injured badly before your eyes, it makes you want to help him, doesn't it?"

I don't know what to say.

"I know it makes *me* want to help him, even though I'm his brother. As a doctor I can't stand to see someone get hurt like that. Jain can't stand it. Sean can't either. The whole community was wounded when Steven was shot."

I wait and there's only a long silence. There's not a lot to say.

"Well go to sleep, honey, and think about it. If I cared the way I think you do I wouldn't wait another day without letting him know about it. We don't live forever. I lost my wife five years ago. You never get that time back, my dear."

I've listened to every word and I say, "I hear you, Dr. Mack."

We go back to the kitchen and I want to say good night to Sean. I hope I didn't hurt his feelings.

"Solved it, Mack?" he says.

"Not really a problem. Standard human crush."

"Brandy, I hope I didn't embarrass you by asking you out," Sean says.

Mack laughs and looks at him curiously. "You did what? What'd she say, Sean?"

"She said she's not free."

"Yeah, you're in trouble for sure," he tells me. "I'll have to give you a hand."

†

S&M

I quit ripping the IV out, so Mac's got me down to one restraining cuff on my right bicep to keep me from escaping. It's nice to know I can reach over and rip the tubes out any time, but we have an agreement now so it's under control. I can roll over and sleep on my side now; it's nice.

When Mac's shift ends at 6am he hangs around and parks himself in the easy chair. I can see the wheels turning. Brandy is right on time and gives Mac a cheerful Good Morning while she takes my vitals, but she doesn't bother exchanging pleasantries with me.

She knows better now and I like it better this way, now that she's respecting my boundaries. Don't speak unless you're spoken to, and don't look at me unless you have to check my temperature.

She heads to the kitchen for tea and when she brings it Mac asks her to give us ten minutes alone. She leaves and shuts the door behind her.

"Steven, I want to talk about business. Is it too early for you? I could come back after I catch some sleep."

"What's up?" He just finished a four-hour shift with me and I'm surprised he didn't bring it up sooner if he wanted to talk.

"Look, I really want to work with you, buddy and I'd like to be done with the hospital. I know this can work. You were right about sickness and wellness alternatives. I'm so stoked about incorporating Ayurveda and yoga into traditional physical therapies. We've got a lot of experience between us.

"We can build something really awesome here. I want to start a private practice. Jain is hot for it and he's willing to invest a big sum as a partner. We like your ideas. This shit here," he points at the tubes and the restraints, "this is temporary. I'm trying to plan ahead.

"We get it. Healing doesn't happen in a hospital bed. We're going to get you up in a few days. A little yoga to start and then some serious therapy. Have you ever seen Jain in the gym?"

I can't say I have.

"He's as serious as you were. Benches 275 for reps. Have him take his shirt off some time. We're going to put in all the gear and weights by the pool outdoors."

"No way!" I'm getting interested and excited.

"As soon as we get you out of intensive care, we'll get someone else in and you can start working with us doing therapy. You know a lot and you're going to learn a lot more going through your own rehab. Jain will drop in day after tomorrow to talk to you about the equipment."

"Outdoor gym?" I smile. "Brilliant. No fucking shoes."

"No shoes, baby, if you don't want them. Free weights, racks, benches, pulleys, whatever you need to get your body back. Make a list and we'll build it."

"Mack, I love you! This is good stuff."

"Nice to see your lights are back on. But here's some more business. We're going to build the staff up. Two doctors, two nurses, two therapists. We've got the doctors. We need one more therapist. I want to talk to you about the nurses."

"We've got two now."

"Well that's what I'm wondering about. Do you want to keep them? I can tell you've got issues with Brandy. If you can't talk to her, you can't work with her."

I roll my eyes. True enough.

"Also, I wonder if she feels comfortable working here, whether she wants to stay. Sean asked her out last night. I like Sean but I wonder if that's workplace sexual harassment. What do you think?"

Mack is up to something is what I think.

"He's much too old for her," I say.

"Not the point, Steven. She told him she wasn't free. I just wonder if there was something else – I mean, I asked her if she had a boyfriend and she avoided answering. I wondered if she was seeing one of your friends or something, maybe you had some issues with that. Can you enlighten me?"

"Hell if I know, Mack, I don't even know her. I don't know who she sees. She has a boyfriend?"

"I don't know. She said she's not available but that's all. Maybe she's just blowing Sean off kindly. I was hoping you could give me some advice, brother. Would you have a few words with her and just see if she's comfortable with the situation here?"

"Mack, you put me in a bad spot. I just now got her trained to ignore me as much as possible. I like it that way."

"Come on, Sim. For me. This is business, baby, we gotta sort the staff out. Just ask her if Sean bothered her and if she wants to keep working here. That's it. Then let me know your take."

He hasn't ever called me Sim before. He's playing his hand very smoothly.

"Okay, I'll talk to her, but just a few words. And then we can go back to ignoring each other unless we have actual business, right?"

"If she's comfortable with that," he sighs and goes to the kitchen to get her.

"Brandy, Steven wants to talk to you about your job. He's my business partner as well as a patient, so I value his opinion, okay with you?"

"Please, how can I help?"

"Good morning, Brandy." I say with a smirk. "We're just wondering if you like working here and what we can do for you."

Her face melts from concern into amazement. She stammers a little and I realize she doesn't know exactly what to call me.

"Um, Mr. Mack, sir. I love it here. It's my first real nursing job and I'm so grateful for the training and the chance to work in a private practice. Working with Dr. Mack and Dr. Jain and Sunny, I couldn't dream of a better place to work."

I note she doesn't list me as one of the dream colleagues she gets to work with but I'm still a patient – and not a very nice one.

"Cool. So did it bother you when Sean hit on you yesterday? Is that a problem?" It's such a pointed question, it's surgical. She does another instant transformation, from enthusiasm to humiliation in a heart tick, and she blushes scarlet.

"Uh. No, it's fine. He's a nice guy but I'm not interested. I said no and I think we're both okay with that. It won't be a problem. I promise."

"Cool," I say again and stare into her eyes. She drops her gaze but then looks up right away and holds my eyes without blinking. I focus on her left eye and she still doesn't back down. Hmm. How much heat will she take from me?

"So who's your boyfriend, Bran?"

She swings away from me and looks at Mack as if for protection or an answer and then she just shakes her head softly. Something's up between them.

"Bran?" I continue, putting a little tease in my voice. I feel like I'm sticking pins into a butterfly and I like it.

"You're not free?"

She's speechless. I give Mack a smile and roll my eyes towards the door. I hold up one finger and he nods. He understands me: get out, brother.

She watches him leave and shut the door behind him and she gets really small and helpless suddenly. Then just as quickly she seems to pull herself together, standing a little taller and looking me purposely in the eye.

"Brannnnnn???" I draw it out really sexy. I just want to keep teasing her until she cries. I haven't had so much fun in weeks. My day is going pretty good considering it's so early and I break out my best lady killer smile.

"You're not free?" I growl softly. I'm going to turn her into stone before her shift even starts.

She turns white again but keeps looking in my eyes. And then she says, straight from her soul, "Not unless you break my heart, Sim."

It shocks me. There's no boyfriend. I'm the one she wants. Well, well. I look like warmed over death, but I own her. Then I remember she's seen me in better days. I used to be pretty hot.

Fuck me dead. I own her. Even though I've been so mean to her. Then an amusing thought occurs to me, maybe it's *because* I've been so mean to her! Does she like that? Even more fun.

But I'm done teasing her for now. I'm just going to sign off on this and deposit it in the bank. She's got balls.

"Then I guess you're never going to be free again, baby." I hiss. It's not a promise; it's more like a death threat or a life sentence.

I roll over and pull the edge of the sheet back in an invitation. "Hold me, honey." It's not a request. She kicks her shoes off and climbs in next to me, IV and all, and I wrap my free arm around her tightly. She smells so good and feels so soft. I just hold her and squeeze her. I'm done talking to her.

The door opens and Mack comes back in the room. His jaw drops. He's been gone two minutes and I've got the nurse in bed with me. I've never been in bed with a woman before. I've never done it that way. Beach caves, back seats, floors, furniture, but never beds before. I must look happy though because he shakes his head and smiles in approval.

"Mack, go get some sleep," I say. "I've got your sexual harassment under control."

I just hug her and don't let her get up for the whole shift. At a quarter to ten, Mack comes back in quietly and taps me on the shoulder. We must have fallen asleep like that.

"Shift change, Sim," he says. "Time to let her go." He seems very happy with me. "Nurse, would you please update his chart before you go?" There's a boatload of sarcasm in his voice.

I rub my eyes and grin at him. I'm not speaking to him. He set me up. This is some kind of perverted prescription, but I feel it working. I feel damn good this morning.

Brandy gets up and takes my pulse, temperature, blood pressure and oxygen levels. Everything's beautiful, she tells Mack, except his pulse rate is a little higher than usual. He laughs. She leans down for her shoes and I grab her arm to stop her.

"Bran," I say nicely, so nice I don't recognize my own voice, "it would be nice if you worked barefoot when it's your shift."

She smiles, cradles the shoes in one arm and pulls off her socks. "My pleasure, Sim." She has beautiful feet.

Sunny walks in at 10 sharp and looks at Brandy's bare feet and then at my self satisfied smile and then she frowns at Mac who's still laughing. She says, "I don't even want to know about it."

†

MACK

It's a quarter to six am and I hear Steven stir. His breath is hard and ragged and when I check his pulse it's racing. His eyes shoot open and he stares at the clock and blinks.

"Good morning, brother," I say. "Good sleep? What's going on with you?"

He looks at me, then the clock and he's actually panting and his heart is pounding.

"Hey, bud, take it easy. I've got your Norco. How's the pain? Try some pranayama, okay? Slow and easy breaths."

He takes a deep inhale through his nose and holds his breath to the count of 8 then blows all the tension out his mouth, and smiles at me, then the clock.

I take his vitals and update the chart and ask again, "Bad pain?"

"No, its average. It's under control. No Norco right now, Mack. I've got stuff to do."

"What's got you going then?"

He doesn't think twice before he answers. "Shift change," he yawns.

Oh, man. I roll my eyes. He can't wait to see me go. I hear a tap on the door and Brandy comes in barefoot.

"Hey, take it easy on the nurses, man. I mean it. I don't want to lose them."

"Me neither, Mack. I'll go really easy," he purrs.

He pulls the sheet back a little and she crawls in without a word. He hugs her like a pillow and shuts his eyes.

"Really easy," he sighs.

I check his pulse again and it's dropped to almost nothing.

†

S&M

I'm not talking to her, just holding her. When I open my eyes, she's staring at me. I want to show her something. I'm going to turn her into melted butter, but really easy. I'm a man of my word.

Tantric sex is so subtle you can do it without anyone else knowing but I *want* her to know. I gaze into her left eye, look into her soul, and smile just enough to give her trust.

She watches me and doesn't say anything. Then I start really gently bringing my attention to my first chakra and visualize the color red. I barely move my lips to form the mantra "lam", tongue against the back of my top teeth then lips together, but I don't make any sound. I'm breathing so slow it's almost imperceptible.

Her eyes dilate but she holds my gaze. I'm turning on sexy like she's never had in her wildest dreams but I'm not going to *do* anything. The best way to teach someone is to show them, not to do it for them. I'm not even going to kiss her.

I put my attention on my second chakra and visualize orange. I put my top teeth on my bottom lip and then close them for "vam". No sound at all. I put my free hand very lightly on her tailbone and I can feel the electricity building up.

The third chakra is tough for me because of all the trauma and injury, but I move my hand to the back of her waist, think of yellow and mouth the power chakra seed, "ram".

I try to feel her prana and pull it into me, into my navel center, into that dead part of me. I feel something stir a little in my stomach, a twinge of pain, life coming back. She's really good for me.

Then very slowly I move my hand behind her heart and imagine I'm sending green light into her heart like a lantern at sea. I feel my heart jump. I mouth the mantra "yam." And I feel a jolt run through her.

And with that it all just shoots through me so fast I have to close my eyes. I grunt with pleasure. Orgasm number one. Then it comes again, my whole body, not my sex organ, it's my whole being coming.

I open my eyes again and smile at her. She's melting. "Ham," I breathe the word and see blue light and put my hand on the back of her neck. Now I'm just rocking with orgasms, I can't stop them. Not that I want to; I've been missing this.

There is a world of difference between an orgasm and ejaculation. Without the latter, the former just doesn't stop coming. It's a Tantric trick that changes the rules of the ball game. Control the finish line and you can keep driving all day. This is definitely an improvement over morphine.

I feel the energy pouring out of her heart and down my spine and I'm visualizing it rising steadily up her spinal chord and back down mine. I feel little shock waves coming off her and I'm just bouncing off the walls now without moving a muscle. She's definitely getting some orgasms but not what's she's used to having. Not the Old School kind that wipe you out and finish you off.

I put my hand on the back of her head and mouth "om" but now the sound is escaping out of me as everything goes white inside my head. I hear us breathing "AhOhOohMm!" the primal sounds of human pleasure as the voice rises up the spine. It's no coincidence it's the sound of Om. The whole universe is coming.

My eyes are closed and I'm breathing in time to her, easy, slowing it down. I feel her pleasure and her confusion because she doesn't know what's going on here at all.

I whisper, "Feel nice, baby?" And then I put my hand back on her tailbone and slow it way down. And I start it up all over again.

When I finally stop she takes a deep breath. I've barely touched her but I've fucked her soul. Then I just hold her some more. This can go on and on for as long as I want but I told Mack I'd go easy on the nurses.

"Steven," she breathes. "What are you doing?"

"Nothing, honey. I just lit you up like a Christmas tree. Feel nice?"

I've got it under control. I can do it all day or I can stop anytime. When you have so many orgasms, the cravings are gone. The desperation and drive are gone, but the interest is always there. I love it like beautiful music. And that last song lasted about 45 minutes. But apparently she's not into transcendence yet. She's squirming against me and begging for more with her eyes. Women can be so demanding if you let them in.

"That's good for now, nurse," I scold her. "Calm down. Take a deep breath. Breathe through your nose."

"I'm confused, Sim. I thought you were – "

"Dead?" I laugh at her.

"Not interested in women. Nick said you weren't straight."

"She said what? How do you know Nick?" I'm pissed and shocked at once. My cosmic afterglow is starting to disintegrate.

"I stayed with her for a week after you were shot. She said you're celibate and you like to be mean to women, kinky."

I can't believe what she's saying. I'm going to thrash Nick if I ever see her again. I thought we were close. While I compose myself I give Brandy the stink-eye. After what I just did with her, now she's attacking my manhood.

"Of course, I'm celibate with Nicky, she's like my sister! But I'm not nearly as mean and kinky as she is!

"But I can't say I'm very straight. Straight sex, Old School sex, it can be pretty dull. I like it more interesting. More intentional." Shit, I'm actually brooding now. I can't believe she didn't like that. I like it a lot and I'd like lots more of it.

She takes that as an invitation to start me up again and starts running her hand south of my bandages.

"No. Stop. I'm not going there."

"You *are* celibate."

"It's just not appropriate for that kind of sex here and now. My brother would kill me for one. And you would be fired. You're supposed to be working. I can't take advantage of you like that. End of discussion."

"Then why did you start all that Om stuff with me? You *are* a mean, kinky bastard, Steven Mack!"

"I wanted to get close to you, not hurt you, Bran. I wanted to show you what I like without us having to pay the consequences. You didn't like?"

Oooh, she's mad at me and she's just getting more aroused by the rejection. Now it's getting a bit more interesting. I roll over on my back and give her a dangerous smile, my best.

I pull my right arm against the restraining cuff to show how really powerless I am to hurt her.

"Where's the other cuff?" I ask innocently.

She gets up and pulls it from the shelf and shows me.

"Look, Bran, the only way you're going to get me to do it *your* way is rape me, honey."

She looks shocked and then she looks hungry as a wolf. Well, let her learn. Old School sex doesn't last more than 15 minutes and just creates more desire and cravings. Most of the time it takes more out of you than it gives you. But as long as she keeps it interesting, I'm happy to play with her.

She puts the cuff on my left arm and tightens it to the bed rail so I'm pinned flat on my back and can't move.

"Tighter," I say. "If you're going to do it, take control."

She tightens it more and I grin. She's in trouble. I'm playing her so hard. She's definitely not in control of the situation. I am.

I say, "Honey, you know there are going to be consequences for this kind of behavior, don't you?"

She gets on top and starts kissing me and getting her hands below the waist, stroking my sex, being very gentle and careful not to put any pressure on my ribs and stomach.

I can't say it's not nice. It's pretty beautiful, especially with her fire and anger and hunger. It's not like she can really rape me because I've just given her Tantric soul sex for an hour. She's already mine.

But like I said, it's all over in about 10 minutes. We're done. Spent. Cashed out and exhausted. She looks really guilty and gets up.

"Are you going to leave me like this, baby?" I tease her. "Aren't you going to wash me? Or are you quitting your job?"

"I'm sorry," she stammers. "I'm supposed to be taking care of you. You need bathing."

She takes both the cuffs off and arranges all the stuff she needs to do a bed bath. She's back to nursing and I'm back to teaching her yoga. And I'm only just starting to teach her what I want her to know.

Most Tantric techniques are intended to get beyond sex as a goal and back to pure intimacy with your partner. One simple technique is to bathe each other without any sexual context, just intention and love.

She starts to focus on how much I need a bath. I'm pretty dirty now. The doctors don't know how to do a bed bath and the nurses are just figuring out their schedules. I tell her how much I appreciate her. Now she's back on the track I want her to take.

"Was it okay?" she asks.

"Just beautiful, Brandy. Thank you for giving me that."

"So you liked it? You're okay with straight sex?"

"If you're thinking I've never done that before, you're a funny girl."

"You're not a virgin?"

"Not anymore than you, sweetheart. Don't believe everything Nick tells you. She's just a friend. She doesn't get the details, just the dirt.

"What I really like to do though, I can show you next time, honey. We'll put two and two together, Old School and New School. But let's take it easy, Bran. I'm a sick man."

†

S&M

Just before 10 in the morning Brandy is sitting on the foot of my bed barefoot and cross-legged and I'm teaching her the koshas. She's a good student. I don't hit her or anything like I did when I was teaching DJ. She's studied anatomy, neurology, physiology and psychology and she grasps it easily. She's going to be a Tantric legend.

Sunny comes in at 10, the perfect punctual Pitta, and checks my chart. Brandy hasn't filled anything in.

"What's going on, Brandy? Why haven't you done any vitals?"

Brandy flushes and just says "Sorry I forgot, Sunny. See you at 6 tonight, Sim." She kisses me softly on the lips. Oh, she's so transparent.

I say, "Get some sleep, honey" as she runs away.

Sunny can read it. "Listen, buddy," she says harshly. "If you think for a minute..."

I interrupt her.

"If I think for a minute – which? That you want me, too? Or that you're going to fix my lunch?"

Oh, God, she explodes in Pitta fury. She hauls off and whacks me across the face as hard as she can with a closed fist.

"If you think for a minute you can get away with this...."

I interrupt again. "Nice shot, Sunny. You hit really well. I bet we could be friends."

Now she's furious and she punches Mack's extension into the phone. "Dr. Mack. I need to see you in IC, NOW, please!"

Mack comes in NOW, because his office is across the hall.

"What did I do?" I ask them both in all my genuine innocence.

Sunny starts in on him. "Look Dr. Mack, I came to work up here to help Brandy. She's my best friend and I can't keep..."

I'm having a good time interrupting her this morning so I go for gold. "Sunny, of course you can't keep... *yelling* like that or you'll wake up my wife."

She's stunned. I smile. "I was just asking about lunch. Have we got any tahini?"

Mack crashes into the bedside chair. "Steven? What the hell? I said go easy on the nurses, brother."

"Mack, they're killing me. One raped me and the other punched me in the face. Not that I minded either one, but I'm the one behaving here."

"Your wife? Your wife?" he stammers.

"Yeah. Brandy. She took advantage of me, Mack. But I'm sure she'll do the right thing. Would you get Sean to take care of it tomorrow?

†

BRANDY

I can't shake it. I'm playing it over in my mind again and again. I've only been on the job three days and now -- what did he say? There would be consequences. What does he mean? Fired? Pregnant? I can't believe that it happened like that.

Then Sunny comes up the stairs and stares at me. I can't face her.

"Brandy," she says, "what went on? Did that SOB do anything? You can talk to me."

I just shake my head. If I don't tell, maybe it will go away.

"Brandy, he's on drugs and I don't believe a word he says. He said he doesn't want to embarrass you in front of Dr. Mack, but that you'd tell me in private. Did he do anything?"

I burst into tears. The truth is bad and I can't say it. I was bad and I liked it so much, I'd do it again. Here and now.

But I try. "Sunny, he told me not to...but he's so sexy and sweet, I did it anyway. He said there'd be consequences and he didn't want to take advantage of me and I... "

"You what?"

"Put the restraints on him and..."

"Oh, shit."

"I did it anyway. Took advantage of him."

"Shit. Shit. And I punched him in the face. Damn, we could both be fired. Except he told Dr. Mack he loves us and had a fun morning. He said he didn't ask for any trouble but it was good.

"And Brandy, he said you're getting married tomorrow. Is he that stoned?"

"What? He didn't say anything to me except there would be consequences. *Is* he that stoned?"

"Pretty much, I think. I'll go face the consequences for us both right now. I'll tell Dr. Mack he's telling the truth. I'm on shift till 2, then we meet with Dr. Jain for training.

"If we're still working here, I'll come up and get you. But right now I've got to make him a tahini and fig jam sandwich on whole wheat. You sure know how to pick them, honey."

†

MACK

Except for some shakes and a low-grade fever when I came on at 2am, he slept like a baby and seems at peace. It's dawn. His eyes snap open at 6 sharp. It's uncanny how precise his body clock is now.

He smiles and yawns and rolls over, his first night free to move with no restraints because he's been so well behaved. Relatively under control, compared to what? I wonder. Compared to the nurses?

I offer him two Norco and he takes it; then I ask if he wants tea. He nods. I'm back in ten minutes and he's watching the door.

"Where's my shift change, Mack?" He's anxious.

"There's none right now. I'll work late and Sunny will start early."

He gulps and spits tea with a haunted look.

"Where is she? I want her."

"She's not working." I let that sink in to let him know I mean business, then soften it up. "Not today. After what she did yesterday, I told her to take the day off and think about it.

"I thought it was a harmless crush. And you play so hard to get these days, I thought... Well, I'm shocked."

"But Mack, I want her. She was really nice to me."

"I don't feel comfortable about leaving her alone with you. I've got to think about this too. It's a business."

"Can't I just talk to her?" he begs.

"Maybe you should, but not alone. She's in the kitchen, sulking."

Two days ago, he wouldn't talk to her or look at her or let her touch him. And I talked him into it. I owe him this.

When I go into the kitchen again to get her, she's buried face down in her arms on the table. I've hurt her.

It's against the core principles of my practice, both medical and spiritual, to harm anyone, to cause unnecessary pain and suffering.

The first principle of yoga is "ahimsa", not harming. There are a lot of things to learn on the path of yoga, but Gandhi taught that if you only practiced the first principle, not harming another, everything else would follow.

Hippocrates taught the same principle as the core of medical practice: *"I will do no harm. There is art to medicine as well as science.... warmth, sympathy, and understanding may outweigh the surgeon's knife or the chemist's drug."*

She's crying and I put a hand on her shoulder. "Come on, Brandy. He wants to see you. Stop crying, honey."

When we go back into IC, Steven has raised the bed to sitting position for the first time. He's let the sheets drop below his waist, but with so much dressing wrapped around his wounds he's as good as fully clothed.

"Come here, beautiful," he puts his arm out. He doesn't mention her tears but he sees them.

She turns back to me for permission. She's afraid to go near him now.

"Just sit next to me, honey. No big deal," he says.

I motion to her that its okay and she sits on the edge of the bed. He puts an arm around her and she starts crying pitifully. "Shush," he says. "Listen to me," and she stops on a dime.

He's not looking at her. He's looking me straight in the eye.

"Mack, listen. Don't punish her. I was just trying to teach her a few things about – control. And she lost it.

"You know me. I can be very suggestive. She would never have done a thing if I hadn't made – certain suggestions. The same with Sunny, she wouldn't have hit me if I hadn't been – suggestive."

"Suggestive? You mean lewd?"

"No. I don't want to hurt them. I was trying to teach them a little about self-control. I made some suggestions. I'm usually a pretty good teacher. I'm sure I can do better, but I'm feeling really sick."

I don't know what to say. He looks serious and very centered.

"What do you mean, suggestions?"

"She was so out of control. I'd really like to help her work on that. She's an awesome student. Tell him, Bran. Why did you put the other cuff on me?"

She looks up at him and then says very softly, "You asked me where it was."

"And then?"

"You said it should be tighter if I wanted control."

"And?"

"You said there would be consequences. I'm sorry."

"And I'm not," he says giving her a squeeze.

"I wondered if she would cross the line for me and she did. Same thing happened with Sunny. She wouldn't have hit me if I hadn't suggested she wanted a piece of me. She made herself very clear.

"Very amusing, the little nurse sucker punch she has. I knew she had it in her. It would be another story if she had a gun but she didn't hurt me."

He stops to consider a passing thought. "By the way are there any guns in the house, my nonviolent brother?"

I shake my head.

"And I presume with your bachelor cooking skills, there's no knives in the kitchen sharp enough to hurt me?"

I laugh. "Where are you going with this, brother?"

"Then I'm safe enough with Sunny in the house. But I was wondering if Bran's going to marry me today. Do we need a shotgun wedding?"

"You're not serious," I say.

"Like a heart attack, brother. You're the best man. Get online and fill out the confidential marriage license for me. No blood tests are required if you've already compromised your partner.

"Sean can do the vows. I think around sunset would be nice. It would probably have to be in here since I can't get out of bed yet."

Then he turns to her and says, "Are you going to come or what, Bran?"

†

JAIN

I drove up the mountain after lunch to see what I could do to help the girls with their study and talk to Steven about the gym gear. When I walk in, Mack's on the phone in his study. Steven is lit up like Christmas.

"Hey, Jain, man, I'm getting married. You're invited."

"You're engaged? When's the wedding?"

"At six," he says.

"Six? What date?"

"I don't know. What day is it, baby?" he laughs. "Today, man! Mack is throwing a party for me, he's taking care of it now."

"Are you in any shape to be getting married today, bud? I didn't know you even had a girl friend." Hell. I don't know what to say. Who's pregnant is my first thought.

"Is it that girl of yours Nick down at the beach? She said...." And then I really don't want to repeat what Nick said about his sexuality.

"Hell no. Nick is a sister. I'm going to marry Brandy."

And Sim is Sim and he's so happy about it, I'm not sure I want to mention that he only really met her 4 days ago. So all I say is "Wow."

"Can we do the gym plan now?" he changes gears so fast I wonder if Mack switched his medications. "I've got a list."

He points to the bedside table and there's a complete list neatly written out in very feminine handwriting:

- flat bench with incline
- Olympic bars (2@)
- Squat rack with safety bars
- Overhead pull-down

-    Fixed barbell set 20 - 60 pounds
-   Free weight set 5 – 60 pound dumbbells
-   Full Olympic weight set 5, 10, 25, 35, 45 pound 4 each (480 pounds total)
-   Power mats 15 square feet
-

"Did I miss anything, you think?"

"Four collars for the Olympic bars. A decline bench. Otherwise, it's pretty good, Sim. Did Brandy help you with this?"

"I dictated," he smiles.

"I'll bet you did."

"She did a really nice party list for me, too. No guests are coming except our staff, but I asked Mack to have Crystal from the Nest come up and tend bar for us and bring all the gear for Margaritas.

"Sean's going to escort her, but I don't think he knows it yet. I felt bad because he asked Bran out first, but I don't really feel too bad because he'll really like Crys. She's a knock-out. He's too old for Brandy."

I hold up one finger to stop him. I need a minute to process all this so I go across the hall to Mack's office. He's on the phone putting in a big order for Mexican food delivery. He already has a drink on his desk and pushes the bottle across to me.

"No kidding," I say when he gets off the phone. "Our patient is feeling a little better today?"

He finishes the glass off and pours another three fingers. "No kidding. Our patient got laid yesterday."

†

SEAN

Mack calls. It's my day off but he said it's urgent.

"The king of pain requests your presence and services this evening and has a to-do-list for you. Are you ready for this, Sean?"

The way my life has been going, I'm very ready for Sim's kinks. Have at me.

"Pick up Crystal, the bartender at the Nest, and help her shop for the party stuff on the way up. She has the list. Plan on sleeping over. You're going to want a few drinks."

"What's up, Mack?"

"What's up is Steven and Brandy. You're apparently performing a marriage ceremony. I got a license on the internet."

Why am I not shocked? I would have married her if he hadn't, but it was pretty clear to me that night in the kitchen she was hard in love already. Oh yeah, Mack was going to give her a hand. I'm pretty impressed.

Crystal is beautiful. How she knows Sim is beyond me. He's just not a bar rat. She says she knows him from the beach. If I had a dollar for every woman who knows Sim from the beach, I'd be at the beach all day myself.

She's thrilled to have the extra work. Mack's paying her top dollar. But she's also a little confused. As far as the town knows, Sim vanished into thin air. The only witnesses outside are Nick, DJ and me, and we're not the kind to talk. In fact DJ and Nick have been totally in the dark since the first days.

The word on the street is almost legend. Crys says they all talk about him at the bar. Some say the dealers scared him off, some say he drowned, he's on drugs, he joined an ashram, he got some babe pregnant and he's run off, or he got a real job and moved to the valley.

The yoga studio cancelled all his classes with no reason given. But the most popular story, the one that DJ has perpetuated, is that Sim is surfing down in Mexico, drinking tequila with Sammy Hagar. It's a good enough story to get passed around.

No one seems to hit on the truth, that he's hurt and nursing back to health at his brother's house on the mountain. Crys has sworn to secrecy and she's a pro. A good bartender knows there are certain things you just don't discuss in public: sex, politics, religion or anything confided over a shot.

But there are also some things that need to be told and she sees a lot more than she cares to see at the Nest.

"We're losing the Point, Sean," she says sadly. "That was Steven's fight. He always said to pick your fights carefully. Half the boys are using drugs, a quarter of them are hanging in the bar all day and the rest are hiding under the bed. It's really gotten ugly down there."

"No really, we've got it, Crys. We don't quit that easy. Just don't bring it up today. He doesn't know how bad it is. He's got to heal before he can fight.

"Oh, and don't be shocked when you see him. He's wrecked. I'd say he's lost about 40 pounds. So be sure to tell him how beautiful he is."

"Same old Sim," she says. "He never gets tired of adoration." She laughs. "He used to start the yoga class by asking the question 'what part of Divine perfection is missing here?' And he meant in the world, but I would always think to myself, 'not a damn bit missing with you.'

"I'm sorry he was hurt but he picked that fight. He'd kill for peace at the beach."

"Yeah. Crazy boy. We haven't seen the last of it."

We pull up at the Mack house and I help her carry in all the party gear, liters of good agave tequila, Grand Marnier, fresh citrus, ice, a half dozen bottles of Carneros champagne and Mack's favorite bourbon.

Crys arranges it all in the kitchen and then cracks a bottle of champers and pours a glass carefully into a flute.

"Where is he?" she asks and I take her down the hall.

She kisses him on the forehead and hands him the glass. "What part of Divine perfection is missing here?" she asks him and he laughs.

"I'm not supposed to drink, Crystal," he says. "I'm on drugs." Then he makes a face at me and says, "Shit. The police. Don't say anything."

I take my police hat off and put it on his head. "It looks really good on you, Sim. I mean it looks kind of epic."

He looks at Crys and she nods with enthusiasm. "You look like a rock star, baby. You should get married in that hat."

"Well, I'm going to," he says. "Sean?"

"Yeah, keep it. It's yours. I'll bring you some handcuffs next time I'm up here."

"Sorry I can't be a better host but I'm stuck in here. Crys, get the party started and give them hell for me."

†

S&M

I get married in Sean's cop hat with my beautiful girl sitting on the edge of the hospital bed. She says she's got a surprise for me, but I'm kind of fading fast, cause Crys has been generous with sneaking the champagne into my room. She says champagne couldn't hurt me, but no to the tequila.

The ceremony is short and to the point. Done deal. I asked Sean to do it in as few words as necessary and legal. Mack, Brandy, Sunny, Sean, Jain, and Crys barely fit in the room with me so I don't want to drag it out.

I'm enjoying the dull roar of the party noise coming from the lounge room and I know Crys is rocking the house. Brandy comes back into the room and sits next to me again and she looks – hmmm, she's wasted. There goes the honeymoon, I think. Not that I'm in any better shape.

She leans over and whispers in my ear, which is silly because there's no one within hearing distance. She's just trying to get in my ear, that close. She doesn't even know me. She has no idea where I'm going to take this.

"Sim?" she slurs, "we are moving out, baby."

"We're moving?" I'm surprised. "Why?"

"We're being kicked out the house. For all the bad behavior. Past bad behavior and all the stuff we haven't even started yet."

Hmm, maybe she does know where I'm going with this after all. My imagination kicks up a notch.

"Where we going, baby?" I ask innocently.

"Pool house." She says.

"The pool house?"

"It's a surprise. Mack said you need more privacy. Or maybe he does. I'm not sure, but it's very pretty. Sunny and I fixed it up today. It's got a real bed, not a hospital bed."

Nice, I think. I like the pool house. It's got a shower and a little kitchen. And it's far enough away from the main house that she won't have to whisper. I could make her scream in the pool house.

Mack comes in with a couple more drinks and hands me some champagne.

"Your last drink tonight, brother. We're going to wind the party down early. We'll pick it up again in the morning. I've got the house next door for the night for our guests. Jain and I have made an offer on it. We need more space."

"And you're kicking me out," I laugh. "The pool house?"

"Oh, she told you? It's a wedding present. You'll be outside with the animals where you belong, closer to the gym and the pool. Seriously, wait til you see it. It's hot."

"Now?" I ask and down the champagne.

"Now. You need your beauty sleep. Let's move you." He leaves the room and comes back with Jain. Jain picks me up like I'm a bag of laundry and carries me out the back door and through the yard. I'm grateful he doesn't carry me out through the party. Mack opens the door and I'm stunned. The room is gorgeous and the bed is where I want to be right now. A real bed. A really big bed.

Mack pulls the covers back and Jain sets me down easily. There's water by the bedside and a multi-line phone.

"My office is on extension 1. My bedroom is 2. Kitchen is 3 and the nurses' room is 4. Not that you need to call them. Is there anything I can have your wife bring out when I evict her from the party?"

I shake my head. "No. Thanks, Mack, Jain. I've got everything I need. Everyone will still be here tomorrow?"

"Yeah, we'll have brunch by the pool. Don't bother saying good night. We're not done yet, okay?"

As soon as they walk out the door, I pick up the phone and dial 3. Crys picks up.

"Crys, I bet Brandy is not that far from the bar. Can you put her on?"

Brandy is definitely even more toasted that earlier, but she can do this one little thing for me.

"Sweetheart, would you please bring my hospital bed restraining cuffs over when you come? I miss them."

Then I get an outside line and call the hospital. I'm just sober enough.

"Hey, I'm sorry to call so late. Can I talk to records? Well, just leave them a message for me. This is Steven Mack. I was discharged a few days ago. I need to get my records updated.

"I know you can't do it tonight but I'll probably be out in the morning. First, I just got married today but my wife isn't authorized to make medical decisions for me until I say so. Just put that in there.

"Second. I've got a lot of drug allergies I need added to my record. Dr. Jain is my surgeon, he's aware of it but I want it in my records just in case. Good. Morphine. Norco. Fentanyl. Sufanil. Codeine. Any narcotics, opiates, pain killers. You got any I didn't mention? Yeah, add those too. I can't handle the stuff. Thanks.

"That's it. I just want it on record so I don't get some in an emergency by mistake. Have a great night, thanks."

†

BRANDY

I wake up in the beautiful little pool house at dawn, very hung over and happy. But when I reach over to see if Sim is awake yet, something is very wrong. His skin is dripping with sweat, but he's shivering hard as if he's freezing to death. I shake him lightly but he's unconscious.

I don't know how long he's been like this. No one came on shift after I came in and I've been sleeping all night. I grab the phone and punch in Mack's study, then the kitchen, then I finally get an answer when I call his bedroom.

"Mack, could you come, please? Sim's really sick. I don't know what's wrong."

He simply hangs up and is in the door as I'm wrapping myself in a robe. I explain I just woke up and found him like this. No one checked on him during the night. And I was dead drunk but I don't remind him of that.

"Brandy, get Jain. I haven't got the phones turned on in new house yet. Run, honey."

Jain's sitting in the little kitchen next door with a cup of coffee and the house is quiet. He's barefoot and bare-chested but when I tell him it's urgent he doesn't bother to dress.

All I can tell him is that Sim is shivering and sweating and passed out cold. "What about his meds?" he asks. "When did you give him the last shot?"

"I didn't. We skipped the Norco at 6pm because he wanted some drinks. Sunny usually gives him something at 10 and Mack does the harder stuff between 2 and 6. Last night, we all were in bed by 10."

When we get back to the pool house, Mack is checking his eyes. They're pinpoints. He looks up at us for answers and Jain says, "It's withdrawal. I think the last shot he had was 2am yesterday, about 30 hours ago. Unless you forgot that one, too. None of us checked on him after the party and he skipped meds all day. He's been causing enough commotion to keep everyone distracted."

"So what's my best plan here? Put him back on the drip or give him a hit or both? I don't want to kill him today."

Jain shakes his head and lowers his voice so I barely hear it. "Buddy, you have a lot more experience with narcotics that I ever want to have."

"I know, I know it's a problem. I just want a second opinion. I'm thinking of some morphine and if he starts calming down, put him back on a drip."

"Have you thought of getting an ambulance? He looks bad."

"It's too far, Jain. But if you wouldn't mind getting one of the EMTs on the radio for advice, I'd be grateful. I'm going ahead with Plan A. Morphine."

"What can I do, Doctor?" I ask. I feel like I'm invisible standing there in my robe. At least I'm not getting blamed for this. Not yet. I'm too scared to even think about the consequences.

Jain is on the phone patched through to an EMT and trying to explain. "No not an overdose. The opposite. He's been on very high doses of narcotics for post-op, fentanyl, morphine, Norco, we're rotating them trying to keep the doses down.

"He's just gone off them all cold turkey yesterday. No, this is not the kind of thing we usually see in emergency. I'd know what to do with an overdose."

He's listening carefully and turns around to watch Mack coming back in with the needle. He motions to Mack to go ahead with Plan A and then continues on the phone.

"Yeah, we fucked up on this one, Jake. Two doctors and two nurses and he's played us all against each other. I'd say it's been about 30 hours since he's had any medication. He's in shock or a coma; we just found him a few minutes ago."

He puts the receiver down. "There're coming up. No point in moving him but they want to give us a hand checking him out. He said Plan A is good, but go really light. Also, some oxygen. You can get that Brandy, then help Sunny get some food out for the guests. Juice, coffee, champagne if there's any left. You look like you need some oxygen yourself. Just go outside and sit down."

†

SEAN

Jain's gone when I wake up and Crystal is sitting at the table across from his half full cup. "Looks like he left in a hurry, Sean," she says.

"Good party," I say. I can see Sunny and Brandy out on the lawn next door setting out pitchers of juice and plates. "Let's go, I'm not done yet." I offer her my arm and she takes it with a smile.

"Never too early," she says.

There's something wrong with the way the girls look. Brandy has that frozen fear on her face that I saw when I first interviewed her.

"Trouble," I whisper to Crys. We see enough of it in our normal workday that we can usually stay cool in the middle of the worst shit storm. I wonder how long it will take the nurses to get the same kind of hard shell.

"Brandy, let me help you with that," Crys offers as she starts setting plates. "What's the problem? No fun on the honeymoon?"

Jain comes out of the pool house and sits with us. "God, where is that coffee?"

"Tough morning?" I ask.

"Yeah. Sim did a reverse overdose on us. The EMT's are on their way up. He's starting to look a little better, but I don't think he's coming to brunch."

"He's always the life of the party," Crys laughs. "I'm so sorry honey, what a nightmare," as she puts her arm around Brandy. "Is he okay?"

"Just really sick," Jain adds. "Is it just me or does anyone else get the impression that he thinks he can walk on water?"

My hand goes up first, then Crys. Brandy and Sunny look at us, surprised. They don't know him that well yet.

"I'm pretty sure he can't be killed, Jain," I joke. "Or at least I think *he's* pretty sure he can't be killed. Some Tantric deal he's got with the devil."

I see the EMT's coming around the side of the house, so I walk over to the pool house to say hi. Jake's been around a lot down at the Point and there's a younger new guy with him.

I shake Jake's hand and say "It's Sim."

"Hey, Sean, that explains everything. Sim's private War on Drugs," Jake laughs.

"And on Western Medicine. This kid does not make a good junkie. Trouble is they've been treating him for a couple of weeks with hard medicine and his body's getting used to narcotics."

Mack has a couple pillows under Sim so he's propped up a little bit with his eyes open and dilated. "Hey, Jake," he says when we come in. "I'm not going in the ambo. I just moved in here last night. I'm married, man."

Jake sits down and holds his wrist, checks his pupils and asks him a few easy questions, where is he? What day is it?

"Don't know what day it is," he says. "I've been in bed forever."

Then Jake sees the hospital restraining cuffs on the bedside table and picks one up with a laugh. "What're you doing with these?" he asks.

"Souvenirs," he says. "What I'm *going* to be doing with them is a more interesting question."

Jake smiles and puts it back down. "Dr. Mack, I think he's doing a lot better than this morning. What's the plan now?"

"I don't know," Mack says. "I'm trying to blame myself for this but the more I think about it, the more I realize he's been telling me this all along. And I can't even blame him. I guess we stop here. Or try to work out a plan to take him off drugs slowly."

Sim laughs, "We stop here. I kicked the plan out the door."

"It's not that easy, brother," Mack says. "I've done it before. A few times." He looks a little ashamed. "Occupational hazard. When my wife was dying..." He drops it. "I wasn't injured like you but it was still not an easy thing to do."

"Did you have two doctors, two nurses, an EMT, a cop and a bartender to help you?" he smirks. "This is going to be fun." He is definitely feeling the morphine.

"Fun? You could go into cardiac arrest or traumatic shock."

"You won't kill me," he says. "Pain is inevitable, but suffering is optional. I'm tired of kicking the tires, Mack. I want a fair fight."

"Dr. Mack," Jake interrupts. "You haven't really got a choice. We ran Sim's medical file on the way up and it specifically prohibits all those drugs. So technically, that last shot of morphine you gave him was malpractice. It's on his permanent medical record as 'do not administer' along with a very long list of opiate derivatives and painkillers. It was just updated at 8am this morning."

"And now I've got to start all over again," Sim complains. "I was just about 20 hours into it before I got sick and about 30 hours before you got me stoned again. If you don't want to do this, Mack, Jain will sit with me. Or Sean, or hey, Jake, you want to baby sit me for a couple days? They've got really good parties going on."

"Sure, Sim. I'll stay for a while. I won't kill you, buddy."

"There. Done. One EMT. One doctor. Mack you've got drug issues, take a break from me. Keep the nurses out of here for a few days, too. Put my wife back in with Sunny and let them cram for their tests.

"Give me a few days to clean up. I've got enough privacy here to peel the paint off the walls if I have to. I don't want to disrupt the house."

And considering he doesn't want to disrupt any of us, he's managed to reorganize all of our lives today. Again.

I say good-bye and tell him I'll check on him tomorrow. "If you feel good enough then, there's something important I want to talk about. The Point Guard needs your help." I hate to tell him the PG is being fucked in the toilet.

Then I go back out into the sunshine to see if Crystal is ready for a ride home. It's a long way down the mountain so we start planning how we're going to take the beach back. I'm guessing that in another week or so S&M will be ready to kick some sand into someone's face.

†

S&M

Mack is not happy with me and gives me that horrified stare of disbelief he has when I beat him at chess.

"Take a break, brother, I've got this," I say in consolation. "Just let me borrow Jain for a few days and you go play with the nurses, work on the new house. Get some more phone lines installed. It's amazing what you can accomplish with a phone."

"You're laughing now, little brother, but you're going to start getting really sick again in a few hours."

"I was already sick for 10 hours on the fentanyl. This time it's only a little morphine. I shouldn't be as bad."

"It doesn't work that way," he says. I wish he didn't know so much about drugs.

"I'll write home," I laugh. "Go away. I don't want to see anyone for a while except Jain, Jake and Sean."

Jain is lost in thought but he looks pretty pleased with himself. He asks Jake to stay with me and motions Mack outside. They're gone twenty minutes and then he comes back alone.

"I've got some hospital business to take care of first, Sim. I need to have Jake take me down in the ambulance and pick up a patient. We'll be gone for a few hours, so you've got no one to stay with you until around sunset. What do you want to do? You're running the show now."

I'm fine with that. I'm in a sewage ditch halfway between hell and high water and feeling pretty well balanced all things considered. I can wait a few hours for the horror movie re-run.

"I want Brandy to stay with me until I start getting sick. Then I'll kick her out and wait till you guys get home. She looked pretty scared this morning. I want to make sure she's okay.

"And tell everyone to please stay the fuck out of here till you get back. I just got married."

A little while later, Bran comes in cautiously. She's got that ghost girl expression on her face again. I owe her an apology, so she's really going to get a good one.

"You're only going back in the house for a few days," I start. "I don't want to scare you again, I don't want you to see me sick, okay?" She nods.

"You're not being punished for anything you did last night. That was my choice." I smile at her kindly until she relaxes, and then I give her a mean look.

"But you're going to be punished for what you did the other day," I tease her. "Honey, you need to be taught a little bit of self control and I'm a very good teacher."

She inhales really hard and I feel myself warming up with waves of pleasure. "What?" she says innocently. "You said it was good."

"I said there were going to be consequences. You fucked me like a wild animal, girl. You need to learn some discipline. I've got just enough time to start teaching you before I get sick again."

I reach over for the cuffs and hand them to her. "Start with this."

"How?" she asks. "This isn't a hospital bed, there's no rails to attach them."

"Take the split ring off your keys and hook the cuffs together. Then wrap them around the headboard. Do you think you can do exactly what I tell you to do and nothing else? Cause this is a test of how serious you are, baby."

I give her my sweetest smile because she looks a little scared and nervous. She should be. She doesn't even know me.

"Yes," she says, but she doesn't move. "I haven't got my keys, Sim."

I just smile brighter with all my teeth. Surely a smart little straight-A nursing student can figure this out. I don't say anything else. There are no hints on this test.

Suddenly she jumps up and says, "I'll go find something," and runs back to the house. I haven't got all day. This is only hardware, it's not the important stuff. I can't wait.

She comes back in a few minutes with Sunny's car keys and starts pulling them apart and rigs the cuffs up the way I asked. I'm getting extreme waves of pleasure just watching her behave.

"Wrists okay?" she asks because rigged this way they won't reach my biceps.

"Wrists are better," I say. "I'm not going to touch you. It's part of your punishment."

When she touches my wrist I get a hard jolt and a warm rush from my hips to my heart. I know what's coming. At least I hope so. She pulls the cuffs really tight, but it's fine because the hospital kind are padded and don't make marks. I'm burning.

"Don't do anything unless I tell you to," I repeat. "Nothing else. See if you can behave today. Lock the door, baby. Take off your clothes.

"Now when I tell you to kiss me, I mean kiss me with love, not lust. This is going to be the simplest sex lesson you've ever had and maybe the most important. Just a nice sweet kiss and no more. Try one."

She kisses me perfectly on my lips, no Frenching, no tongues, but a really beautiful kiss.

"You're going to get straight A's, sugar," I laugh. "Now kiss me right between my eyebrows on my forehead chakra and see if you can feel where it goes."

She kisses me again, light but long. I can feel it all the way to my toes and if she's paying attention, she should feel the same. "It goes everywhere," she says. I laugh again with pleasure. "My mouth again." She kisses my lips.

"Now my throat chakra," I put my head back and come before she even kisses me there. "My mouth again. Easy, baby." I can tell she's getting worked up and she gives me a little tongue with it.

"Kiss my heart. Can you feel my heartbeat with your lips?" She moans a little.

"Mouth again." We're half way through my chakras and she's doing all right.

"Belly". She kisses my navel and looks up. I lick my lips instead of repeating myself and she comes back up and kisses my mouth with a big French kiss.

"Now my cock. Go easy. Just a kiss." We're getting towards her final exams.

She gives me a very gentle kiss, looks up and asks "mouth?" I nod.

"Sweet. You are so beautiful like this, so controlled. Now put me inside you and listen to me." She does it very slowly with love and care.

"Now just stop," I say. "Just don't move. Don't kiss me. Just feel me. Feel us."

We lay like that for a minute and she doesn't move. I can feel ripples of prana racing up and down my spine and the sweetness of her embrace.

"Can you feel me coming everywhere, honey? Can you feel my heart beat? Can you feel my love without me even *doing* anything to you?"

"Yes," she says. "How long do we stay like this?"

"Until you can feel me inside you permanently wherever you go. Until you can feel me when you're at the kitchen table. When you're trying to sleep alone tonight. Till you can feel me when you breathe. How long will you wait?"

"Always," she says. She's passed her first lesson. It's worth the wait. I keep her there for a quarter of an hour detention without moving except for some soft kisses on the top of her head as she purrs against my chest.

I look at the light fading on the window and know I'm going to be turning into a monster when the sun goes down, so I ask her to bathe me before she goes.

She goes into the bathroom and gets a pan of warm water with soap, some washcloths, a big bath towel and my sweat pants. I know I'm going to sweat this thing tonight.

When she's done she tucks me in and kisses my third eye and winks. She whispers, "I can still feel you inside me, Sim."

"Go away, honey." I say. "Wait for me."

†

BRANDY

Mack is in the kitchen sulking when I go in to help Sunny with dinner. I put my arm around him and kiss his forehead. He looks shocked, so I wink at him.

"Now you've got all my attention, big brother," I tease him.

"Brother-in-law," he corrects me. "And no I don't. Jain's bringing in a new patient tonight, so you'll probably have more things to do than feel sorry for me. But you look happy again, Brandy," he adds. "Sister."

"I don't know anything about a new patient, but it's been crazy here. Tell me."

"I only found out a few hours ago. Jain has a patient who had emergency surgery ten days ago. She wasn't expected to live. Its turns out she has no medical history at all, never been sick, but she had an accident, broke some ribs and pneumonia set in.

"The strange thing is she wouldn't see a doctor until she was almost dead. She hates doctors, hospitals, drugs. It turns out she's a yoga therapist and was trying to treat it herself with botanical medicine and Ayurveda. Almost killed herself. Now she's desperate to get released and we've got a free bed.

"She reminds me of my brother and I have very mixed feelings about it. But Jain thinks she might turn out to be the second therapist we need. So I agreed to see her. They're on their way up. Running late, too, because of all the discharge papers."

The kitchen phone rings and when I pick it up it's Sim. "Where is my EMT?" he asks. "It's getting dark in here."

I whisper, "They're just a little late, baby. Close your eyes. I feel you in the kitchen. Do you want one of us to come over?"

"Never mind," he says. "I'm going to strip the wallpaper off," and he hangs up.

A half hour later, we see Jain and Jake roll the new patient around the back of the house on a gurney. When Mack opens the sliding door, Jain waves him back.

"Plan B," he says. "Never mind her, get me the wheelchair."

I roll the chair out and he lifts her and helps her into it carefully. "Don't hold dinner," he says. "I'll call." Then he pushes the chair to the pool house with Jake leading the way.

†

NAT

I'm tired and drugged and in a lot of pain, but I'm so grateful to be out of the hospital and up on the top of the mountain that I never want to lie down again. All the way up the mountain, Dr. Jain has been telling me about this place, their stories and dreams, and the twists the universe has thrown at them.

The two brothers intrigue me. One is practicing medicine and the other is doing everything in his power to escape it. But as the story unfolds, I learn that the younger brother is very much like me, powerful, injured and drugged.

He's a very well known yoga teacher. I've never met him, but he's a renowned Tantric with a very wild reputation. Dr. Jain says he's refused all medication and is very sick so we need to get back there as soon as possible.

I'm so grateful that he's taking me up there. I think that there's no reason for a man to suffer through this. I tell Dr. Jain I'd rather work tonight than crawl into another hospital bed. I know I can help him. Let me show you what a yogini can do, please I beg him.

They wheel me into a dark bedroom behind the house and turn on the lights. He's curled up on the bed shivering and sweating and he actually snarls at us when we come in.

"No. Turn them off," I say. "Get some candles." There's enough ambient light from the yard that we're safe in the dark. Jake goes to the house for candles and comes back with them. He says Dr. Mack asked with sarcasm if we needed incense with that too.

"Absolutely, if he has some champa that would be great," I say and Jake goes back. I don't intimidate that easily.

I light some candles near the bed and look at him. He looks back with pure cold steel blue eyes and says, "I said no fucking nurses, Jain."

"I'm not a nurse, Sim. Look at me. Who am I?"

He looks into my eyes, first the right and then the left and holds my gaze. "Who are you?" he says.

"I'm Nat," I say. "Do you know yoga nidra?"

"Yes. Tantra," he says.

"Well, baby, your prana is totally screwed up from the drugs. Nidra would be a very good bet for you right now. Unless you like to suffer. Are you game?"

"Who are you?" he asks again. He's still shivering, but this time he asks without the venom. I'm speaking his language.

"I'm Nat. Do you trust me? Do you know how to do yoga nidra? I can plant you deeper than any drug known to man if you want to rest."

"Yes. I know how," he says.

Jain is watching me like I'm a witch. I'm much better than that.

"Good. Set your intention, Sim," I say. "What do you want?"

"Strength," he answers without a second thought.

"What kind of strength? Physical?"

He laughs through the pain. "The only kind of strength worth having, integrated on every level. Body, energy, mind, heart and spirit. The whole kitchen sink."

"Beautiful," I say. "Put the intention of strength in the center of your heart. I've got you. Show me how you do nadi shodhana."

He breathes in through his left nostril, holds his breath, then exhales through the right. Then reverses it. He doesn't even use his fingers to hold his nose; he's doing the advanced pranic version. His breath is ragged and choppy at first, but after a few rounds it settles into a smooth deep rhythm, getting deeper and the pauses lasting longer. He knows his shit.

"Now put your palms up, honey. I've got you. Let go. Put your attention on the right side. Right thumb, index finger, middle finger, ring finger, little finger, palm of the hand, back of the hand, wrist, forearm, elbow, upper arm, shoulder..."

I began the litany of his entire body part inventory. It's such a simple practice that it's deceptively powerful. Science calls the phenomenon "rotation of consciousness" where the body parts are mapped across an area of the brain in a particular order. Rotating attention in the hypothalamus calms the mind.

Yoga teaches it's much simpler than that. He puts his attention on the parts as I recite them and it takes him down though the koshas. As the mind focuses and then moves onto each body part in sequence, it becomes less preoccupied with it and lets go of the physical layer.

Once the attention is off body parts, the prana flows more freely. Then the mind can happily turn off and allow consciousness to go far deeper, where healing happens, into the wisdom kosha and then deeper into the core of the soul.

With a willing advanced practitioner, I can turn his lights off in less than ten minutes and keep them off. He stops shaking. He stops breathing hard. The sweat stops dripping. He's breathing like a baby before I even finish the body parts. Then I polish him off.

"Take a step down into your heart, honey. It's dark but there's light coming up from the bottom of it. Take another step. The floor of your heart is covered with gold. Keep going. The deeper you go, the brighter it becomes. It never stops. Take another step. All your strength is burning down there.

Steven is so deep now he could be dead. "Now stay down there, baby," I say. "Stay down until I wake you up." I kiss him on the forehead and look at Dr. Jain.

I put a finger over my lips and motion toward the door, then put a hand on Jake's shoulder and signal him to stay. Dr. Jain writes "extension 1" on a notepad next to the phone and gives it to Jake, then he pushes my chair out into the night air. At the top of the mountain, the sky is so thick with stars that the Milky Way is almost consumed.

"How the hell did you do that?" he says. "Hypnosis?"

"No, just some really good yoga he already knows," I smile.

"So he's unconsciousness now, without any drugs?" Jain is properly blown away.

"Not a bit. He's totally conscious. He can hear what's going on around him. Yoga nidra is conscious sleeping. The fun part is that he's aware that he's sleeping. He's healing. You should try it sometime. It takes a bit of practice, but he sure was easy."

"So that's all there is to it?" Jain asks.

"No, it's just the beginning of a really long night. He's probably good for three hours max. Why don't you introduce me to Dr. Mack and we'll let Jake watch for a while?"

†

JAIN

I knock on Mack's office door. The door is seldom closed, but I realize this is the first chance he's had to kick back in weeks. He doesn't open the door for a while and when he does, his eyes are dilated. The bourbon is still on the shelf; he's doing bigger things.

"Bad time?" I ask. I tug his shirt sleeve up high enough to let him know I know. There's more than one mark on his arm.

"Just took the edge off, Jain. I'm good enough. Come in." Then he smiles at Nat and puts his hand out. "Thank you for coming up. How do you feel?"

"Tired but very, very happy to be here," she smiles. "Your brother is a remarkable man. I hope I get a chance to work with him."

I help her out of the wheel chair and onto one of the big leather couches. She pulls her feet up under her and sits cross-legged yogi style. Mack starts laughing.

"Candles and incense?"

"Oh it gets worse than that, Doctor," she says. "Pranayama and nidra and mantras. I'm hitting him with the whole kitchen sink. Abhyanga tomorrow. My specialty is botanical medicine. I can put more plant extracts into him through his skin than he could ever ingest. It would actually poison him if I gave him that much orally. But through the skin it goes directly into the tissues instead of through the digestive system."

She pauses as if wondering if its safe to say more and then she laughs. "But you know that. The skin is the largest organ of the body. Although most men would argue that fact."

"Mmm." He seems to know what she's talking about. "And how is he now?"

"Sleeping like a baby," I say. "She took him from the cold sweats to sweet dreams in ten minutes. I wouldn't believe it if I hadn't seen it."

"I couldn't have done it if he didn't already have that training, Dr. Mack. Dr. Jain says you were Steven's teacher."

"It was a long time ago," Mack says. "Steven kept it up and took it further and I started working in the hospital. Eight years ago, when I was his age. I'm really tired of it, burned out. I want to do something different."

"I want to help you do something different," she said. "It's rare. It's hard getting work in the medical field doing what I do. I'm sure Steven has to water down his teachings to work at the yoga studio, too. Private practice is the key. Does he want to go back to teaching yoga or what?"

"No, he wants to work with us but we're fighting each other now. I'm mainstream and he's beyond the box. My idea was two doctors, two nurses and two yoga therapists. That way we can take on medical patients but then transition them from disease care to wellness care."

"And my idea," I add, "is that we have two teams. Standard medical care in this house with the intensive care unit, Dr. Mack and the two nurses, kind of a medical halfway house from the hospital. And alternative therapies and wellness care in the new house. Steven will be the head of that side and he'll have a medical doctor, me, and another assistant therapist. Maybe you?"

"I like that," she said. "It's brilliant. So what do you need from me?"

"Well, first your ideas about what kind of services, what kind of wellness facility we should have. Steven's been too sick to work with us much on that. But he did design a gym for physical therapy. What would you need?"

"Oh," she drools. "If I had a shopping list for a wellness center? First a lab with an apothecary. Meditation and yoga space. Massage area. Weights are a great idea. I saw the pool, and the property up here is therapy on its own. First I would do the lab. By the way Steven's going to be needing that as soon as possible. I can give you a list of botanicals I need if you'd like."

Mac is looking a thousand percent better and he gives a big sigh. "What kind of salary are you looking for?" he asks.

"I think I'd pay you to work on this project," she laughs. "I'm dead serious. He's going to be my boss?"

The phone interrupts and Mack picks it up. "Yes," he says. "Right away."

Then he winks at Nat. "That was Jake. Your boss has just come back from the dead."

†

NAT

Back in the pool house, Jake is trying to get him to drink some water. Dr. Jain tells Jake to go see Mack about a bed and some sleep and we'll take it from here. Then he sits down in the corner and watches me, waiting for some kind of miracle.

I take Steven's arm in my hand and put three fingers on his radial artery to feel what's going on. All three doshas are erratic and he's breathing like a wild animal. He opens his eyes and stares at me.

"Maybe you shouldn't be touching me," he says threateningly.

"I'll be touching you a lot, honey, I promise you," I threaten right back. "I'm just checking your pulse. Tell me. Why are you awake? I didn't ask you to come up yet."

"It was black there, too dark. Nightmares. Voices. Animals. I couldn't stay down there any longer," his voice is like a frightened child.

"Then don't go back down there. Stay awake with us. Dr. Jain is here. Look at me. Why are you breathing like that? You know how to breathe. Look at me."

He's losing control. He tries to breathe slowly but it's just a spasm of air.

"I'm going to touch you, baby. Here." I put my finger on the right side of his nose and close off the right nostril so he's forced to breathe in through the left side. Then I move my finger to the left side and wait until he exhales and inhales again. I'm patient. I keep it up until I see the pranayama taking effect and his breaths becoming longer and slower.

While I do it, I start singing to him in Sanskrit, the Gayatri mantra.

Om Bhur Bhuva Svaha. Tat savitur varignam. Bargo Devasya Demahi. Dyoyona Pratchordyat

His eyes get wide and dilated and his breath softens.

"What is that?" Jain asks.

"Its just an ancient blessing. He knows it." I sing it again a little softer, a little slower. Again. Again. Again. I see his lips moving with the mantra.

Then I whisper it in a simple English version.

Om. Earth. Heaven. Awareness. Everything around us is sacred. Surrounded by divinity, we are all protected.

"Look at me, baby," I whisper. He looks carefully and then his eyes shut and his breath falls into a little snore.

"And that?" Jain asks.

"Actual normal human sleep," I whisper. "It's only midnight. Wait until he hits Vata time. It's going to get a little wild."

The beautiful moon is waxing again and nearly three quarters full. The yard is full of light and we let the candles sputter out. I am having one of the best meditations of my life as I sit for two hours in a wheel chair in the pool house on the top of this mountain watching over this beautiful soul.

Instead of using a mantra, I meditate on the sound of his breath, ujayii, the raspy snore of victory. It must be contagious because soon Dr. Jain is snoring softly in synch. I'm feeling so blessed to be sitting here keeping vigil over both of them.

I'm just waiting for the wild Vata hours from 2 until 6am. There's no doubt in my mind that it's coming. It's why I'm here. It starts kicking in like clockwork just after 2am.

First he starts tossing from one side to another, then his breath gets hard, short and heavy. I feel his forehead and he's burning up, dripping sweat. I feel his pulse and it's rampant.

He starts talking in his sleep and it's just senseless stuff. He's talking about seaweed and rock reefs and dings and broken glass. He's talking about vampires and lemons and bourbon and nicks and brandy and guns and needles. I try to wake him and get him focused but he's beyond reason.

Jain starts up from his nap and listens. "Now what?" he says.

"I can't work with him like this," I admit. I need his attention. "He's delirious. It's hell boiling over. I saw it coming."

"So what do we do?" he says. "Sedative? Sleeping pill? If you can't work with him, then what?"

"Ahimsa. It's the first tenant of yoga and the basic philosophy of Hippocrates: no harm. You know the oath? 'There is art to medicine as well as science.... warmth, sympathy, and understanding may outweigh the surgeon's knife or the chemist's drug.'"

His eyes are narrow and he winces. "Warmth and sympathy?"

"It's a very big bed, Dr. Jain," I say. "I suggest you lie down. Sometimes the best thing you can do is to hold someone. That's what I plan on doing now."

"All right," he says. "Hold him. We don't do that much in med school."

He lies down on Steven's left side and puts an arm over him. I get on the right side and put my hand in Steven's hair and pet him like a child. Between us, he can't toss anymore. He kicks a few times and yells a few choice obscenities, then surrenders to our human shackles. We're not letting him go. After a while he quiets down and sniffs. He sniffs a lot like an angry boy, then eventually he drifts away.

I can see Dr. Jain's eyes in the dark. "Ancient yogi practice?" he whispers.

"No, it's an ancient human practice. Sweet dreams, Doctor."

†

NAT

It's a beautiful peaceful sleep for a few hours until dawn. I'm tired, but I feel a sudden surge of pleasure jolt through me and feel him kick hard. I don't want to open my eyes yet, so I wait. I feel it again, his whole body jerks hard. I think he might be having convulsions so I open my eyes.

He's staring at me. His eyes are half closed and his lips are curled back baring his teeth in a smile. His smile gets bigger when he sees me open my eyes. He groans with pleasure.

"Fucking orgasms," he laughs. "It never stops but it's really strong when I wake up. I'm a morning man."

I'm not even touching him but I can feel his sexual energy vibrating through me. He can't move at all because Dr. Jain's arm is clamped around him in a bear hug, pinning his arms down. Jain's sleeping without a shirt and his bicep is huge, extraordinary. Steven is helplessly pinned and seems amused by his plight. He's stuck.

"Maybe you shouldn't be in bed with me," he muses and he groans again with a smile of pleasure. "Aren't you afraid? I could hurt you."

"Dr. Jain will protect me," I say. "I thought it was better than tying you up," I tease.

"Oh, sweet no," he laughs. "Nothing's better than that. Is that Jain holding me? How charming."

"You had a rough night, honey. But you seem pretty good right now."

"I'm always good in the morning," he smiles and he squirms against Jain's bicep but can't get loose. "Who are you?"

"I'm Nat, honey. I guess I work for you now."

"Your first day on the job and you're in bed with your boss? How amusing is that?" he moves his elbow and tries to poke it into Jain's ribs but he can't get any traction. "Let me go." He kicks and manages to wake the doctor.

"What? Oh, shit, Sim," Jain says and yawns stretching his arm overhead, releasing him.

In a heartbeat, Sim reaches his free arm around me and puts his hand on my tailbone. I come so hard it shocks me and I jump out of the bed as fast as I can.

"Sweet Jesus," I say. "Do you treat all your employees like that?"

"Maybe you shouldn't get in bed with me, Nat," he repeats. "You don't even know me. Who the fuck are you?"

"I'm actually a patient here. Dr. Jain was my surgeon. I came up last night in the ambulance. He told me about you and I thought I could help. I'm a yoga therapist and I've heard a lot about you. Do you remember last night?"

"I remember I was planning to knock the walls down. Some really bad dreams. Hmmm. Some chanting and candles. I remember a little bit. You were here last night?"

"Yeah, we did yoga nidra, pranayama, mantras. You were doing really well for a while. Then around 2am you got delirious. So we decided to just hang on to you. May I?" I point to his wrist, trying to show some respect for his boundaries before I check his pulse.

"Sure."

I take his wrist and put three fingers on his radial artery. His pulse is smooth as a Swiss watch. He's watching me very closely and smiling.

"Are you finished coming?" I joke.

"As far as you're concerned I'm finished. As far as I'm concerned it's never going to stop."

Jain gets up and pulls his shirt on. I must be staring because Steven starts laughing at me. Jain's been my doctor for nearly two weeks but I've never seen him like this. His chest and shoulders are a work of art. I blush.

"Yeah, I used to look like that, too," Steven sniffs. "But Jain's going to be my personal trainer. We're going to build a gym by the pool and use it for rehab."

Jain corrects me. "We're already doing it. They delivered the equipment yesterday afternoon. It rocks, man. If you feel up to it, you can come out and watch me take it for a test drive."

"You're going start without me? Traitor. Better not let her watch. She'll turn to stone."

"Sim," he says. "We're your team. Me and Nat. We work for you now. Mack's signed off on it unless you don't want her. We got the gym in yesterday and Nat's going to start on the apothecary and lab today. We've got the whole house next door. Done deal. You're the boss. Get up and start running the show unless you plan on being sick forever. Can you stand?"

"Can I stand?" he laughs. "Good question." He tries to sit up. "Nah. Shit. I'm going to be sick," he tries to throw up but there's nothing in him.

"Well, maybe tomorrow. Let's work on the lab plan. Can you help Nat with that?"

"Dunno. What's the plan, Nat?"

"Right now?" I say, "I want to work on what's most important to you."

"Thanks, honey, but I'm married. What else have you got?"

"Be serious, Steven. I know what you want. I can have it delivered before lunch."

He's curious now. "You can have what delivered?"

"Strength," I say. "Body, energy, mind, heart and spirit. The whole kitchen sink."

He's stunned. I've hit on his intention and whether he remembers it or not, it's at the level of his soul. He narrows his eyes and stares at me and asks for the billionth time, "Who the hell are you?"

"I'm Nat. I'm here to help you get strong and you're going to help me do the same."

"How?" he says.

"For starters I want to infuse you with medicinal plants to heal you. I think I know what you need, but it would help if I could see your injuries to see how much I need."

His gaze darkens and his mouth hardens in a frown. "I don't think you should be looking at me anymore, Nat. Or talking to me or touching me," he threatens.

I roll my eyes and look to Dr. Jain for help. He steps up to the plate.

"Sim. Let's take a look. You don't need the dressing any more. I'd like to see how it's healing. And she can't work through all those bandages."

"Fuck you, Jain," he says.

Dr. Jain takes a deep breath and blows it out. He looks at me and I can read his mind.

I stand up. I'm a little wobbly. "Sweetheart," I say to get Steven's eyes on me, then I turn my back to the bed and do a slow strip tease with a little bump of my hips and pull my shirt over my head.

There's a deep fresh scar from the back of my heart all the way across to the side of my right breast where Jain cut me open and two big holes at the side of my ribs where they pumped my lung out. I know its ugly. And it hurts.

Jain says, "Gee, Nat, they didn't clean that up very well, did they? There's still glue on it. The nurses here get straight A's in wound care. We'll make it beautiful for you."

I pull the shirt back down and turn around. "Can you beat that, baby?" I smile at Sim.

"You win, Nat," he says with a little shock and awe in his voice. "Go ahead and take a look."

Jain helps him turn on one side and unwraps the bandages gently, then turns him over and does the other side. It's nothing short of horrific but it's clean. The nurses get straight A's.

His stomach and ribs are scarred and burned from the gunshots, but his back is much worse, as if a bomb exploded behind him. From below his heart to his waist, it looks as if he's been patiently pieced together like a puzzle.

Jain apologizes. "I'm not a cosmetic surgeon. I was just trying to save his life. My best work is on the inside, his organs, but there was so much trauma and tissue damage it was the best I could do."

What I need to know is how big the wounds are and how deep. And now I see. It's massive. The worst part would be the internal concussive damage where the bullets ripped through the soft tissue and the shock waves reflected from the bones. The scars are much, much more than skin deep.

"You're going to be very expensive, boss," I say. "The helichrysum costs $50 a dram and you're going to need buckets of it."

"The hell what?" he asks.

"Helichrysum. The most powerful healing plant oil, very hard to get but you need it. What's the budget here, Jain?" I ask.

"None," he says. "Even if it costs more than fentanyl or morphine, it's got to be better. Drugs kill the pain but they don't heal anything. Order what you need and have them call Sunny for payment authorization. I'm serious about that. You're setting up the lab and we've got the funds. Shit, we just bought the house next door for the wellness side of the business."

For starters, I want rosehip and almond carrier oils, and the very dear helichrysum, about $500 worth if they have that much available, to heal his scars and deep tissue.

I want frankincense and myrhh to ease the pain, palo santo for cellular detoxification and jatamansi to calm his spirit, help him sleep and help release subconscious trauma.

I also want sandalwood for its powerful calming, uplifting and sedative properties. It's also very beneficial for injuries and inflammation.

Then I remember that if Jain and Sim are serious about bodybuilding they'll need sweet birch oil to help them recover faster. Rich in the same compounds as aspirin, it has a long history of use for sore and fatigued muscles. Mixed with helichrysum it will turn them into iron men.

I want this sickness to end now. I want to see him strong. It's not simply about detoxifying his body from the narcotics, though that's a serious concern. It's about removing the cause of the pain in the first place, repairing the tissues, erasing the trauma and calming his spirit. He needs to rebuild his strength in all five koshas before he's whole again. This is the difference between wellness care and disease management.

I call the little apothecary in Saratoga and talk to the owner, Sage. I tell her what I'm up to, setting up a private lab in the mountain for the doctors. She knows me and immediately offers a medical discount of 25%. When I tell her how much I want, she adds another 10% quantity discount.

When I tell Dr. Jain how much we've saved, he says to call Sage back and double the order. Then he goes back to the house to talk to Sunny about payment authorization and get some breakfast. I add two portable massage tables to the order. We've just bought $2500 worth of botanical pharmacopeia essentials for about $1600. For that kind of quantity they're happy to send a courier up the mountain to deliver it before lunch.

"That's a lot of medicine, Nat," Sage says. "I really appreciate your business. You must have a lot of patients up there."

"Not really, there's just two and I'm one of them! But the other one is a very special patient who needs a lot of care. We're going to need a lot more helichrysum next week, so see if you can source some more for me, honey."

"Who's the patient?" she asks, curious about who would buy thousands of dollars worth of botanicals. Dope dealers spend less on their habits.

"Mmmm, it's confidential but I trust you, Sage. You probably know him. Steven Mack."

"You've got S&M? The yoga teacher? I heard he was dealing heroin in Mexico! I didn't believe it but he just kind of disappeared. The stories they're telling about him are wild."

"Well don't let on that you know any better, Sage. He's just very sick and it's important no one knows where he is."

Steven's been listening to my conversation. "Tell Sage I love her," he laughs.

†

S&M

When she hangs up she's excited and starts pacing around the room looking for space. There's not much room to work.

"We'll put one of the tables in the new lab," she says, "but I want one in here for now. I don't want to move you yet. The big house is close enough but there's not the kind of privacy you need for this."

I'm giving her a little predatory warning smile, but the truth is I'm really starting to feel sick again. I haven't got anything left in me to even tease her. It's 10am and my body is heating up as it switches gears. Pitta time.

She sits down in the chair by the bed and studies the room. She hasn't had much chance to see it in the daylight yet. "I know better than to give you a massage in your bed, boss," she jokes. "I'm a quick study." She laughs and then her eyes go to the bed headboard just above my pillow and the laugh cuts short.

"Um," she says. "Have they been -- " She stops. I know she's looking at my beautiful hospital bed restraining cuffs hooked on the headboard.

"Restraining me? Not recently," I say. "Not since I started behaving."

She seems a little stunned as if I've been the victim of Chinese torture. She bites down on her lip hard.

"It's not what you think, Nat. I'm just playing with them now." I put both of my arms over my head, cross my wrists and give my biceps a little flex, what's left of them. "Just having a little fun." I wink at her.

That seems to shock her and she starts looking nervously around the room. I get the feeling she wants to run and hide. I want to show her the best hiding place on the planet.

"Nat. The kitchen," I say and she turns to look at me.

"The kitchen? Too small for a massage table," she says. She's clearly upset.

"Through the kitchen, baby. Trust me. Go through the back door."

Then I wait because she is going to forget everything about the cuffs in about three, two, one. I hear her open the back door and then the silence is deafening.

When I used to live up here, my favorite place was the back of the pool house. I'm not sure what kind of shape it's in now, but that's where Mack used to teach me yoga.

Behind the pool house, the mountainside falls away into deep forest below as far as the eye can see. There's no yard behind the house, but there used to be a yoga shala, an outdoor room on a deck overhanging the treetops, with a tinted plexiglass shade roof. There were flowering shrubs around its edge, jasmine, bougainvillea and hibiscus. It reeked of perfumed flowers when we sat back there to meditate. Sometimes it reeked of marijuana too when I was young and sneaking a smoke behind Mack's back.

Mack grew herbs out there and some stunning orchids. There used to be a big cement Medicine Buddha sitting near the edge. One of his hands was holding an apothecary bowl as an offering to heal mankind and the other hand held the branch of a flowering herb.

I remember how happy I was when I was stoned watching the heavy yellow orchid blossoms bowing at his feet. I liked to pick up the orchid petals and pile them in his little bowl and stick stems of herbs in his hand.

The only thing missing was a lotus pond and I'm betting she could have one sent up the mountain if she felt like it. I'll bet she could grow some of those $500 medicinal plants out there, too, if it crossed her mind.

She's gone a long time. Long enough to fall to her knees or sit on her ass and invoke the sacred deities that surround the shala like sweet Tibetan butter lamps. I hope it's still nice out there. It's my dream office. It ought to work just fine for therapy.

I wait a good twenty minutes and when she doesn't come back, I find the strength to sit up, put my feet down and take a few steps holding onto the wall. I haven't been on my feet since that day on the beach.

I pray I don't fall as I inch my way towards the kitchen. Fortunately the pool house is a very small place. I make it to the kitchen and the back door is open. The smell of jasmine is overwhelming.

I hold onto the doorframe and feel my head spin. It's beautiful out there, epic. I haven't been outside for so long. There's no rail around the deck and I know I can't go out there safely. The mountainside drops off so steeply one wrong step could take my life. But I wouldn't mind dying that way.

She's sitting in lotus position on her ass just as I thought, watching the divine perfection of the mountain. I just want to sit down without falling down.

"Nat," I say softly, "help me down. Please."

She comes back to the world suddenly. "Oh, Steven, I'm so sorry. I shouldn't have left you alone. Are you okay?"

"Just help me sit down," I say, pointing to the deck. I'm thinking of the Teaching Buddha with one hand on the Earth and the other hand open for blessings. The Earth is my witness. I want to sit down and touch the ground so badly. I want everything. Earth, Heaven, Consciousness, everything around me is sacred.

She takes my arm and helps me down to the ground before I fall down. But it's a long way down and I kiss the wood of the deck with the side of my head as I pass out.

†

JAKE

No one answers when I knock on the pool house door. Dr. Jain asked me to bring all the packages over for Nat and to sit with Sim for a few hours while he takes care of some business.

When I open the door, the bed is empty. I call out "Anybody home?" and I hear Nat's voice.

"Jake, out here. I need help." I follow the sound of her voice to the kitchen and out the back door. Sim is lying on the deck. I kneel down and start checking him. He's unconscious and has a cut over his right eye, not bad but a little blood."

"What did you do, honey? Punch him?" I tease her. "I'll bet he deserved it."

"No, he came out here, passed out and hit his head. Of all the things I know about healing, I know what I don't know. I don't know if I can move him if he has a head injury. I didn't want to leave him to use the phone because it's dangerous out here. I'm glad you came, Jake."

"Well, if he passed out before he hit his head, he probably just fainted so it's not a concussion. We could X-ray him to be sure, but unless he shows any symptoms, I wouldn't put him through all that ambo and hospital drama. Let's see."

I take his chin in my hand and turn his head and wipe the blood off. It's a very superficial cut with no sign of bruising. He opens his eyes and looks at the sky. "Bitch," he says. "I've missed you, mother." I know he's not talking to either one of us.

"Hey, Sim, let me get you back to bed."

"No." he says firmly. "Just help me sit. I want to sit here."

I help him sit up and he crosses his legs and sighs. "It's all I want," he says and looks out over the top of the redwood trees below. He seems okay.

I remember the packages and ask Nat where she wants them.

"You really are Santa Claus today, Jake. One of the big boxes, a massage table, goes to the new house. Just leave it outside for now. The other one comes out here. Can you set the table up for me? The rest of the packages go in the kitchen for now. I also need a couple of sheets from the house.

"Leave him on the deck where he can't hurt himself. We're going to be working out here anyway. It's his new office."

I set the table up and get the sheets and teasingly ask her if she needs some incense with that. She laughs and waves her hands at the flowers and pine trees surrounding the deck. "This is the incense," she says. "And as if this weren't enough, just wait until you smell the medicine."

†

NAT

Jake sits with Steven while I unwrap the packages in the kitchen. They are so very small and precious, it's hard to believe these little bottles cost so much. But as I open the bottle tops to blend the oils their fragrances are intoxicating. I find a few bottles that I didn't order, samples that Sage thought I'd like.

This first one I open is so seductive I put everything else aside to examine it. Like a fine wine it comes with "tasting notes". It has a beautiful sweet, woody fragrance with subtle citrus notes. And I note it's simply a blend of three of my favorite oils, Palo Santo, Frankincense and Sandalwood. The notes read:

'The Spirit Blend is the perfect combination to assist meditation or yoga practice and, emotional support. Some of it's the more important healing benefits are anti-anxiety, mood enhancing, nervine calmative, euphoric and cleansing and clearing to the mind. (Floracopeia)'

My job just got simple. This is the perfect blend for him and I don't think I can improve on it except to dilute it in the champa almond carrier oil and spike it with a big dose of the honey sweet helichrysum.

I pour the oils gently into a big shot glass I find in the kitchen. The mixture is possibly the most beautiful and interesting smell on the planet, rivaling even the forest behind the pool house.

The boys are both sitting silently on the deck when I return. I sit down between them and hand the shooter to Steven. "Don't drink it, honey, it'll kill you. Just smell."

His eyes widen as he starts taking deep breaths of the fragrant oils. "Fuck me," he swears. "Sex in a glass."

"Well, just keep breathing it for a minute. It works just fine with direct inhalation. But the real magic happens when your skin drinks it into the tissues and cells." I reach over and dip my index finger into the glass and anoint his third eye. Then I put a drop on my own forehead for focus.

I take the glass from him and put it on the ground. "Come on, let's get you on the table." Jake and I each take an arm and help him to his feet. He weighs next to nothing. "Lose the pants, Steven," I say and he drops his sweats and kicks them off without arguing. We help him onto the table flat on his back and cover his lower body with a sheet.

Smell is the most primal of the senses and is associated with the lowest chakra. The fight or flight instinct is linked to smell; it can either induce panic or wellbeing. Although the deepest benefits of abhyanga are created by absorbing botanicals into the skin, the heady scents begin the healing process as they draw the mind into the plants energy and information.

Smell, taste, sight, touch and hearing all combine to create wholeness and health in the lower chakras so that balance and integration can manifest in the higher chakras. The most powerful medicines have traditionally come from plants for millennia, but simple botanicals are only the raw ingredients. We can only absorb so much through the digestive system. The distiller's art has created powerful extracts from the essential oils.

"Do you know abhyanga, Steven?" I ask as I start gently rubbing the oils around the fingers on his right hand.

"Yep, yoga oil bath," he says. "I like almond oil."

"Good, so you know it's not a traditional massage, it's a means of trans-dermal absorption. Usually it's just done with simple fragrant oils, but we're taking it to higher ground. I'm adding very powerful medicines so that the base oil carries them through the skin into your cells.

"The healing qualities of the plants allow toxins to be released from the body and nourishment to be absorbed by the tissues. It's one the most important weapons in my arsenal."

"That's not been a big part of my practice," he says. "Never really got into it much except to keep my tan beautiful. I don't know why not."

"I can tell you why not," I'm working my way up his right arm and shoulder, following the same physical pathways as the nidra practice. "You never really needed it."

The fragrance of the oils are inspiring me. "There are eight ancient branches of healing and you've probably never needed to know about any of them. Internal medicine, pediatrics, gynecology, protection from demons, wounds from weapons and injury, poisons, aging and impotence.

"You're young, strong and healthy and haven't needed medicine until now. So you've focused your yoga practice on transcendental sex. Poor boy."

"Ouch," he squirms "That makes me sound really shallow."

"Consider it a blessing," I say. "Now you're forced learn about healing injuries and wound care. Trust me, transcendental sex is a lot more fun."

I start on his left fingers and work my way to the center of his heart. "But this is going to make you a better teacher. That which doesn't kill you makes you stronger, as Nietzsche wrote."

Then I start working on the scars and burns below his heart, slowly, easily. As much plant oils as I put on his skin, it disappears as a parched earth drinks in the rain.

"Nat?" he asks quietly. "Why didn't I learn how to teach this? The Medicine Buddha has been sitting here for a decade. Why didn't Mack go down this path? How did we miss it?"

"My favorite word, baby: 'Yet'. Mack hasn't gone down that path yet. You don't know how to teach it yet. But the door is open and you've both walked in."

I work my way down his lower abdomen, thighs, knees, calves, ankles, and give a lot of love to his feet. I think of the Buddha with lotus feet. Every bit of him is divine perfection. Then I turn to Jake, watching the whole procedure with a mix of interest and jealousy. I've used the whole glass of oil. I put one of Jake's hands on Steven's heart and go back into the kitchen to stir up some more medicine.

Steven's whole attitude has changed since he's come out here, as if the knock on the head shook him awake. But intuitively, I know it's the effect of the most illusive and pervasive element of the natural world: space.

We study the four elements of the body in Ayurveda, the same elements that pervade nature and botanical medicine: earth, water, fire and air. But often we forget the fifth element because it is so subtle that we take it for granted.

Akasha, the element of space, permeates the universe and holds us in a way that allows movement, change and life. Without space, the universe would be cemented into place, dead. On the deck of the yoga shala, above the forest top, face to face with the sky, space is so predominant that it's like an overdose of nectar. Space is wrapping us in a blanket of healing.

Jake helps me roll him over on his stomach and I realize I'm just starting. He makes a horrible grimace when he sees Steven's back, but I put a finger up to his lips and shake my head. Then I put an oiled finger on his forehead for focus.

Steven's got surfers lats, wings like a swimmer, lean and detailed like a carved deity. The beauty of his back is only accentuated by the damage. Weeks in a hospital bed have softened and shrunk the muscles but it's still a beautiful sight. It's all I can do to keep from crying as I rub the oils gently into his skin.

"I think I'm starting to see you a little more clearly," I tell him, "now that I've seen your office. You had me a little worried there for a minute."

"I'm sick, Nat," he groans. "If I were myself, I could really give you something to worry about."

"Is that a threat or a promise, Mr. Mack?"

"Both. By the time I'm walking, you'll know every hiding place on the property, or wish you did. But I won't molest you, Nat. I'll just harass you. I'm married."

His back is drinking the oils as fast as I apply them so I add a few more drops of straight helichrysum directly to his scars.

"Fair enough," I say. "Just so you know, the largest muscles of your body are here." I pull the sheet down and expose his cheeks. "So this isn't harassment, its why doctors like to give you injections in your ass. You can diffuse a huge amount of medicine into the body through the glutes."

"Sure, Nat," he says, "Eat your heart out, honey."

I roll my eyes and Jake starts laughing when I put my hands on his hips and butt cheeks. "Damn, Sim," he says, "you smell so beautiful it's dangerous. If you weren't married I think..."

"Don't think, Jake," he warns. "You might hurt yourself. I love you, too, buddy, but you're not getting any."

I finish the back of his legs and we turn him on his back again. There's not a drop of oil, not even a sheen on his skin.

"What now?" Jake wonders.

"I think we'll give him another coat." I start again at his finger tips. After the second coat on both sides, I take him through yoga nidra so the medicines can do their cellular work. He drops into deep conscious sleep.

"Jake, just stay here and make sure he doesn't get up for at least ninety minutes. I'll be back. I've been up all night and I've got to go see a doctor about a bed."

†

S&M

I dream of the ocean and of the long boas of seaweed dancing in the green light underwater. The image of the sun is etched on the surface far above me and its rays scatter like jewels of citrine and sapphire underneath the waves as they peel around the point.

I can sit down here forever, legs wrapped around a boulder, holding my breath and meditating to practice staying calm in a big wave wipeout. In this dream though, I'm pinned to the ocean floor flat on my back in sivasana, the corpse pose. I weigh so much that nothing can float me back up to the surface. I don't even need a rock to hold me under. I'm made out of cement. I'm the Teaching Buddha, lying on the ocean floor.

On the top of the mountain I can see my brother, the Medicine Buddha, sitting on his deck with a bowl full of drugs in one hand and sticky ripe cannabis flowers in the other. He's waiting for me with his medicine, but I'm hiding at the bottom of the ocean. I've been hiding underwater for eight years.

A beautiful fish circles above me and I can hear her singing my name. She swims up to my face and gives me a fish kiss on my forehead. Now I can see it's not a fish at all, but a mermaid with long streaming green seaweed hair, singing to me in Sanskrit. Om bhur bhuva svaha, she sings.

Earth, heaven, consciousness. She's forgotten to mention the ocean. Maybe a fish doesn't know about the ocean because it's so immersed in the water. Or maybe consciousness is the ocean. I like that better. The ocean is consciousness. I am so deep in it that I don't know it.

"Come up," she says. "Come up." I'm not sure if we can breathe if we both come up out of the ocean. I want to stay down here with her. Then she blows a kiss on my lips and I taste the air. I *do* know how to breathe.

"Steven," she says softly, "how do you feel?" I open my eyes and see Nat. I feel really nice. She kissed me. I feel rocked to the core of my soul and all of me is on the same page. But I also feel the powerful plants working in me, twitching pulses of blood and nerves around my ribs, rushes of energy in my feet and hands and smooth waves of orgasm snaking up my spine exploding in my forehead.

"I feel – ooh" I can't put a word on it at first. "I feel like– sea glass, I guess. I feel like all the edges have been polished off. I feel as smooth as glass."

"Good," she laughs. "Dr. Jain is here. We let Jake go home tonight. He'll be back in the morning and Dr. Jain will start your physical therapy then."

"Hey, Sim," Jain says. "You look absolutely stoned. I want whatever you're having."

"You absolutely do," I say, a little dreamy. "You absolutely have to have some of this. She can teach you some Tantra, Jain, and a little of the botanical witchcraft she's got. She's mad. I love her. Thank you for bringing her up here, brother."

"She needs some sleep, buddy. I can stay with you tonight. I got some good sleep today and she's loaned me a book on chakra therapy that I can read while I baby-sit you.

"Na.na.na.nah!," I insist. "You need direct transmission from a Tantrika, Jain. You can't learn this shit from books. If you're going to work with us, you need to learn this. I don't want to be the one who has to show you where your chakras are. Go get some lessons, baby."

I can see my beautiful assistant blushing. I'm handing her Jain on a plate.

"How about you, Sim?" she asks. "Jake's gone down the mountain. We can't leave you alone."

"Sweetheart, I don't need a doctor right now. What I need is a nurse."

She looks concerned. "Are you okay, honey? What's wrong?"

"That's the wrong question. 'What's right?' is what you should be asking. Whatever you gave me, I feel like fucking the universe tonight. I want Brandy. I want my wife."

"Oh, brother," she sighs. "I didn't think the champa would hit you that hard. But it's a sign that your body is getting stronger, so it's a good thing, baby."

She punches the nurses' extension into the phone and hands it to me. Sunny answers. "Sunshine," I beg, "Can Brandy take care of me tonight? I miss her so much. Please. With sugar."

Sunny laughs and hangs up on me, but after a few minutes Brandy walks in. "Can I stay?" she asks. I nod at Jain and point to Nat and then the door.

Jain says, "Gym at 10. Board meeting at noon. Get some sleep and call if you get sick. I'm on extension 5 now." Nat kisses me on ajna chakra and they're gone. I hope Jain gets some tantra lessons tonight.

"Lesson two, Beautiful," I smile at Brandy when they're out the door.

"I've been waiting, Sim," she says. "I feel you all the time."

"What I'm thinking is we should try something very unusual. Something I haven't done since I was a young punk who didn't know anything better."

I'm feeling like Shiva, the first yoga teacher, with his original student and consort Parvati. There's nothing I want to do more in this world right now than to teach her everything I know. It may take a long time, but I don't mind. The journey is the whole point. Which is why I married such a good student. I know divine perfection when it hits me in the face.

She pulls her dress over her head and gets in bed. She's got nothing on underneath. "My God, Sim, you smell like paradise."

"Yeah, I'm a very expensive whore right now. What I'm thinking is pretty wild even for me: plain old school straight sex. No hardware, no kinks, just see what kind of mileage we get. A proficiency test. What do you think? Just slow and serious. How late can you stay up tonight, honey?"

"All night. Forever."

"That's my girl. But I've got therapy and a board meeting tomorrow so let's just go half the night. Don't rush me. Just behave yourself, sweetheart."

I put my left hand on her tailbone and pull her close. I don't bother with chakras or mantras. I just let her take me slow.

†

S&M

Bran washes me and helps me into my sweat pants and I feel pretty hot, rested and excited about the therapy. When Jake shows up at 10 to get me, he has the wheelchair, but I want to walk.

"No, buddy," he says. "Dr. Jain insists you save your energy for the iron. Have a seat."

Brandy wants to come with us but I say not this time, it could be ugly my first time out. "We'll walk you to the house. I want to see my brother before I go."

Mack is in his office. He's surprised and jumps up to greet us.

"I just need a minute alone, Jake." He shuts the door. Mack just stares at me then says, "You look good, Steven. Two days. I'm impressed. No shakes? Not sick?"

"Yeah, I'm still getting sick but I'm much better, thanks. And that's all I wanted to say was thanks. I'm blown away."

"I'm sorry if I caused any unnecessary harm, brother."

I interrupt him before he can go too far down that path.

"Mack, you did the best you know how. It's not what you did, it's why you did it. You never left my room in the hospital. You never left me alone up here. And the pool house..." I can feel the tears coming but I don't care. "The shala is still there, the medicine Buddha, the herbs and flowers. It's the most healing space on the planet. You gave me that again. And you gave me that a long time ago, too." I sniff a little and give him a grateful smile.

"Do you know what I've got at my house down at the beach? On my deck, there's a Teaching Buddha, a little different from this medicine one. Teaching Buddha has one hand on the Earth and the other hand held up to pour out blessings. They could be brothers.

"I've got to go work out with Jain now. But thank you for you and for bringing me home, for bringing Jain up and thank you for Nat, God bless her hands."

"How about Brandy?" he laughs.

"That goes beyond the thank you department," I smile. "Get me out of here before I start kissing you."

Jake wheels me out into the yard by the pool and I see Jain doing bench press reps with 225, four forty-five pound plates on a forty-five pound Olympic bar. My heart sinks. I don't think I can press the empty bar. Then I send my shrunken ego out the back door. You can't get from here to there otherwise.

The little gym is compact and lethal. It doesn't take much to wreak mayhem on muscles. And why is Nat here, I ask? Jain says she's going to coordinate the weight work with yoga and show him a few things

"Can you stand?" she asks. "Tadasana. Mountain pose."

I push up from the chair and plant my feet perfectly parallel. I know how to stand. I know how to breathe. I'm seriously ready to tear the walls down and get back to my life.

"Hasta Utthanasana," she instructs. Sky-reaching pose. The sky is a bloody long way up there and my lats are destroyed but I go slow, arms wide with my palms up. When I can't reach any higher than my shoulders, she puts her hands under mine and pushes my arms up slowly. My palms are still a good two feet apart and I can't bring my hands together.

"That's fine," she says. "Do a couple more, nice and slow. Whatever you can do right now is where you are today. How about Utkatasana?"

"No way in hell," I say to the chair sitting pose. It's enough to just stay on my feet.

"A couple inches, whatever you can do," she encourages me. Jain watches me do a pitiful air squat and winces.

"I've got this, Nat," he says. "Start him with just a negative squat to the bench. Here," he shows her. He stands me next to the bench and puts his hands under my arm pits. "Sit down, buddy," he says. I squat down a little and he holds me and eases me down so I don't crash on the bench. Once I'm sitting, he lifts me back to my feet. "Like that, okay? Just negative reps for now. Five times is good." He's doing most of the lifting but my legs are remembering how to work.

Jain loves me. I'd like to tear the weights up for him, but it's only going to get ugly here.

"Lats," he says. "pull downs. Just ten pounds."

I reach my hands over head and grip the bar, but when I pull it down the pain is excruciating. I don't much mind pain but this interrupts my world. I let go of the bar and the little iron slab comes crashing down on the stack of weights. It's really bad form. I'd be kicked out of a gym for less.

"Again," he says patiently. "This time wrap your head around it."

So I know what's coming and I wrap my mind around the pain and pull the bar down to kiss my heart as I arch my back, but it's not any better. It's a horror show.

"One." he says. "Give me five."

I give him two and let go of the bar.

"Don't tell me we built this gym so you could do two reps with ten pounds, Sim. If I have to, I'll get some hand cuffs and fasten you to the bar until I get five."

I start laughing hard. He knows me better than my brother. It's going to hurt no matter what. I pull the pin from the stack and move it to twenty pounds. It's not the weight that hurts, it's the movement through space.

I give him a perfect eight, breathing smoothly through my nose, ignoring the red hot iron knives cutting through my flesh. I can feel Nat's eyes on me like the most powerful balm on my muscles. She sees my strength and I feed on her attention. I walk on water. I set the weights smoothly back onto the stack instead of letting them crash. Control. Intention. Will. I'm driving now.

Jain laughs. He puts his hands on my shoulders and gives me a squeeze. "You know, buddy, they gave us some t-shirts when we bought all this equipment. I didn't think you'd want one because you hate shirts, so I gave them to the girls. But I thought I'd pass the message on. They read "Pain is weakness leaving the body."

I fasten my eyes on Nat. She knows everything I know. The world is pain, so said the Buddha. Pain is optional, arising from ignorance and confusion. Physical pain is a messenger from the flesh to the mind and that which doesn't kill me makes me stronger. This little twenty pound stack can't kill me or do me any harm. I move the pin to thirty pounds.

I like this new mantra. Pain is weakness leaving the body. I give it eight reps and watch all the weakness in me going to hell.

†

S&M

We hold the first official board meeting for the wellness center in the living room of the new house. Jain, Mack and I are the Directors and equal partners. Mack nominates me to be the corporate President, Jain the CEO and he'll be the CFO. Since he's got the nurses on his team, they'll do all the administration and accounting. My team will do education and therapy. We all agree on that.

We've got our core staff, two doctors, two nurses, two therapists, just like we planned and we all agree these are the people we want to keep.

"So, Mr. President," Mack jokes, "What shall we call this business? Got any ideas? Mack, Mack and Jain, Inc. sounds like a law firm."

I haven't given it much thought but I want something that says healing, yoga, surfing and enlightenment all at once. "Without going all kinky into Sanskrit, I like Surya, the Sun. So Sunrise Wellbeing would be cool for me."

"I'm good with that," Jain nods.

"You're too easy," I joke.

"You have no idea how easy I am, buddy," he winks.

Mack laughs at us. "I'm good with that, too. Sweet. I'll have Sunny mock up some logo designs for us. We'll get the lawyers to draw up the papers and incorporate effective today. I think the proper order of corporate conduct is that the President runs the meeting, but I've got an agenda item if you don't mind."

"Shoot," I say. "I don't really have anything planned."

"Sean wants to meet with us to discuss a community project in partnership with the police department. I thought it would be okay to invite him to talk about it. He's having coffee with the nurses right now. Should I call him over?"

"Absolutely. We need coffee, too. Do we have any corporate minions to serve us some lunch? I'm ravenous."

Mack calls the kitchen and asks if Sunny minds sending Sean over and fixing coffee and sandwiches. He puts his hand over the phone and asks, "Egg salad or tahini, Mr. President?"

"Both," I say. "Lots of sandwiches."

Sean comes in and shakes hands all around. "Looking good, Sim," he says. "You're finally up."

"Your floor, Sean. Tell us how we can help the department."

"Thanks. I've been meaning to talk to you about this but you had your own problems. I didn't want to add to it. But now things are getting better up here.... and terribly bad down there."

"I think we might have made a big mistake by hiding you and keeping the story out of the papers. I wanted to protect you but it's backfired in a big way."

"Yeah, it's kind of funny. I've heard the rumor that I'm now a notorious heroin dealer in Mexico. That's a laugh. Nat heard it from Sage at the apothecary."

"It's all over the place. Crystal said the story started spreading through the bar a few weeks ago. You've got a mansion on the beach in Oaxaca and you're working with the Zetas cartel up in Sonora."

"Not my style," I laugh. "I'd be more inclined to sell pot out of Nayarit. Nice islands offshore."

"Well however bullshit the story is, the cartel is now actually controlling the point. And most of your old crew thinks you're working with them. And there goes the neighborhood. The girls won't even surf there anymore. And the Point Guard is history. They're all shooting smack and dealing to the tourists. Gangs drive in from San Jose to get a piece of it. The department has lost the battle. We don't have the community on our side anymore. It's filthy dirty with drugs down there."

"Ouch," I say. "So that's why I got shot, to get my crew out of the way?"

"Most likely. And I've been thinking a lot about it and talking to Crystal. We need to tell the truth and take the beach back. It's only been a few weeks so it's not all the way to hell yet. But we've got to go big and hit it hard. You know the old surfer mantra, 'Go hard or go home.' That's what I want to do with this."

"I'm in, Sean. How do you want to do this?"

"Well, Crys came up with this idea the night of your wedding and we've been talking to a few people. I've got connections at the local paper and they are dying to break the story. I made a deal to give them an exclusive interview if they run it on the front of the Sunday paper. That way everyone and their mother will see it."

"Wow," I say. "Front page."

"Front page Sunday paper. Very important. Everybody's sitting around drinking coffee over their brunch reading the local paper. The gossip is going to hit town like a bomb."

"So what's the story going to be? I'm alive and bench pressing 20 pounds?"

"No this is going to be totally 'in their face' news. The reporter and photographer will come up here on Friday to interview you and the staff and write about the wellness center as a private invitation only training facility. No word of where it is, just a website contact form. We'll say you're training a team of surfers for a community challenge. We're taking applications."

"Not a bad idea, even if we aren't."

"Aren't yet, buddy. Keep that thought going down the road. It's a project I've been thinking about.

"The best part is not the interview, though. This is Crystal's brain child. We go down to the point on Saturday and just create a major scene before the story breaks and get some more photos.

"I mean we take a lot of squad cars and go down there with lights and sirens and park illegally all over the top of the cliff and do a live press conference. Staged but impressive. The story's already written, we're just going to turn heads and get attention. Crys got the idea from your cop hat.

Dress like a freak in the hat and handcuffs and get out of the police car and make them think they've seen a ghost. No shirt, all your kinky gunshot scars and you're coming on looking for revenge with the whole police department backing you up. We'll have enough cops there to protect you from the thugs, and we'll have a lot of guns out for show.

"The bar's going to go wild with gossip and then the story will hit the front page the next day. Bam! We got their attention. We'll let everybody know which side you're on. Crys wants to call it the Steven Mack Attack."

Sunny comes in with a mountain of sandwiches and two pots of coffee. I'm going to need a lot of egg salad if I want to look good next week.

"We got any steroids up here, CEO?" I tease Jain. "This could get fun."

†

NAT

I'm working in the new lab, just off the kitchen of the new house, mixing up my newest science project, the bodybuilding blend. Brandy helped my cut some sprigs of orchids and pine branches out on the shala and arrange them on the window still. There's a dance of sunlight filtering through the redwood trees behind the house and there's enough space, privacy and warmth in here for the ambience we need.

It's a beautiful little lab, probably at one time the pantry for the kitchen, with glass door shelves along one wall which I'm filling with amber bottles of oil. The massage table is in the center of the room and there are neat stacks of sheets and towels.

I can hear the guys laughing in the next room as they finish up their board meeting. It sounds like they're done with their business and just enjoying each other's company. I peek into the room and Steven waves me in.

"All done but for the food. Tahini, honey?" I've already eaten so I shake my head, but I sit down at the table with them.

Jain winks at me and I feel it hit me in my sacrum. I've got to concentrate. I look into his left eye and see his soul, warm and sweet. Then I look at my boss and get another wink. Mack is smiling like I've never seen before and licking jam off his fingers. I wonder what's gotten into them. They seem so relaxed. Then I wonder if they know.

"I'm looking for a guinea pig," I say. "Someone who's been lifting weights."

Jain and Steven raise their hands at the same time. Jain says, "No you first, Mr. President. By all means, you go first. What are you up to, Nat?" he smiles.

"I've got a new birch and helicrysum blend with rosehip oil. It's supposed to help your muscles repair and rebuild faster. A poor girl's steroid concoction. And I've got the new lab set up for a test drive. Open for business, baby."

Steven pushes up on the table and winces a little. "Negatives, Jain," he swears. "Funny how they can sneak up on you without warning. I'm definitely ready for this."

I take his arm and walk him into the lab. He whistles. It's a beautiful space and already filled with the heady scents from the little diffuser.

"Nice work, Nat," he says. "Are you trying to get a raise?"

"You know the drill, boss." He toys around with the draw string of his sweat pants like he's not sure if he wants to lose them, but I know he's just being a bad boy. "Boss? Please?"

I pick up a sheet and hold it in front of him for modesty.

"Oh? Getting shy now?" he says.

"Never," I tease. "I could shock you."

He strips and lays on the table and I cover him. "Try me," he says.

"Tantric sex lessons," I whisper in his ear. Then I start working on his right hand and fingers. "I shocked myself."

"No way. Jain?"

"When we left last night, I didn't want to sleep in IC so we came over here. There're two spare rooms. But I was so tired, I didn't feel like being alone. I asked him if he'd just curl up with me."

"And?"

"He said it would be hard to just hold me. And I said I hoped it would be hard. He was just as easy as frosting on a cake. So I showed him a little transcendence."

"Good girl," he smiles. "He's going to be a very good student."

†

NAT

The nurses have gone down the mountain to shop and pick up some more oils for me. I've taught them both how to do abhyanga on me. My scars are clean and less painful now. Between us, Sim, Jain and I, we're going through hundreds of dollars worth a day, but the results are extraordinary. Sim's bench press is up to 95 pounds for a single and he's pulling the lat stack with 60 pounds. I can tell it's painful for him but he just blows through it.

So I'm just checking on him because he's all alone taking a nap. He's really so beautiful I have to leave my heart parked outside. He stretches one of his arms overhead and yawns, smiling into my eyes and then a wave of energy makes him groan.

"Oooh. That's what I'm talking about. Abundance doesn't stop coming," he grunts with pleasure.

I put my hand on his wrist, tight. "You know, baby, that gesture you made the other day?" I take his other wrist in my free hand and raise it over his head so I have both wrists crossed against the headboard and hold him tight. "Do you know how disarming that was?"

He grins and his teeth flash like a dozen suns rising. "It was meant to be. You know what I like," he says. "Why are you so sweet to me?"

"It's what I do," I say. I'm intoxicated with him. I don't really know what he likes. It's a little crazy for me.

"I'd love to tie you up," I say, "but what's the point? You're already my prisoner, aren't you?" Two more jolts hit him in succession and I feel it resonating through me as well.

"What's the point?" I say again and it's not a question. "Sex is an expression of love and trust. Otherwise, it's just an act of loneliness and fear. I've got your love and trust in my pocket."

He has another orgasm and I let go of him. God, he's so easy.

"It's the thought, Nat," he smiles. "Thought creates intention and desire. The rest is just energy."

"And you've got enough sexual energy to burn the house down, my friend," I tease him. He doesn't need anything from me except a clear mirror reflecting back what he already feels.

Then he shuts the flirting smile off and looks at my face closely like he's assessing a piece of art.

He's got me pinned with his steel blue stare. "Nat," he says "I wonder if you can help me out with some, um – physical therapy. I trust you, honey."

His eyes are glazed with passion and he nearly chokes on the words 'physical therapy.' To tell you the truth, he's scaring me.

He says, "I wonder if you'd help me. I miss ....."

As beautiful as he is, I don't want to go further.

"Steven, stop it. It's just not happening." I think I know what he wants.

"Look, baby, I'm not talking about sex. I'm talking about play. I just wonder if you'd do some things for me."

I think I know but I wait to hear it from his lips.

He winks and smiles at me. "Hit me, honey."

It's a game changer. I work for him. He's also my patient. And he wants to play at some kinky stuff where I won't go.

"No thanks. No way." I say and I'm halfway to the door.

"Nat, I thought you might. I had a friend, Nick. Mmmmm. She – oh shit I miss Nicky."

I turn around and may have turned to salt. I'd do anything for him and he knows he can coax this out of me if he plays his hand carefully.

"I'm not talking about sex, honey. I'm talking about pain. What kind of twisted pervert do you think I am if I don't know the difference?"

He's broken the ice with a hammer and his laughter sends a chill down my spine. If he were begging for sex I would have gladly paid him for it. But he's just freaking me out a little.

"Not happening," I say. "Ahimsa. 'No Harm'. Not to you. Not to me. You teach this, Sim. Rule One. Do no harm."

"That's why I'm asking *you*, Nat, sweetheart. I don't want to get hurt. I trust you, baby.

"I'm sure Sunny would like to whack me into next week, but I'm not into the emotional side. I'm not into domestic violence, injury, damage, suffering. Its not complicated. I just want a little simple pain without all the emotional baggage. Pain is weakness leaving the body. That which doesn't kill me makes me stronger."

He crushes my emotional baggage as he gets out of bed and pulls on his jeans. I don't think my English can express his details with any justice. I can't help but stare.

"Don't you think you have enough pain already, hon?"

"No," he says. "This is all wrong, this constant crap everywhere. I want the optional kind. Controlled. Intentional."

He zips his jeans. He slides the belt out slowly like a pro, smiling and biting his tongue. He should have been a stripper; he's missed his true calling. He folds the belt in half and tests it across the palm of his hand. It smacks. It works.

"Nick always used a surfboard leash. It never left a mark or did any damage. But I'll bet a belt will work." He laughs. "I'll bet its been done before."

Why I'm still in the room talking to him about this bothers me.

"Ahimsa," he says. "It will really hurt me if you say no. I trust you, baby."

I don't answer so he starts pouring sugar and sweetness all over me.

"Look, beautiful. I know you're not shy. And this is not complicated."

He puts the belt into my hand and closes my fingers around it. Then he turns his back on me, putting his hands against the wall. "Come on, honey. Give it a shot. What have you got?"

He spreads his back muscles like a body builder, making himself a bigger target, but the sight of his beautiful skin with all the gunshot scars below his heart tears my own heart open.

"Sim, no." I say.

He turns and sees the tears in my eyes and his face falls into cold fury. "Look, Nat. I'm not crippled. I'm not wounded. I can walk on water. I'm fucking immortal. Just hit me and see how strong I really am. Damn it, girl, I'm just trying to have a little fun here. You're killing me."

Then he mutters under his breath. "Where is Nicky when I fucking need her?"

I'm standing on the starting line and don't want to step across it. I have a feeling this is going to hurt me far worse than its hurts him. But he's asked me so sweetly. He wants this. I swing the belt and bring it down easily between his shoulders.

He doesn't move for a minute. Then he drops his arms and turns around slowly. His eyes are burning into me.

"Nat. Shit. Did you even put a drop of intention into that?"

I feel guilty. I've put more effort into slamming a car door.

"Get serious, Nat. Quit wasting space."

He twists his lips so I see teeth on one side and a frown on the other. He's not happy with my performance. Then I see his upper lip twitch hard like a mad dog. He stops talking to me and turns his back again, hands against the wall.

This time I lay into him with all the tea in China. I can feel the blow vibrate back through my arm and body and it sends a rush of fear and adrenaline down my legs.

I admit, its not a cold shot. There's an element of fury and proving my point in it. He flinches hard and starts to laugh.

"Shit, woman. You're not supposed to hurt me! You're not very good at this, are you?"

I'm shaking with fear. Every instinct in my body tells me I'm in danger, that he's going to come at me and hit me back. But instead, he puts an arm around my shoulder and gives me a squeeze as he takes the belt away.

"Let me give you a few pointers," he says like a patient yoga teacher correcting my posture.

He smiles sideways at me and then tears into the wall with the belt full force and laughs.

"I can take the paint off the walls, baby." He snarls and I can actually see the damage where he's hit the wall.

"Or," he continues, "I can put a little love into it and pull it back so it just stings without causing any damage." He whips the belt against the wall hard but pulls it back sharply so it makes a cracking sound. There's not a mark on the wall.

"See what I mean? You don't want to take my skin off, Nat. It's all in your mind. If you intend damage, you'll cause it. But if you play, it's game on. Put some intention into it. Try again, honey."

He turns his back on me again and I can see a wide red welt rising where I took the paint off. I want to do this right. Nice. Hard. Intentional. This time I hit him hard with loving care and precision.

He turns around with a smile of admiration and appreciation. "There you go, baby," he says. God, I'm proud of myself. What the hell am I doing here?

"Give me a second, Sim," I go over to his bed and untangle the leather cuffs from the headboard. He's watching me and then he turns all thirty-two teeth on me at once.

"Game on, baby!" he laughs.

†

S&M

By the time the girls get back from shopping, I'm lying by the pool working on my tan. Nat is working on my back with helichrysum, birch, sweet myrhh, and frankincense infused in champa almond oil. I smell like a French whore.

I'm not talking to her, but I'm proud of the way she crossed the line for me today. I wouldn't trust my wife to do that. Brandy is still an amateur in the transcendence department and I don't think I'd like her to hit me. I don't want to get my sex and my games all mixed up. It's too complicated.

Jain comes over and pulls up a deck chair and smiles at Nat.

"Some people have it all sorted," he says. "What do I have to do to get the royal treatment?"

"Just ask me, Jain," she says. "I've got two hands and they're not going to be on him all day."

"Please." He begs.

He's watching her hands on me and I guess I've got a pretty hardcore welt across my back that he notices.

"What's up with that?" he says and he puts his hand on my back to feel it.

"A tactical error, Jain." I volunteer. "No medical attention required."

"Are you sure, buddy? It looks like a burn. Or – "

"No," I say. "It was a mistake. Nat put some arnica on it for me. Is it a nice addition to my scars? I can't really see it."

"It's pretty sweet, Sim, if you're into that. As a doctor, I'm not really that fond of scars."

"I hear you, Jain, but we can't survive on candy. You'd get sick after a while. Hey, I think I've overworked my assistant today but she's got some game left in her. Take your shirt off, lover boy. It's your turn."

I push up on my elbows so I can watch this. He's taking his shirt off like a twelve-year old boy in a locker room but he's built like an atom bomb; she is loving every inch of him.

I get up and wink at Nat. "Thank you, baby. He's all yours," I say. "I'm going to go molest my wife."

I find Brandy in the pool house making the bed. She picks the cuffs up off the dresser and says, "You've been playing with these?"

Nah. I don't think she needs to know what games I'm playing, so I just say, "I think it's your turn." I put one of the cuffs gently around her wrist and pull her close to me. I know I smell intoxicating and the fragrances are turning me on full force.

She looks at the cuff and says, "I don't think so, baby. It's not for me."

"Oh, yes," I insist. "I know you're going to like this. Look what you're doing to me already just thinking about it." I take her free hand and put it on me and see her eyes go big with excitement.

"You know, baby," I add, "how the old surfers' mantra goes? 'Go hard or go home.' I want to show you hard today." I kiss her with everything I've got and I know it's money in the bank now. She'll do anything.

"Follow me, honey," I command her. I pull the futon off the sofa and drag it through the kitchen and out onto the deck and she follows me out. Then I lock the kitchen door from the outside. What's the point of a sanctuary if you can't bolt the world out?

"I hope you're not shy about doing this in front of the birds," I tease her because this is probably the most secluded and private spot on the property. I pull her dress over her head and then hold the other cuff out to her. "I won't do anything without your permission," I add.

She gives me her wrist and she's looking a little wild. I put the other cuff on her. "More control lessons, Sim?" she asks.

"Mmmm. I'm not going to attach you to anything, just lay down."

I start stripping really slow for her as she lies on the futon. I haven't got much to take off so I make every bit count, unfastening the belt buckle, pulling it slowing out through one loop at a time, running the leather through my hands slowly and damn, I start thinking about Nat tearing into my flesh with it, hitting me the wrong way.

I'm running a little bit hot and on the edge of control. I unfasten the button and unzip the jeans so she can see how hard I am, but I can't bother taking them off. I take a deep breath and lie down and pull her wrists over her head. Then I kiss her softly on the mouth with my lips closed. I pull my head back and look her in the eyes. She's wild with passion.

"Your turn for chakra lessons, baby," I tell her. I kiss her forehead long and slow. Then her mouth again a little harder. Then her throat and back to her lips, just like I had her do for me. She starts groaning. When I kiss her heart, she puts her hands down with the cuffs around the back of my neck and holds me there tightly. I can hear her heart pounding.

I'm in no rush to get anywhere. I can make this last all day. I've got all the time in the world to kill and no mercy at all. I kiss her belly button and put my tongue in it, then give her a huge long French kiss on the mouth. When I kiss her sex she digs her hands into my hair and pulls it.

"Don't hurt me, baby," I scold her. "Behave like I taught you." Then I'm back to her mouth and push my cock hard and deep into her first chakra. I don't move for about a minute just to tease her.

"Please, Sim," she begs. "Please, baby."

"Can't you feel me?" I tease. "I'm right here."

"Yes, but please don't stop yet. You said hard. Show me hard, Sim."

"Are you begging, baby? What's my name?"

"I'm begging, S&M, please. Please teach me some more."

"Well, since you're begging so politely, I'll do whatever you tell me to do, baby, as long as you tell me to do it. Hard it is."

As private as it is back here, I have a feeling they can probably hear her screaming all the way down in Saratoga and for sure in both houses. But I don't really mind much. I'm still on my honeymoon.

†

S&M

The moon is full again. It's been a month since I was shot and it feels like an eternity. We're sleeping outside on the futon on the shala deck. Well, trying to sleep but it's impossible to close my eyes with all the stars glittering and dancing in the moonlight.

I wonder if I can hear the high tide sucking on the rocks ten miles below and I listen for it, but instead I hear cars coming up the steep road. Big engines at a steady pace, cop cars I think. I wonder why they're sending more cars up at this time of night. It's after 2am.

I feel a cold rush of adrenaline down my legs and know something's wrong. Then I hear car doors slam, four times, and voices from the house.

"Bran, honey." I wake her. "Can you go see what's up?" She gets up, naked in the moonlight and wraps herself in her beautiful kimono and then she's gone. More voices, then a long silence. She doesn't come back.

I go back into the bedroom and dial 1. Mack picks up and says, "If you're up you probably should come over. Fair warning, though, it's very bad."

I'm shaky. It's my worse time of the night, Vata time, but it feels good to walk. I step off the path onto the grass and feel it wet with dew between my toes. How bad can anything be under this blanket of ancient stars and galaxies? Because we are surrounded by divine perfection, we are all protected.

I'm humming the Gayatri mantra as Bran comes out to meet me. She takes my arm without a word and I keep singing, but when we get to the house and I see what's going on, I stop breathing.

Sean is standing there with Mack and two other officers. Between them is DJ in handcuffs with his head down. It doesn't look like they're playing cops. I just stand in the doorway bewildered. My first thought is how did he age so much in a month? He looks rough and dirty and hard as nails.

But when he looks up and sees me, he starts crying like a baby. "Sim." He chokes on my name, then tries it again. "Darrell's fucking dead."

Sean is the only one in the room with any composure. The other two cops look decidedly uncomfortable being here.

"Good news or bad news first, baby?" he asks. "Cause there isn't a lot of good news."

"Fine," I say. "Go there then."

"We think we've got the guys who shot you." He nods toward one of the officers who produces some mug shots from his clipboard and hands them to me.

"I'm not sure if that's good news," I say. "Now I can't get a fair fight."

I pass the photos to Brandy and she breaks out crying. "Yes, that's them," she sniffs.

So the good news is you don't need police protection any more. They're in jail for the long haul on three felonies. Attempted murder, conspiracy to commit murder and murder in the first degree. And that's the end of the good news.

"Murder?" I ask.

"Okay. Here we go down the long road of bad news. They shot Darrell. Same guys, same time and place as you, full moon high tide on the beach by the stairs. Except this time there was no one down there to help him.

"There were witnesses on the cliff but by the time anyone could respond, it was too late. I'm sorry, Sim. You know I loved him. It's fucked."

DJ is watching me like a dog. He's stopped crying but he looks like he's waiting for a whipping.

"And him?" I ask.

"Two counts of felony narcotics possession and intent to sell. Heroin. Resisting arrest. He's looking at prison time, Sim."

Now I'm ready to belt him, handcuffed or not.

"What the fuck, DJ?" I hiss at him. "You're working with the guys who shot me and killed Darrell? You..." I dig deep but can't find words strong enough to hurl at him. He won't look up.

"It's worse than that, Sim. Your beach house is drug central. That's how the rumor got started that you're down in Mexico working with the cartel. I didn't want to do this, but it was getting too heavy and we had to shut it down. Most of the Point Guard are using and dealing and they all think they're working for you, thanks to this little shit."

I'm standing at the starting line and there's a fire burning in my feet and rising up my spine. It takes everything I have to walk across the room and stand in front of DJ without beating the shit out of him.

He's concentrating hard on his feet and sniffing and I realize it's not from crying, it's a junkie sniff. I take his arm and inspect the tracks along his veins. Then I laugh and hold my own arm up next to his. The marks and scars from all my IVs look like a road map compared to his. His eyes widen with interest but he keeps his mouth shut.

I see a fresh tattoo above the knuckles on his right hand, a gang mark. It's a 36. Christ, I think, that's my street, 36th Avenue. "Getting an early start on your prison tatts, honey?" I snarl. He says nothing but shakes and sniffs.

I take his chin in my hand hard and raise his face inches from mine, forcing him to look into my eyes. He looks at me with such an intense mixture of fear and love that I feel a knife going through my heart. He's waiting for my worst and I can't raise it.

"Sean, let's talk in the office. You, too," I tell DJ and let go of his face. "The rest of you go back to bed. Brandy, baby, go to bed."

She comes over and kisses me. DJ's eyes go wide with shock, as if of all the events of his world crashing apart, seeing me kiss the ghost girl tops everything.

†

SEAN

Sim leads us into Mack's study and locks the door behind us. He doesn't say a word but sits down in Mack's big chair and tips his head towards the couch. We sit but no one speaks. Sim puts his head back and inspects the ceiling for a minute with long steady breaths. Then he looks at me and holds his wrists up together.

I take a cuff key on a neck chain out of my pocket and toss it towards him on the desk. "I told you I'd bring you a pair to keep," I joke. He doesn't laugh.

He picks the key up and grimaces. Then he gets up and unlocks the handcuffs on DJ and snaps both cuffs on his own left wrist like a bracelet. He puts the key chain over his head and hangs it next to his silver handcuff necklace and sits down again.

He's still not talking and his silence is more menacing than any hard words. This is a side of him I've never seen before: hard, mean and cold. No wonder the gangers wanted to see him dead.

I throw an envelope on the desk and he pours the contents out: a big wad of cash and a silver cuff necklace. He fingers the necklace then tosses it on DJ's lap.

"Put it back on, baby," he says.

DJ is speechless.

"You're welcome," Sim says. "I don't think you should be talking anymore either. So, Sean?" he turns to me. "Why the fuck is he here?"

I explained that we arrested him yesterday, arraigned him today and I personally bailed him out tonight but I can't put him back on the street. "Would you take him?" I feel stupid asking but it's all I've got.

Sim starts laughing a mean laugh. "Would I take *what*?"

"Lock him up, clean him up, put him under house arrest, under medical supervision."

He stops laughing and glares at me. "Sean, we have pharmaceutical drugs up here that make your stepped on street heroin look like candy. I don't think he needs to be here."

"Sim, it's his only chance. If I can get him into rehab and cleaned up by his court date, we might keep him out of prison. It's a heavy charge but he's young and it's his first offense. There's only a slim chance the judge would give him the opportunity when it goes to court, but if he's already voluntarily in treatment, we have a much better chance.

"We can still win the war, Sim. Darrell's dead. Billy's been suspended from the pro tour. I can give you a list of all your friends losing the fight. I don't want to have to arrest half the county. And if I put him back on the beach he's as good as dead."

"Are you staying over, Sean?" he asks.

"If you need me to. Otherwise, if you take custody, I'd love to go home and sleep."

"Then go home, Sean. We'll talk tomorrow." He shows me to the door and points his fist to the floor in a shaka. "Thank you, brother," he says.

†

DJ

Sim shuts the door and stares at me. I'm ready for him to hit me but he just shakes his head and sneers.

"I guess you're going to be getting those Tantra lessons after all, little brother," he says.

He puts his arm around my shoulder and walks me out of the back door into the night. We walk across the grass to a little house at the edge of the mountain and he opens the door.

There's a candle burning and the room is bright with moonlight. The girl is curled up in the big bed and she sits up when we walk in.

"I know him, Sim," she says. "He was at Nick's house."

"Oh?" he teases me. "You got into Nick's house? I'm impressed."

I'm stunned. I'm still waiting for his anger. It's like a gun with one bullet in the chamber and I don't know when it's going to fire.

"Don't get too used to this, honey," he says. "You'll be staying in Mac's house after tonight. But for now, I think you need to sleep here. With a nurse. You're going to be a sick fuck."

He points to the bed with the girl in it. "You take that side. Don't touch her. Get some sleep. And don't worry, I'll beat the shit out of you tomorrow."

Part Two: FIRE AND ICE

*"Some say the world will end in fire, / Some say in ice.
From what I've tasted of desire / I hold with those who
favor fire.
But if it had to perish twice, / I think I know enough of hate
To say that for destruction ice / Is also great / And would
suffice."*

~ Robert Frost

Part Two

FIRE AND ICE

†

BRANDY

Before the sun even rises, I wake up confused. I have my arm around his shoulder and he's dripping wet and shaking. I remember the morning after our wedding and how sick he was. I thought he was better now. And then I'm fully conscious and I realize it's not Sim, it's the other one, his young friend who slept with us last night.

"It's okay, honey," I whisper so I don't wake Sim. "We're going to help you." I climb out at the foot of the bed so I don't have to disturb either of them and get a cool wet washcloth from the bathroom for his forehead. And then I notice how dirty he is. It's not just that he needs a bath; he's got fresh cuts and scrapes all over him with thick dirt embedded in the dried blood.

He's got dirty tear stains still wet on his cheeks and dried snot beneath his nose. I guess he may be about 21, but right now he looks like a twelve year old boy throwing a temper tantrum. I start washing his face gently with the cloth, taking some of the grime off and he hisses at me.

"Fuck off," he says. "Don't touch me."

That makes me laugh, in spite of his plight. "And don't talk to you? And don't look at you? Right? You sound like someone I know. Sim's right here sleeping. He wants me to help you. I'm a nurse, remember me from Nick's house?"

"Sim's going to kill me," he says and a huge shiver runs through him. "I'm a dead man."

"Why should I bother?" Sim growls from the other side of the bed. "You're doing a damn fine job of killing yourself for me, DJ. I can just sit back and watch."

DJ freezes at the sound of his voice. I pull the sheet back a little to assess the mess and see the needle tracks on his arm. I look closer and see that the long dirty scrapes along his forearms have sand and rocks in the cuts like he's been dragged behind a car.

"How did you do this, honey?" I ask.

He doesn't answer me. His eyes are nailed shut and he's breathing like the planet is running out of its atmosphere. I try to wash some of the dirt off the cuts and he yells at me to stop.

"What happened?" I try again.

"I fell," he says and then sneers, "resisting arrest. I went down the fucking cliff the hard way."

I pull his shirt up and see his rib cage and groin are all scraped up as far as I want to look. "Get your fucking hands off me. Fuck off," he hisses.

"Sim," I beg. "He needs medical care. Can we get him out of here?"

"Please," he says. "I know exactly where this is going. I don't need to see anymore. He's got a one-way ticket to hell. It's definitely Mack's specialty from here: needles, hits and drips. Get him out of here, please. I can't be around this right now."

"Can you help me get him back to the house, Sim?" I ask.

"No, I can't," he says. "I've got some important business. Mack will take care of it." He gets up and walks through the kitchen and slams the back door behind him.

It's barely 6am. I call Dr. Mack's study first, then his bedroom. I hate to wake him, but he's my boss.

"What's up, Brandy?" he asks. "The new guy?"

"Yes, sorry but he needs to move to IC. He's sick and he's injured. Can you help me?"

"Wow," he says. "I'm surprised Steven let him stay. He's not helping you?"

"No. He's busy in his office."

Dr. Mack breaks out laughing. "He's busy on the yoga deck? Okay, I get it. I'll bring Sunny over and give you a hand."

They bring the wheel chair in and help DJ into it. Sunny raises her eyebrows at me and rolls her eyes when she sees he's been sleeping in my bed.

"This brings back memories," Mack laughs. "Steven didn't get quite as dirty when he was that age but he was a wild one."

He squats down and looks at DJ's eyes and feels his pulse. "Jeez, little brother, I think we need to slow you down a little. Do you know where you are?"

DJ's face is ashen and his mouth twitches. "Out of jail," he says.

"Do you remember me from the hospital? Sim's brother?"

"Yes. Can you fix me?"

"That's funny, DJ. I'm going to fix you good. We'll talk about it. Let's go."

I wheel DJ into IC and Dr. Mack says don't bother with sheets and blankets yet, he's filthy. Just get him on the bed and put him out.

"DJ, is that what I should call you? Do you have a name?" he asks.

"David. No one calls me that."

"Do you consent to medical treatment, David? Are you 21?"

"Yes. Yes."

"Just a few more questions. Sean said you've been using heroin. Street drugs. How long since you took any? How much did you take?"

"I was in jail yesterday. Before that we had a lot. I didn't count."

"Okay, I want to give you something else now. It's about fifteen times stronger so I'm only going to give you a little bit. It's nothing like what you're used to shooting but you'll like it.

"This will let your body transition from the crap you've been getting on the street to something purer, the medical stuff. Then I can work with you on that, Okay?"

"Okay, please," he sniffs.

Dr. Mack draws a lot of fentanyl into a needle and says, "Have a good sleep, DJ. We'll see you later, little brother."

He finds a vein and injects it and waits with his fingers on DJ's wrist. In seconds, I can see DJ's panic begin to subside as his face passes from pain to serenity to totally gone. He sucks air a few times then he closes his eyes and barely breathes.

"Okay, ladies," he says. "Show me what Jain taught you about cleaning up wounds. He's not going to be screaming at you any time soon."

We undress him and it's a little embarrassing because he's so young and very beautiful, but at the same time he's so banged up and cut and dirty and it's what we do.

None of the cuts are lacerations and there's no stitches needed anywhere, so it's just a matter of getting the dirt out of the cuts and cleaning him up. It helps that he's unconscious. We give him a bed bath and decide he doesn't need any bandages or dressing. We just want to keep everything clean. Then we roll him on one side and back over while we change the sheets.

Dr. Mack is watching us carefully. He leaves for a few minutes and comes back with some clean sweatpants. DJ's jeans are ripped and filthy. At first I think we should throw them away but then I realize once they're washed they'll be a boy's hardcore fashion fantasy. I'll wash them.

"Good job," he says. "If you didn't already work for me, I'd hire you again. Now set up a morphine drip and take all his vitals. Really be strict with that, okay? One of you check in with me every four hours. He's going to be critical for a while so I'll stay with him myself."

†

S&M

It's another perfect day on the top of the world, as long as I've got the door locked and bolted. I don't do well with anger so I try to ignite it and burn it off like a toxin. For the first time in weeks, no one is sitting with me, injecting me, training me, massaging me, talking to me or fucking me. I'm just here alone on the deck of the shala breathing.

The Medicine Buddha is watching over me with his bowl full of nothing and I think sometimes nothing is the best medicine. Possibly the most powerful healing begins when you come to the point where you quit trying to fix things and just sit with the way it is. Sometimes it has to come to the point where you are giving up for you to stop and look at it instead of sticking your finger into a dam of denial.

I sit on the deck cross-legged and stare at space for a long time before I can rein in my attention. I start with my body, the layer made of food. It's just a smashed up, scarred and painful outer coat I'm wearing. It's not who I am. I feel the pain clearly and acknowledge it for what it is, sensations doing their healing work.

I accept it. Things could be worse. I have all my fingers and toes and I'm rather fond of the welt on my back, Nat's autograph. The rest of it, the gunshot scars, smashed ribs and deep trauma in my back are souvenirs. I'm alive.

Next, I assess my prana kosha, my energy. If I let my anger flow, I can feel the prana turning white hot and dangerous. It's already so erratic from drug withdrawal that it can hurt me, and everyone around me. So I sit with it and smooth it out and coax it with pranayama. I sit with it as long as it takes for it to quiet down. I do 99 rounds of pranic nadi shodhana, breathing in through the left nostril and out through the right. In through the right out through the left, holding it for long counts between each breath.

Then I assess the level of my mind. That's an easy one for me now. I won't let the pain and hatred penetrate my mind. I keep it open with witnessing awareness, one hand on the ground to teach me. The earth is my witness and I am a witness of the earth. I refuse to judge him. It hurts me to see his pain, but it will teach him and make him stronger. My prana is protecting my mind like a moat around a castle.

The fourth level, my wisdom, is smooth. And that protects my soul. I close my eyes and watch my breath, now slow and smooth through both nostrils at once.

This is yoga. And I didn't even stand up.

Om Sim Namah.

I am a ripple of consciousness in the ocean of space.

†

JAIN

Mack calls around nine thirty and asks what my morning is looking like. I'm drinking coffee with Nat, just taking it easy.

"We're training Sim at 10. What's up?" I ask.

"We got a new patient late last night. Remember the kid who came into emergency with Sean? Sean brought him up in handcuffs around 2 am and they weren't playing cops. He's a full on junkie. I thought you might take a look when you're done with training. Maybe Nat has some remedies."

"Sure, Mac. We'll be over before noon."

"And don't be surprised if Steven doesn't show up for training. He's been in time-out since dawn. I imagine he's pretty pissed about it."

"Okay." I hang up and pour another cup. I don't want breakfast so I can train on an empty stomach, but the coffee helps warm me. "There's another junkie in the house, Nat. A really young kid. Mack wants us to check him out. He thinks Steven might blow the gym off today, but I want to train anyway. Are you coming?"

We take our cups out to the gym and sit on the benches for a few minutes. The sun warms my muscles and I feel like going really heavy today. Maybe a max rep on the bench. A short and sweet workout if Steven doesn't come out to play.

Nat is watching the pool house and I see her eyes shift. "Oh, he's coming all right," she laughs. "He's coming all over the place."

I turn around and see Steven strutting slowly across the lawn barefoot with his porn star walk. He's got his cop hat on, jeans, no belt, no shirt, and he's swinging a pair of real police handcuffs in his right hand. The smirk on his face says "I dare you to fuck with me" as clear as sunshine.

I start laughing. It's a pretty good act. He doesn't crack a smile, just walks up to me and drops the cuffs at my feet. "In case you need to fasten me to the lat bar today," he says. "Let's go hard, lover boy. I've only got five more days."

Nat puts a hand on his shoulder and inspects the welt on his back. "It's healing up nicely," she says. "It's almost gone."

"Too bad," he says. "I liked the way it looked. We might have to do something about that." He gives her a mean smirk and I wonder what's up. "How are your studies going, Jain?" he sneers. "She's a pretty good teacher, isn't she?"

I really can't answer that without being indiscreet, so I say nothing. He turns back to her and puts his face a little too close to hers.

"We won't be needing you this morning, teacher. I've been doing yoga for three hours on the deck. Why don't you go check on the new patient?" he hisses. "He's really shocking."

She smiles and gives him a kiss on the cheek and heads towards the house. "Go hard," she says.

"Oh, Jain," he sighs when she gets out of earshot. "Can you handle her? She's a nuclear bomb."

I blush. I really don't want to talk about sex with him.

"Handle this," I say and point to the bench press. The bar is empty and it's a good warm up weight for him. He's in a manic mood and he's so intense it's absolutely surgical. He lies down on the bench and aligns his hands with careful measure from the ridged grooves on the bar, plants his feet flat on the ground and arches his back.

He lifts the bar as seriously as if it had a hundred pounds on it, in competition form, rest pausing the bar on his chest for a split second before he drives it up. Perfect twelve reps. The bench press doesn't bother him as much as the lat pulls because it uses the antagonist muscles to his injuries. His arms are getting solid again.

I take my turn with a pair of 45's on the bar and try to copy his perfect form. Then we strip the bar and put a couple 10's on for him. Again, perfect form. It's mad to be proud of a 65 pound bench press but he smirks. We go five rounds. He works up to 105 for a single and I want to try 275. I haven't lifted that much in a while, but I've done it before.

I lie down on the bench and square my body up to the bar. Sim's spotting me. If I get in trouble I know he can't get 275 pounds off me, but I feel confident. I push the bar off the rack and lower it to my chest.

Just as I'm starting to drive it back up, Sim says, "Can I be the best man?"

He breaks my concentration so completely that I lose control and the bar won't move. I'm pinned with 275 pounds of iron on my chest.

"Fuck!" I scream. He can't lift it off me but he walks casually over to one side and pulls one of the plates off. The bar tilts to the other side and the weight crashes on the ground instead of on me. My whole body is shaking in shock.

"Sim, you dick. You could've killed me."

"Probably not," he says. "I was just wondering if you want to have a shotgun wedding or what? You know she works for me. I love her. What are you going to do about it?"

†

MACK

Nat comes into ICU earlier than I expected, a little after 10. I'm happy to see her. I need help. DJ is a little delirious but still conscious. It's been about four hours since I hit him with fentanyl and now I'm thinking about knocking him into next week with a little morphine. He looks so much like Steven that it breaks my heart. I just hate to see the guy suffer. He keeps telling me he wants to kill himself or wants me to kill him.

Nat sits next to his bed and takes his wrist. In a heartbeat, DJ turns on her with venom.

"Don't touch me," he hisses.

"Okay, baby," she says letting his arm go. "I'll just talk to you, okay?"

"Fuck off. Don't even look at me. Go away."

She looks at me for a clue and I know exactly what's on. I've heard it from Steven for years.

"DJ," I say. "I'll tell you what. I won't let her look at you or talk to you or touch you for now. But you have to make me a deal. Talk to *me*. Tell me what's going on and then I'll give you a hit so nice you can spend the rest of the day in Disneyland. Fair enough?"

"Yeah," he says. "Tell you what?"

"Where's the pain?"

"Do you know the koshas?" he asks.

"Of course. I taught your teacher."

"Then you know I've got pain in five places. Five very fucked up places. One, my body is ripped up but that's the easy part. The drugs help bury that. Two, my prana is wrecked. It's like a seizure and I can't control it. My nerves are burning up. The drugs are causing that and nothing can stop it. Three, my mind is fucked. I'm going to prison. I'd rather die. I'm scared. Four, my conscience is screaming at me. I screwed up. My best friend hates me and Darrell is dead. It can't be fixed. Five, I've lost my teacher and my karma is permanently screwed.

"I wish I were dead. I don't want to go to back to jail. Send me one-way to Disneyland. I don't want to be here anymore."

"Okay," I say. "So we know what to work on now. By the way there's no such thing as permanently screwed karma unless you kill yourself. As long as you're here, we can sort it out." I can see Nat's eyes wide with interest. She's getting a lot of intake without actually interacting with him.

"So what happened at Sim's house?" I ask. "How did it get so screwed up?"

"Help me out a little bit, doc," he says. "It's a long story. My nerves are one fire."

I put a little morphine in the needle and ease his pain. He sighs and sucks air.

"I was there when S&M was shot. Sean told me to stay at the beach house with Darrell and don't talk. It was fine for a few days but then we didn't hear anything. The boys were looking for him. I lied and said he surfing was in Mexico. I didn't know if he would ever come back, if he was hurt or scared or crippled. I didn't know. I heard bad things.

"One day a couple of the boys came by and asked if they could share the house since S&M was gone. They had a lot of cash and offered us $1,000 a week. They were local guys. They didn't move in but just hung out, meeting people, dealing. They had everything.

"They gave me junk and I liked it. Free, as much as I wanted. It felt good and I forgot how fucked the neighborhood was. They said we were the kings of 36th Avenue and we got these '36' tats. S&M almost killed me when he saw it.

"I learned how to shoot up and I've been stoned ever since. But Darrell left last week. He said the house was out of control and the Point Guard was useless. He must have gone to talk to Sean. On Sunday night the police turned up with a warrant and kicked the door in.

"There were only a few of us there and the guys split out the side door. I ran out on the back deck and tried to escape down the cliff but I was too fucked up and did a face plant. They arrested me down on the beach.

"Everyone else got away. There was a shit load of heroin in the house worth heaps of money. Someone must have known Darrell talked because they shot him the next day when I was in jail. I screwed up. I wish I were dead. Help me out, doc."

I watch Nat but she's not allowed to talk, so I imagine what I would say if I were her, a yoga therapist. It's not too far a stretch. I'm starting to feel a new calling and an old one coming back. I simply go through his koshas from the outside in to heal him by teaching.

"First, DJ, your body will heal. Second, we can help you settle your prana. Nat's been working a lot with Sim on that. The amount of narcotics he was on after surgery was epic. We know how to deal with that. Third, get your mind off prison. You're here because Sean asked us to help keep you out of there. Get your mind on that. You're dead if you go to prison. The guys who murdered Darrell are in there. They know you.

"Fourth, that's a tough one. You need to talk with Sim. That's personal. But you wouldn't be here if he hated you. You'd be in jail. He took legal custody. He put you in his bed and had his wife look after you last night.

"Fifth, your soul is only suffering because you know what bliss is and you've lost the plot.

"Do you still want me to give you an overdose or do you want us to help you?"

DJ doesn't say anything for a while. He's on his way to the Magic Kingdom. But then something hits him like a poke in the ribs and he looks up at me and laughs, "I slept with his wife. I don't even know her."

†

NAT

When I walk back to the house, the boys are sitting on the grass soaking up the sunshine waiting for my special bodybuilding abhyanga. I wave them over and they follow me into the lab.

Steven kicks back in the chair and says, "Him first. He went harder." He gives a little evil laugh, picks up the tiny bottle of Spirit and inhales it deeply.

"How's the junkie?" he snarls.

"I'd like to talk to you about that, boss. He's a real train wreck but I can't work with him. He's suicidal and very drugged right now. I tried to touch him and talk, but he wouldn't let me. He told Mack not to let me even look at him. How can I do any kind of therapy? And what is the deal with that? It's the same thing you said when I tried to help *you*."

"I probably did. It's something I taught him. Something Mack taught me."

"Why? It's like putting up a brick wall."

"I'm not sure I want to tell you why, honey. It's a long story."

"I'll tell her if you don't," Jain volunteers. "I've known him since he was twelve, Nat."

"Jain, you're fired if you continue," Sim warns.

"I'm the CEO, buddy. You can't fire me without a board meeting," he laughs. "Steven was a very bad boy, Nat."

"Okay, okay! I'll tell it. You don't know everything anyway." He inhales the bottle of Spirit again with a wicked smile, as if the memories of his behavior taste delicious. "When I was eighteen I was a little loose. I mean very, very loose. I didn't know any better. Is that a good enough excuse? I think the word is promiscuous. Any girl, any time, anywhere. Beach caves, back seats, carpets, fields, furniture, wherever. Furniture not involving a bed is always interesting," he sighs happily.

"By the time he was twenty he'd fucked every available girl in town," Jain adds. "He probably has a lot of beautiful children."

"My story, Jain," Sim interrupts. "I wasn't a sexual predator or anything, just a willing victim. Girls chased me. I can't really say they chased me though because I didn't run. I just said yes.

"All they had to do was look at me or talk to me. And if they touched me it went that much faster. A look or a word or a touch can be very suggestive, very intimate. That's all it takes to let someone in."

"Oh!" I get it. "It's about sex?"

"Yes, pure and simple sex. Of course it's about sex. But I never loved any of them and never got involved. I was too busy with the next one and then with her sister or her girl friend. I was into – variety. And I never gave repeat performances. At that age, it was like being a kid in a candy store. And candy makes you sick after a while. You can't survive on it.

"My friends started to hate me. Their girl friends were fair game. And the girls hated me because they never really wanted just sex in the first place. They just wanted entanglement. If they asked for my phone number, I used to give them the number for the welfare department. I was never home anyway. So I got a reputation, well deserved, of being a prick.

"I got beat up quite a bit and there were a lot of threatening phone calls to Mack from various mothers. I got the clap a few times and probably gave it to a lot of girls, but Mack always treated me and cleared it up. Even that didn't stop me."

"Mack used to call him the one man epidemic," Jain adds. "It's a miracle he never got HIV."

"Not a pretty story, I know. But you want to know why DJ won't talk to you. Mack was teaching me yoga, but it wasn't doing me much good. I just did the physical practice, superficial yoga. Then he started teaching me Buddhism. Somehow that really made a difference to me. He taught me the path of enlightenment. I was in a lot of mental and emotional pain in between – uh, fucking everyone.

"He said the only thing I needed to learn in order to be enlightened was not to hurt anyone, including myself. Every time I had sex with a girl I didn't love, I hurt her. Every time I slept with a friend's girl friend, I hurt my friend too. I hurt everyone in town. And he said that all the time I was hurting myself. I hurt so good.

"Mack said I could hurt a girl if I looked at her or talked to her or touched her. I'm sure he was just keeping me off the starting line, but it worked very well for me if I ignored them and put a wall up. It let me concentrate better on my dharma."

"Yeah," Jain adds, "And he was running out of girls he hadn't already had by then, too. It was time to cool it or move to another town." Sim gives Jain a glare but Jain's got his head face down on the table.

"By the time I was 22 I was celebate and teaching yoga. I studied tantra and learned how to control my sexual energy. The more I controlled it, the more powerful and interesting it got. *You* know what I'm talking about, Nat.

"When I met DJ he was fifteen. He copied everything I did. He was like my shadow. I was grateful that he didn't learn all that bad behavior from me because pretty soon the girls started coming after him like he was a pair of new shoes. I taught him to stay away from women.

"I told him he could hurt them if he looked at them or talked to them or touched them. He's probably still a virgin and he can thank me or blame me for that. God help him if he goes to prison."

I finish up with Jain and stare at Sim. Jain gets dressed, but Sim doesn't move to get on the table.

"You know, boss," I say thoughtfully. "I don't know if I should be touching you any more."

He just sits there sniffing the little bottle watching for my reaction. I suspect he's going to need an invitation after that story. So I wink at him. "Lose the pants, boss."

†

NAT

I'm finishing up with some extra work on his feet. I can tell he's wired, wound up and angry and he's been mean all morning. He keeps sniffing on the bottle of Spirit. The combination of palo santo, frankincense and sandalwood is helping to calm his nerves and clean his mind.

"Sim," I say, "I think you better go talk to him."

"Nah," he says. "Let him stew for a while. He's lucky we let him in here. That's some pretty bad karma he planted down at the beach."

"He's suffering. He's suicidal. I want to help him and he'll listen to you."

"Yeah? Well all he has to do if he wants to kill himself is to let Mack keep him stoned and then go to prison in a few weeks. That ought to take care of it."

"That's mean," I'm a little shocked to hear that from him.

"It's not mean. I don't have a mean bone in my body. It's tough. There's a big difference between mean and tough, a world of difference."

"I can't see the difference."

"Mean is cruel. Tough comes from love. He means a lot to me. I want to see him help himself. Threatening to kill himself is just junkie drama. He couldn't kill himself up here unless he held his breath. We haven't even got a knife sharp enough to cut tomatoes.

"If he doesn't fix it, he'll get killed in prison. He won't last 48 hours in there. He's a 21 year old little boy."

He gets up from the table and pulls his jeans on and cocks the cop hat back on his head with the brim backwards. Then he picks up his cuffs from the table and locks them on his left wrist bracelet style. In spite of what he said, he looks mean. He looks dangerous even. He looks like a 28 year old boy having a tantrum.

"Sim, please. For me. Would you come over and ask him to let me work on him a little and see if I can calm him down? I know I can help him. You don't have to do anything else. Please."

"I don't think so, Nat. I don't want to work with the Ice House any more. I'm out of there. I'll work with him if and when he gets off drugs."

"The Ice House?" I'm curious.

"Yeah. Mack's IC and narcotics medical palace. I don't want anything to do with it. You can help him all you want but I want to concentrate on wellness not drugs. And I don't want any junkies in the wellness house."

"Where's your compassion, sweetheart?" I beg. "I'm only asking you to talk to him for a few minutes."

"The last time someone asked me to just have a talk, I got raped and married," he laughs.

"Please, Sim, with sugar on it."

"Oh, God," he moans. "I love it when a woman begs. You're killing me, Nat. But I'll tell you what. I've got something in mind I need from you. You'll owe me if I do this. Is it a deal?"

"Deal, honey. Jain, will you come with us? You haven't met the new patient yet. Mack's going to need a hand with him. We did intake this morning and he's pretty messed up."

The three of us head over to the Ice House and I ask Sim what he calls our new wellness house.

"It's the Fire House, baby," he laughs. "The healing power of Sunrise."

Mack is sitting in the corner scowling when we come in. He looks depressed and maybe even a little medicated, but he's really happy to see us.

"I'm not getting a very good start with this one," he complains. "I don't want to just knock him into next week but he's suicidal. I need help."

Sim walks over to the bed and frowns at DJ. He looks back at me and says, "Okay, you begged for this but it's not going to be nice."

He shakes DJ hard and puts his face down to his ear and hisses something. Then he waits a few seconds and does it again. This time I can hear what he says, "You little fuck, wake up."

DJ's eyes open and he's focused on nothing at first, then he sees Sim and blinks.

"Can you hear me, fucker?" DJ blinks again and nods yes.

"Okay, this is going to be really simple. Either you work with Nat or I'm going to let you go to prison and die. There's no half way. You do what she tells you, you let her touch you and you thank her for it or you're a dead man. Understand?"

DJ nods yes. "I understand," he says. "I'll let her in, Sim."

"Mmmm," he smiles. "Easy wasn't that? I'll try to keep this very simple for you. Quit fucking with my brother by threatening to kill yourself. We can help you do that. Be careful what you wish for, little brother."

I'm starting to see the difference between mean and tough. There's nothing mean about it. It just works. I walk over to the other side of the bed and take DJ's wrist. He doesn't object. I put my fingers on his radial artery and feel his pulse erratic and pounding. I look up into Sim's eyes and he's smirking at me. I mouth, thank you, baby.

"DJ, I'm Nat. I need to look at your cuts and see how I can help. May I?"

"Yes," he says. "It's okay."

I pull the sheet down and he just keeps watching Sim's face. I'm a little shocked he's gotten so easy. The cuts are pretty fresh, but they're clean and crusty enough that I can use oil on them if I'm careful. I can't get the oil into open wounds so I have to make sure I don't rub the scabs off.

I want to use something very calming and grounding on him. He doesn't have massive injuries so I won't bother with the expensive helichrysum. I want to use the same blend Sim has been sniffing, palo santo, frankincense and sandalwood for cellular detoxification, calming his nerves and clearing his mind.

I'll also add a large dose of jatamansi to help release subconscious trauma. It's nice to have such an arsenal of botanical medicine at my disposal. I smile to myself. The Fire House is infiltrating the Ice House.

"Mack," I say. "Why don't you take a break? We'll work with him for a couple hours. Jain can stay, okay?"

"Thanks," he sighs, visibly relieved.

Sim goes over to Mack and puts his arm around his shoulder and grabs his forearm. "Give it a rest, brother," he says. "I mean it. You've had enough."

Then he lets him go and Mack says, "Okay, I hear you."

"I'll walk over with you, Nat," Sim says. "I might learn something."

Back in the lab I show him how I blend the oils, how much and why. "This is very different from what I'm using on you. It's more like the stuff you've been sniffing all morning, for addiction, depression and toxicity, not injuries." I make a really large batch and pour it into an amber bottle. Then I put a label on it and write: "Rx DJ" on it. It should last a few days. I put a ½ ounce of the blend into another little bottle for Sim to take.

"So what can I do in return for you, Sim?" I ask. "What's the deal?"

"Nothing now," he says. "Just save a little time for me on Friday after the press conference."

†

S&M

I've changed my mind now. I want to work with her and we walk back to the Ice House together. Jain is talking to DJ and taking his vitals but backs off and sits in the chair again when we come in.

I go over to the bed and look at him. He's too passive. He's loaded.

"Hey, buddy, we're going to do some yoga therapy for you. You have no idea what's coming. Nat is a very powerful Tantrika. It's okay to let her get close to you. You can't hurt her. She can fix you. The doctors can't fix you like she can. Nat will teach you Tantra, okay?"

His eyes get big and he smiles, "It's about time someone did, Sim," he laughs. "I've been waiting a long time."

"Okay, then. You won't be needing this for a while." I pull the IV out of his forearm. Jain jumps up to stop me and says, "Hey!"

"Oops," I laugh. "Shit happens. We're working with different meds now."

Nat puts an arm on his and says, "It's fine, Jain. It's hard to do massage with the needles anyway."

Jain sits down again to watch.

She pours the oil into two shot glasses and hands me one. I help her get his sweat pants off and we start on his hands. This will go fast with two of us working. I'm pretty sure I know how to do this after all the work she's done on me but I watch her carefully so I can coordinate with her. Circular strokes on the wrist joints, long strokes on the forearms, circular strokes on the elbows, long on the upper arms, circular on the shoulders.

When we get to his stomach I say, "Don't worry, we're not going there, buddy. No medicine on the sex organs, it could burn you." I feel him relax a little but I can't help tease him and teach him a little,

"Your ass is another story, it's the biggest muscle on your body. And your skin is the biggest organ. We're injecting botanical medicine directly through your skin with no needles. The oil is the carrier. Abhyanga, yogic massage is very powerful stuff.

While we're working on his feet, Nat asks him if he knows yoga nidra. I know he doesn't. He doesn't even understand the question so I answer no for him.

"Do you want to teach him, Sim?"

"Sure. Tantra lesson number one. It's a good place to start."

We turn him over and while we're working on his back, I explain the process to him.

"So, DJ, yoga nidra is conscious sleep. The way it works is we take your consciousness down through the koshas so you can work on the really deep layers and release subconscious trauma in your core. Clean out the addiction. You understand?"

"Yes, but how do I do that?"

"Its actually ridiculously simple. Don't worry about how it works, just trust me and follow my instructions. It's going to take you deeper than heroin but you'll know you're sleeping and you'll hear everything around you. You'll feel really good afterwards, okay?"

"Okay."

"Try this. See if you can put all your attention into your left big toe. Say yes when you do."

"Yes," he says right away.

"Good. It should be that fast. Don't try to move the part I say, just put your attention there. Try you right shoulder."

"Yes," he says.

"Great. So I'm going to name your whole body bit by bit and you just follow me with your attention. Before I even finish, your mind is going to get so bored with the details, it will forget about the physical layer and let it go. Then it will let go of the next kosha, the energetic layer. Then the third layer, the mind itself lets go and you've drilled down to your core consciousness.

"You'll still be aware and you can hear everything around you, but it's a deep witnessing awareness. You stay down there until I tell you to come back. About 90 minutes is good for therapy, but if you were healthy 30 minutes would be fine."

"Cool," he says. "I want to try."

We're done with the oil and we get him back in his sweats and cover him.

"You're going to like yoga nidra, DJ," I say. "I can do it all day long. It's my favorite practice.

"We start by setting an intention. Something very specific and important to you, whatever your heart desires. What would you wish?"

"Love," he says without missing a beat.

"What kind of love? Like a girl friend? Nicky?" I wink at Nat who's watching me closely.

"Mmmm, no. More. I want to be full of love and have it come at me from everywhere, in me and around me."

"Oh, yeah, that's better than Nicky, but we can include her in the package, too," I laugh. "So take that intention and plant it in your heart, that you want to be full of love and surrounded by it. An intention should feel good just thinking about it."

"Got it," he closes his eyes and smiles.

"Okay then. Put your palms up and just relax and follow me. Start with your right thumb. Right index finger. Middle finger. Ring finger..."

It takes me about ten minutes to go up his arm, down the right side to his toes, up the left arm and down to his toes, up his spine, around his head and down the front. Before I even get to his third eye, I can tell he's gone. I keep talking to him, walking him down to his intention at the bottom of his heart and tell him to sit down there with it.

Nat smiles at me and puts a thumb up, well done. Jain's seen it done before on me but he's still impressed. He probably thought it was witchcraft when Nat did it.

Somewhere during the therapy, I lost my anger. I've been his teacher for six years and this is the first time he's really made a serious mistake. We let Jain sit with him and go into the kitchen for tea.

I want to know about the intake session and she tells me what happened down at my beach house. The Kings of 36th Ave dealing heroin from my living room is not a pretty story but I let it in without malice. I'm sorry he had to get caught in the middle of it. It's not even DJ's fault that Darrell was killed. He made the decision to rat on the house and knew the risk.

I would have done the same if I couldn't stop it. And none of this would have happened if I'd been there, so I could even blame myself for getting shot. But what's the point of blaming anyone? Guilt, anger and hatred are the most toxic emotions on the planet. We can't get the drugs out of his system without getting the guilt out. I tell her I can help with that.

When the time is up, we find Jain snoring softly in the chair and DJ is still on vacation, very deep, barely breathing. I wonder if I should just leave him down there longer. We wait another 15 minutes and Jain's snores are getting deeper and resonant. I know DJ can hear it and I listen for other sounds in the room but it's just this deep vibrating snore.

I can hear it coming like a distant freight train. The first time it happened to me I was deep in nidra when I heard a neighbor mowing the lawn. The sound vibrations rolled through me with such intensity that it set off a spontaneous roar and I woke myself up groaning with pleasure. I still get turned on when I hear a lawn mower. Who am I kidding? I get turned on by almost anything that moves. Orgasms aren't the goal of Tantra, but they're a really nice side effect.

All of a sudden DJ comes up so fast and hard it's like he hit the ceiling. His whole body jolts and he gasps for air. "What!" he yells. Then it hits him again, three in a row. I look at Nat and we both burst out laughing. He's confused and reaches out and grabs air. Nat takes his hand and holds it tight.

She whispers over her shoulder to me, "Yes, Jain does have a very sexy snore, doesn't he? He's done that to me a few times."

"What did you do to me?" DJ pants.

"Nothing, honey," I say. "You did it to yourself. Welcome to Tantra. You didn't have sex. Sex just had you.

"And you thought all you were going to get was love."

†

JAIN

I must have fallen asleep. I was supposed to be watching the new patient but the heavy workout, the adrenalin from getting pinned under the weights, the sunshine and the massage all caught up with me at once. When I open my eyes, Mack is back in the room and he's staring at the bed. DJ has his eyes closed and he's holding Nat's hand close to his heart smiling. Sim is gone.

"What happened to him?" Mack says. "Where's his IV?"

"Yoga happened," Nat says. "Steven asks you to stop giving him any narcotics unless he gets sick and then only a minimum hit, not constant drips."

"I'll talk to him about it," he says. "How's the patient doing?"

"Oh, he's coming along," she giggles. "Not threatening anymore. I can stay with him a while. He doesn't seem to want to let go of my hand."

I feel a little tinge of jealousy and wonder if she'd go for a man that young. He's fifteen years younger than I am but he's a very good-looking kid. A little rough looking, too, like Sim. At least she's not in bed holding him.

"Good," Mack says. "If you've got a few minutes, Jain, Sean's out by the pool with Steven."

†

SEAN

I'm beat. My shift didn't end until four a.m. and then I barely slept. It's my day off but I told Sim I'd be back up there today. Crys is excited about a road trip and has me stop to pick up a few bottles of cold Carneros champagne because, she says, it's his two-week anniversary and he can probably use a drink after last night. I know I can.

I really don't expect him to be in any mood to celebrate but I'm too tired to argue with her. When we get there, it's not what I expect at all. Sim's out by the pool in board shorts working on his tan and Brandy is massaging his back with oil. He looks rested, happy and his skin is so brown his blue eyes are piercing. The sun is getting low, but we're up so high, he's still catching rays.

He smiles and jumps up to kiss Crys when he sees us. "Oh yes, baby!" he says when he sees the bottles. "Perfect timing." He pops one of the corks, takes a swig straight from the bottle and passes it back to her. "Fuck glasses," he says. "I haven't got anything catchy."

"Not like ten years ago, Sim," she teases and takes a drink. "You used to be the town carrier."

"Shhh," he whispers, rolls his eyes towards Brandy and shakes his head. Shut up. She wouldn't have a clue where he's been. Everywhere. But she's concentrating too hard on his back to notice. Crys hands her the bottle.

"Happy anniversary, honey," she smiles. "Two weeks. Things are looking better than the last time I was here."

I'm shocked to see him in such a good mood and tell him so.

"I'm on a mission, Sean. Job one is to get as dark as an Indian for my photo op. I'm working on it as hard as I can. Are we still on for Friday? We train at 10. And remember, we're on sun time up here. All you Daylight Savings people down there need to adjust. "

"Sure, we'll be here at 11 our time then and we'll do the interview over lunch. I've got Chris Croft, the sports writer, dying to write the story. His slant is going to be the surfers vs. the dealers."

"Oh, cool. Croft surfs; he's a legend at the Point, the perfect guy for the job. I can't wait to see him again."

"And we've got almost too many volunteers from the force wanting to show up on Saturday for the circus. We'll probably have half a dozen patrol cars and there's supposed to be a good swell coming up.

"But what I really came up for – how is our junkie? It was pretty heavy when I left him here last night."

"Mmm. He gave us a rough time this morning but he's going to be gold, Sean. I would have sent him packing but Nat turned me around. She turned him around, too. We're lucky to have her. Now I can focus on kicking some ass."

He grins and finishes the bottle off. Crys pops another one and hands it to me.

"How's my house?" he asks. "I heard the story from Nat as much as I need to know I guess."

"It's locked up and under police surveillance. It's pretty safe for now I think. No one is in there. A few crew came back and were hanging out on the deck but we harassed them enough that we don't expect them back."

"I was wondering if you'd like to move in, Sean. That would send a huge message to the community, having a cop living in my house, huh? The next rumor will be that the cops are dealing heroin for me.

"Crys, you too if you want to stay there. There's two bedrooms if you're shy, but I wouldn't mind keeping one for myself down the road."

"You're kidding," I say and then I realize he's not.

"I won't be staying down there for a while. You'd be doing me a favor, Sean."

"I'd love to," I say and look at Crys. She's beaming. "We could probably work on that one bedroom deal," I smile at her and raise the bottle in a toast. He might not have anything that's catchy but he's definitely contagious.

†

JAIN

Mack and I walk out across the lawn and see them laughing and drinking champagne out of the bottle. It's a good look. I haven't seen Steven look this happy. Ever. He takes a drink off the bottle and hands it to Mack.

"Brandy," he says with a little slur, "go get that mean little red head nurse and see if she'll come out to play with us. I'll bet she could straighten my brother out pretty quick if she wanted to."

"Ouch," Mack says. "I'm doing just fine, thanks." He hits the bottle and passes it on to me. I take a big swallow.

"Nope, big brother. You're probably the sickest guy up here, DJ included. When was the last time you kissed a red head? Or anyone?"

I jump in to save his face by changing the subject. I take a second hit. I need it right now. "Sim, remember what you asked me on the bench press today? Yes. You can."

"Ah-ooh," he howls like a wolf. "You asked her?"

"Uh, no," I admit. "I'll be back in a few minutes." I take the bottle with me and head back to IC. I'm just drunk enough to pull this off, I think.

†

SEAN

"Hey, Sean," he slurs, "I wanna show you something, bud. You gotta minute?"

"Sure, Sim. Where?" He gets up and staggers a little and waves me to follow him to the pool house. As soon as we get in the door, his demeanor changes. He's totally sober.

"Come on," he says and walks me through the kitchen and back behind the house to a beautiful deck overhanging the forest.

"Sit down, bud," he says. There's nowhere to sit but the deck floor. So we sit.

"You're not drunk?" I'm surprised.

"Not in your wildest dreams," he says. "I barely hit that bottle. The fun thing about drinking off a bottle straight is you can't really tell if I drink anything or not. I'm stone cold sober."

"Why pretend?" I wonder.

"I don't want to ruin the party atmosphere. There's too much heartache and tension up here already. And I've got things on my mind."

"Like?"

"I was wondering if I could bail those guys out. How much? I've got money."

"Bail them out? What? So you can take them?"

"Something like that. A little karmic cleanup. How much?" he asks.

175

"No, no, no. They're in without bail. They're history. I couldn't let you do that anyway. They're just young punks, kids trying to get rank by doing a hit for the gang. They're not the ones you want, Sim. If you want to hurt someone, hurt management. Work with me."

He grimaces and then sighs. "Management is really big, Sean. Mex, Centro, South America, it's one of the biggest businesses around. I can't hurt them."

"Yeah," I say. "That's kind of the cosmic joke, isn't it? You can't change the universe. But you can still change things. We can do something here, on the beach, maybe in the whole community. You can help me keep a lot of the crew out of jail, starting with DJ. Isn't that a fair fight?"

"Honestly? If I had any choice, I'd go back to that day and swim in the ocean with DJ and Nick and then growl at Brandy. I don't want to fight. But here we are, brother, here and now. I'll work as hard as you want. Let's go check on the junkie."

†

NAT

He's still holding my hand on his heart, but he's staring at me with a curious look and not talking. I can hear the laughter from the party outside and wonder how long I have to wait until someone else comes in to take over. I've been working since 10 this morning and could use a little break.

DJ pushes himself up in bed and drops his legs over the side.

"I'm not sure you should be getting up," I caution.

"I'm afraid I'm already up, Nat," he growls. "I've been up for an hour." He takes my hand and puts it roughly on his cock. It's up so hard I can feel it pulse.

I try to pull my hand free but he grabs my other wrist and shoves me hard backwards pinning both my arms to the wall. He puts a knee between my thighs and pushes himself against me, holding me tightly in place.

"Sim said I can't hurt you," he whispers. "I don't want to."

Then he covers my mouth with his and kisses me hard.

I start to resist but his hands are staying in place and he's not taking this anywhere beyond an interminable kiss. I have a feeling he doesn't really know anything else. He smells intoxicating thanks to the oils and he tastes delicious. He's kissing me with such an interesting mixture of eagerness and inexperience that my knees start to go out from under me.

For a minute I imagine how much fun it would be to teach him everything he doesn't know. It could take years. I start kissing him back with all my heart and I can feel waves of pleasure rolling between us. He's got a river of raw new kundalini energy kicking up his spine and we've just opened the floodgates. My whole world starts to disappear into an ocean of bliss.

"Oh, shit!" I hear and the spell is broken. I open my eyes to see Jain standing there with a bottle of champagne. He doesn't move but DJ lets go of my wrists and stares at him, breathing hard.

Jain is a good six inches taller than DJ, about fifty pounds heavier and fifteen years older. There's no question about a fair fight between them. My face flushes when I look at them side by side, a man and a boy. Both of them are beautiful.

Jain puts an arm around DJ and looks at his face. There's no anger in his eyes, just surprise. "I'm sorry to interrupt, buddy, but let me give you a little friendly advice," he says. "I don't think she's available. I'm going to marry her."

†

DJ

I sit back down on the bed and my hands are shaking. I need a hit. I'm breathing hard and my heart is pounding in my ears. She laughed when I came so hard, but then she held my hand and sang to me. When I kissed her, she put her tongue in my mouth and it wasn't casual. It was a bomb. And when I touched her it was like a rush of heroin. I've never seen a woman that sexy and powerful at the same time. I want her. I don't even care if I hurt her I want her so bad.

But the doctor's in my way. He was in Emergency with Sim and he was snoring in my room today. Sim's bigger than me, but the doctor's massive. He's been out in the sun drinking with his shirt off and I don't want to get in a pissing contest with him. He looks like he can bench press the house.

"Did he hurt you, Nat?" he asks her quietly. She shakes her head, looking at the floor.

I feel like I'm going to vomit. My nerves are exploding in all directions at once. My mind is confused and my body is on fire. I want to hide under the bed.

She's looking at him and asks, "Are you serious?"

"Yes," he says. "I hope I'm not too late. This guy looks pretty serious, too." He looks at me and I see worry and fear in his eyes. How can a man that big be worried about me?

She looks back at me and laughs. "Oh, he's serious enough to be dangerous, Jain. He kisses like it's the end of the world. I lost my head a little bit there. Do you think some of that subconscious trauma he released was sexual frustration?"

"Blame Sim," he laughs. "Look, DJ. I'm not mad. But maybe you should keep your hands to yourself."

He's not mad, but I'm furious. I want to smash everything in the room. I don't care if he hurts me. I look around for something to hit him with but there's nothing. All the sharp things are put away and everything's locked up. I knock the IV drip rack over in fury and the bag splits open spilling the drugs on the floor.

"Fuck," I scream. I don't know how to fight. The Point Guard always protected me. I reach down to pick up the rack pole for a weapon. The doctor grabs my arm and twists it behind my back and then holds the other one. I try to kick him, but I can't move.

Nat puts both her hands on my shoulders and looks in my eyes. Now I'm the one who's helplessly pinned. I want her to kiss me again, but instead she talks to me like I'm a child. "I love you, baby. Don't make us hurt you. Show me how you breathe. Slow it down."

She tears my heart open. I feel a powerful force like a snake crawling up my spine through my belly and into my heart. My breath doesn't get any easier. It feels like my body is going to combust. Her gaze is too powerful to hold so I shift my eyes over her shoulder to the locked cabinets on the wall. I can see needles and bottles behind the glass doors. It calms me down, just thinking about the warm river of opiates in the same room as me. Mack will shoot up with me like he did last night.

The doctor feels me relaxing and releases my arms. Nat smiles and says, "Are you okay now, honey? I'm still your teacher. I still love you."

"Sure, all better," I say and she drops her hands from my shoulders. As soon as I'm free I take a step back then lunge at the glass cabinets with my fist on automatic pilot. The window pane and my hand shatter at the same time. I feel a massive orgasm shoot through my heart as glass and blood spray everywhere. *Now* I feel all better.

Sim walks into the room with Sean and looks at the mess everywhere, broken glass, blood, spilled drugs and the IV stand on the floor. He whistles. "Jeez, DJ. I thought we had an understanding here, buddy."

The doctor takes my arm and wraps a towel around my hand to stop the blood. "Looks like I get to do some more surgery," he says.

Nat says, "Sim, can he borrow your sex toys tonight? He's going to need those cuffs. With drug addiction, sexual frustration and kundalini rising all at the same time, I think he needs a time out."

The doctor looks at S&M with even more concern than the worried look he gave me and whistles, "Sex toys?"

†

S&M

"Strike two, DJ," I warn. "What do you think Mack's going to do to you when he sees this? Give you a pat on the back and another hit of morphine? He'll probably tell Sean to take you back to county jail until your court date. Actually, Sean, you better get out of here in case he does."

DJ's sniffing again. He's bleeding pretty bad and he can't take his eyes off Nat.

"Nat, what happened?" I ask.

"Uh, he kissed me."

"You *liked* it!" DJ hisses at her, then he turns on me and insists, "She *said* she liked it, Sim."

She blushes and bites her lip. "Well, yeah. It was the best ever, baby. Very tempting. I'm not going to forget that for a long time."

"You better go, Nat," Jain warns. "I need a nurse in here."

"Yeah," I say, "Go off and stall my brother while I get this cleaned up. Be cool and pretend nothing happened."

I unlock the police cuffs on my wrist and put one around DJ's and fasten him to the bed rail. "Is that okay, Jain, or do you need the hospital cuffs?" I ask.

"For surgery? That's way too loose. It'll hurt him. It's no good."

I don't want Mack to see this yet. If I send someone back the pool house for the padded cuffs, he might suspect something. I go up the stairs and knock on Sunny's door. I smile at her innocently when she answers.

"Hey, Sunshine, it's school time. Dr. Jain is going to give you some surgery lessons if you're free. What have you got that we could use to tie down a patient?"

"You're joking, Sim," she says.

"Belt? Scarf? Stockings?"

She glares at me and then realizes I'm dead serious. "There's surgical tubing in IC."

"I knew I could count on you to be so creative, honey. Have you done stitches before?"

Dr. Jain has DJ's hand out flat on a stainless steel table by the bed and he's laying out some instruments. I pick up the rack, get a mop and broom and start cleaning up the glass, drugs and blood. Sunny gets a length of tubing out of a cabinet and ties DJ's arm tight to the rail so he can't move it.

She ties it tight enough that the blood flow in his hand eases up and the veins along DJ's track marks pop up eagerly for a hit. He smirks and looks excited but it fades pretty quickly when no one produces a needle.

Jain just quietly picks the glass out of the cuts. "That's nice," he says. "You managed to obliterate the tattoo. You won't even be able to see it when I'm done."

"What about the morphine, Doc?" DJ whines. "What about the pain?"

"Hmmph," Jain grunts and doesn't answer.

DJ turns to me in panic.

"Hmmph," I echo Jain.

I get the room pretty well cleaned up. You wouldn't know anything hit it except for the missing pane on the cabinet. Sunny has a key so we take the bottles and needles out and move them to another cabinet to lock them up.

"Fuck," he yells. "This is medieval. You can't do surgery without drugs."

"I can't?" Jain teases. "Watch me. In fact, I think you should watch."

I sit on the bed and hold his left arm. "You're okay. Don't be a baby."

"Sunny, get me a local anesthetic, please," Jain says. While she's prepping it, he turns DJ's hand over and takes a good look.

"Do you want to keep any of these fingers, buddy?" He laughs at the horror on DJ's face. "I'm really not going to hurt you. You just don't need morphine for stitches."

He takes the needle and shoots the anesthetic into the four corners of the back of DJ's hand, then holds it while he's waiting for it go numb.

"What were you dreaming of during that yoga sleep?" Jain asks to take his mind off his hand.

DJ thinks for a minute. "I was walking down the railroad track singing. I was singing at the top of my lungs because I liked it so much. People were looking at me like I was crazy but I didn't care because I was so happy I *was* crazy."

Jain starts stitching his hand carefully. "Does that hurt?" he asks.

"Not much," DJ says. "It's only physical."

"What were you singing, baby?" I ask him. I want to see him happy again.

"Ah, you know that old blues song you like?" he sings a few bars.

"I can fly like a bird in the sky.
I can buy anything that money can buy."

"Oh, yeah, that's my song! I love that one!" so I sing it for him, loud and in my best gravely blues voice. It's a power song.

"I can turn a river into a raging fire.
And I can live forever if I so desire."

He starts laughing with pleasure, so I keep going, twisting the lyrics to suit myself.

" I can walk on water, you better believe I can.
I can turn back time just by waving my hand."

"Yeah, that's the stuff, Sim. You rock. But it ends badly."

"How's it end?" Jain asks, taking another stitch.

"Oh," I say, "sexual frustration I guess, the usual blues," and I finish the chorus.

"Unhappy am I with all the powers at my command,
You've got the key to my happiness
And I can't get next to you Babe
I can't get next to you"

We do a couple more versus and then rounds of the chorus to entertain Jain while he finishes up the stitches, bouncing riffs off each other. It's good to hear DJ singing.

"Can't get next to you, babe."

"I've been trying to call all day."

"Can't get next to you."

"Baby, I'm on my hands and knees."

"Can't get next to you."

"Can't find your number, honey."

Jain takes the last stitch, inspects his work and asks Sunny to clean his hand and wrap it.

"The moral of the song, if there is one," I say, "is no matter how much power you have, if you put the key to your happiness in someone else's hands, you're powerless. Love comes from here. I put my finger on DJ's forehead. So does sex. It's already in you and all around you."

I tug on the handcuff key hanging around my neck and wink at him. "Don't ever give the key away."

Jain unties the surgical tubing and I unlock the police cuffs. "You're not really going to need cuffs tonight, are you?"

"No thanks, Sim," he says. "I'm sorry. I lost my head. I don't need cuffs."

"If you want morphine, talk to Mack. We don't do that. I'm going to tell him you tried to get up and knocked the rack over and cut your hand on the broken glass. Which is all true without going into the details."

Jain puts a hand on his arm and says, "And one more thing, DJ. You *did* get next to her. She said it was the best kiss she's ever had. She's probably going to be dreaming about you tonight and I'm just going to have to step my game up."

†

NAT

Jain leaves before dawn for the hospital. He's still doing a shift once a week in emergency, occasional surgery, some consulting and referrals, which is how I was lucky enough to get invited up here. I haven't given him my answer yet but I've made up my mind.

I walk over to the Ice House barefoot in the cool morning air and step off the path onto the dewy grass to feel the prana vibrating up from the earth. All night I dreamed of gardens and perfumes under the starlight. I put a few drops of Spirit and Vata oils on the crown of my head and the sole of my feet before bed for healing sattvic dreams and Jain said I smell like an exotic flower. I massaged his feet with vanilla and saffron oil and I can still taste it from his kisses.

I want to work with DJ during the powerful transition of dawn. We've got unfinished business. I find Dr. Mack in the kitchen having coffee. I pray he doesn't interrogate me about the damage in IC yesterday, but he's tired enough that he's just happy to see someone relieve him.

"He's sleeping," he says. "He had a rough night, so he's medicated but I used less. Sean says he's got to be completely clean before his court date in three weeks. Steven wants him off cold by the weekend so we can submit blood tests and affidavits to the judge."

"I can take him until noon," I volunteer. "Sim's training with Jake today."

"Thanks," he says. "Any more broken glass though, please *please* wake me up."

DJ is sleeping peacefully but when I put a hand on his forehead, he opens his eyes and hums with pleasure.

"Don't you dare get up," I threaten him, "or I'll leave."

"Yes, teacher," he purrs. "I'll behave."

"Good. Because I can't teach you if you don't. It's powerful."

"Hmmm," he smiles. "More Tantra?"

"More Tantra," I sigh. "I can't teach you just enough to be dangerous without finishing it. How do you feel this morning, beautiful?"

"Epic," he says. "I can walk on water today. I slept like a rock on the bottom of the ocean."

"Stoned?" I ask.

"Sure. Sure. Nicely stoned. Mack loves me. Sim loves me. You love me. Feel me." He takes my hand from his forehead and moves it down to his heart. I'm relieved when he stops there but my mind travels a little further down to yesterday. God, I think. He's teasing me. I try to concentrate on his heartbeat instead, his human soul.

"No kisses today, honey. I don't want you to touch me. But I'm going to lie down next to you, okay?"

"Oh, yeah!" he growls.

"I mean it. No touching me. But you'll come."

"A hundred orgasms without taking my pants off? That's what Sim said."

"Today, maybe twenty orgasms, but who's counting," I laugh. "Move over, give me some room."

He does and I lie down facing him a few inches apart. I can feel his heat and smell the champa oil on his skin.

"So this is about your chakras, pranic sex. You already know about physical sex."

"Not really," he sulks.

"It's over-rated anyway," I assure him, "physical animal sex. Pranic sex is much more powerful. And you can always mix them once you learn how.

"Your second kosha, the prana layer, is organized around the chakras. What do you know about the chakras?"

"They're not real. None of the koshas or chakras are real. They're just illusions of separation."

"Ooh, your teacher was really good, DJ! You were listening. They're not real but they're energetic pathways. Just like the line around a state on a map doesn't really exist. It just indicates an effect.

"You've got seven main chakras, but the crown doesn't need your attention. It just flowers. So we're only going to work with six of them.

"Just look in my eyes. Look in my left eye. I'm right handed, so that's the non-dominant side of my brain, my soul instead of my mind. And that's it, just keep looking and follow me. Like we did with your body parts in nidra, I'm going to go through your chakras with you. Put your attention there, listen to the sound and imagine the color.

"The first one is the root. Mooladhara is on the pelvic floor at the perineum."

"The what?" he says.

"The root of your energy, right between your legs behind your sex organs. It's where you felt the adrenalin hit when you decided to punch the door off the cabinet."

"Oh that," he says.

"The 'fight or flight' response happens when the first chakra is disturbed. The feeling of a powerful first chakra is being grounded, standing your ground. If you're not grounded, all the rest of your wiring is crossed. Feel it. See the color red. You'll feel the vibration there if you hum 'lam'. Keep looking into my left eye. I'm with you. Just feel the flow of prana down there, all the way down to your toes.

"Second, Svadisthana." I put my right hand on his tailbone. "From your sex back to here. Mainly in the back along the spine. Orange. 'Vam'. Feel the vibration connecting the first two." He's breathing hard now, so I say, "Slow it down, honey. We want to get further than this. Otherwise it's just animal. Breathe with me deep."

We keep breathing into the second chakra and I can feel his energy starting to come higher. I feel it stronger than a kiss rolling through me.

"The third chakra is Manipura. Power and control." I put my hand on the small of his back. "This is where your energy evolves beyond animal sex. Imagine the color yellow. Feel it right behind your navel in your back. Feel it coming right up into your stomach. Right here. 'Ram', I hum.

"Fourth chakra. Anahata, is your sweet heart. This is where you really start to feel the connection with love. Green. 'Yam'." He has an orgasm through his heart and shuts his eyes even before I touch his back.

"Keep coming, honey, come on. Look at me," I whisper.

"Fifth. Vishuddha, the throat chakra. It's your self-expression and creativity, your voice. Blue. 'Ham'. Feel it all the way from the tip of your toes to your mouth." I put my hand on the back of his neck. I want to put my mouth on his so much but I keep my eyes steady on his. I'm feeding his prana with mine. I want to keep it building.

"Sixth. Ajna, the third eye chakra, your higher consciousness. Violet. 'Om.' Your whole body should be coming through the top of your head now. Nice?"

"Nice fucking insane," he pants.

"Keep coming, honey. Follow the prana. Lam. Vam. Ram. Yam. Ham. Om. Keep it coming. You've got all day."

I guide him through twenty rounds of pranic orgasms and then I hold his bandaged hand and put it back on his heart. I don't want to blow his fuse.

"But I didn't – "

"No. We're not trying to reproduce here. You just want to keep that beautiful river of prana flowing through your body so you've got control. You don't need to ejaculate to have an orgasm or ten or twenty.

"And you don't need me to work on this. Just meditate on it and learn to control it. It's very good for you."

"Nat, it's better than a heroin rush." He blows all of his air out hard through his mouth and stops breathing for half a minute.

"A whole lot better for you, too," I laugh. "If you think your teacher just sits there contemplating the universe when he meditates I've got news for you. He might do that when he's upset, but when he's in tune, he's just humming along with the cosmic orgasm. Om. Sim never stops."

†

DJ

"How's your hand, honey?" she asks as she brings me some tea. I know this shit. Black pu-erh tea, funky, fermented and strong with no sugar, the stuff Sim likes. She puts the cup down on the stainless table and sits in the corner chair.

"Which hand?" I joke. I feel good. Not so stoned anymore but incredibly high. My energy is clean and organized instead of frantic. I can still feel her hand on my heart and her body next to me even though she's across the room.

I try to pick up the tea cup with my bandaged hand but I can't grip it, so I reach over with my left.

"Oh, no," I growl at her. "I don't think I can pin you down again today. Maybe I won't have to this time."

"There's no this time, baby. You promised to behave."

"But you said you loved me. You said you liked it."

"I do. And I did. That's why I'm not kissing you. I like control."

"Have you kissed him?"

"Dr. Jain? Yes, a lot."

"No, I mean my teacher. Have you kissed Sim?"

"Oh no, baby! Not like that. I kiss him every chance I get, but it's always controlled and respectful. He wouldn't let me touch him if I didn't have the right intentions. I might kiss you again if you get yourself organized, but right now you're just dangerous."

"Bummer. You could teach me a lot."

"Well, I will, baby, but you don't know what you don't know. And you really don't need me to teach you how to make out. You already know how to kiss."

Damn. I try again.

"I feel organized now. Show me how you kiss Sim then. I can be controlled."

"You incorrigible boy," she says and looks at the clock. It's 10am. "Not here. Do you feel like getting out of here? I can show you how outside.

"And I'll bet you can walk. You pinned me against the wall yesterday and punched out the medicine cabinet."

I'm good to walk. I'm warm and caffeinated from the pu-erh and I'd follow her anywhere.

She takes my arm and helps me to my feet. A shock goes through me when she touches me. Sim was right about touching. And she made me come just looking in my eyes. It's a little dangerous in a very sexy way.

I've got someone else's sweat pants on, no shirt and no shoes but she says that's fine. We walk out the sliding door into the sunshine and across the lawn to a beautiful pool. Next to the pool there's an outdoor gym. Sim's on the bench press and Jake is spotting him. There's an old sofa on the lawn next to the gym and the ghostly girl from Nick's house is curled up on it watching the boys.

Jake looks up and sees me and gives a hoot. "Look who's coming out to play! Dracula Junior!" he howls. I haven't seen him since we last surfed together, what seems like a million years ago. "I thought you were in the mob now, brother. I heard you did some jail."

Sim finishes his set with 95 pounds and sits up looking at me cautiously then Nat.

"What did you do to him, Nat? He's glowing."

"I don't think he wants to kill himself anymore," she laughs. "Do you know Sim's wife Brandy? She says she's met you before."

I'm stunned, then I remember what Mack said. I slept with her two nights ago when I was sick. She was on the beach holding Sim with blood all over her. She was at Nick's.

Sim laughs, "You can talk to her, buddy, but don't touch her."

Brandy gets up and hugs me in spite of his warning and kisses my forehead. "Good morning. Nice to see you again, beautiful," she whispers, "Have a seat. It's the greatest show on earth."

I sit on the sofa next to her and she puts an arm around my shoulder. Her touch rolls through me like an earthquake and I shake hard.

"Oh!" Sim notices it. "Is he awake or is he dreaming that?"

Nat says, "He's on his own very special recipe of narcotics and kundalini Tantra."

Sim starts laughing. Jake hasn't got a clue what they're talking about, but I do. I can feel the twin rivers of fire and ice raging through my blood, my nerves and my mind. The rivers cross at my chakras and flood my whole being. I feel the chop at the surface of the rivers and the dark peace at the bottom. I'm lying on the reef where the rivers pour from waterfalls.

Sim gets up from the bench and walks over to Nat. His nose is almost touching hers. "Namaste, sugar," he says and then he kisses her, in front of his wife, on the lips, soft and cool without any heat. He doesn't put his hands on her.

She smiles and turns around to me and says, "And that, baby, is how it's done." She sits on the other side of me on the sofa and I'm in a beautiful sandwich. It's the best seat in the house.

"Too bad your hand is fucked," Sim says. "You won't be able to train with us for a while." Then he gives me a mean laugh and says, "Wait. I forgot you're still on drugs. You're under Ice House arrest. You don't get to use the gym. Or the pool. Or the yoga deck. Or the lab. Your life sucks, honey."

He spots Jake on the bench with 225, then strips the weights and puts 115 pounds on the bar. He does one clean rep. Jake spots him but he doesn't need any help and the girls applaud politely.

Then he goes to the lat pull down and sticks the pin in 40 pounds to warm up. When he turns around to put his hands on the bar, I get my first look at his back. It's horrible. He's tanned and his muscles are hard and cut, but there's a good 10 inches of ragged scars covering his lower back below his heart. I feel like throwing up and flash back to the blood and gore on the beach. I feel sick. I need a hit again. I start to shake a little. I need to see Mack.

"I need to go back, Nat," I say. "I don't feel good."

"Not yet," she says. "Sim, can I show him around? I think he needs to walk it off."

"Be my guest," he says. "But remember, house arrest, no amenities." He puts the pin on 60. "You don't like my back, DJ?" he sneers. "You ain't seen nothing yet, honey." Then he pulls the bar down smooth and controlled and I see every muscle in his back working, even the damaged parts.

She takes my arm again and leads me to the pool house. I slept in the bedroom the night before last but I take a good look around. There are fresh flowers on the bedside table and padded cuffs by the telephone. On the shelf above the dresser, there's a police hat and the metal handcuffs I wore up here with another key on a chain. There's one around his neck still, so it must be a duplicate. The bed is huge. I notice the futon is missing from the sofa frame. I'm thinking, I'm alone with her in Sim's bedroom, but I've got two strikes already.

She leads me through the kitchen and out to a yoga deck behind the house. There's a Buddha kind of like the one on the deck of the beach house, the missing futon, a massage table and yoga mats. Flowers are dripping everywhere from the shade roof. The smell of jasmine starts to seriously arouse me.

"Have a seat," she says as she sits down cross-legged. I sit down facing her. "This is your teacher's office. I work for him. Beautiful, isn't it?"

I'm still shaking but I'm feeling a little calmer here.

"He kicked drugs out here. He was much more strung out than you'll ever be. We know how to fix you, DJ, when you're ready. But he doesn't want to work with you until you stop taking drugs. He doesn't want me to work with you either, but I find it hard to say no if you need my help. Just remember, we've got better medicine than Dr. Mack."

She lets that sink in for a few minutes and then says, "Come on and I'll show you my office."

We walk to the house next door, past the gym. Sim is lying on the sofa now with his feet up on the arm and his head in his wife's lap. She's playing with his hair and she winks at me as we walk by.

Nat shows me the living room. It's got a flat screen and a pretty nice bar. "No internet, no television here," she says. "We only watch training videos, surfing, yoga, educational stuff."

There's a huge dining table, large enough to seat a dozen people. "This is the boys' boardroom, corporate headquarters and party central," she laughs, then shows me into her office, the lab next to the kitchen.

It has a massage table, fresh flowers, sheets, towels and a lot of glass door cabinets full of bottles and shot glasses.

"Do NOT punch out my cabinet doors," she warns. "If you want anything, just ask. By the way, my stuff costs a lot more than Mack's narcotics."

"What ya got in there," I ask. "Anything good?"

"Everything good," she says. "Mostly distilled botanicals and carrier oils. Some hydrosols. Some tinctures that are much nicer than bourbon. She unlocks one of the cabinet doors and takes something out.

"Try this. It's the one your teacher likes best."
She gives me a little bottle to sniff and it smells like the
oils she put on me. It smells delicious. It reminds me of
my first yoga nidra when Sim took my mind down to the
train tracks and I woke up with her.

"Can you put some more of this on me, please?"

"Not in here. Your oil is in IC. You're under Ice
House arrest. You heard Sim."

I like her office. It's got high windows facing out to
tall pine trees behind the house so it's completely
private. It's not S&M's bedroom so I'm thinking this is
the place where she's going to show me control. I put
my good hand on the wall and lean in towards her with
my nose close to hers like I saw him do.

"Oh, no, no, no, babe," she says and pushes my
arm off the wall so I have to lean back for balance. "I
said no. I mean no."

"You said you were going to show me," I whine
with frustration.

"No. I said I was going to show you how I kiss
Sim. And I did. I kissed him in front of you, Jake and
his wife. We're all done here, honey. Let's go back and
see how your teacher is doing. I'm sure he wants to have
a word with you."

She gives me the little glass bottle to keep and
says to sniff it as much as I like if I feel disintegrated. I
feel disintegrated a lot so I thank her from the bottom of
my heart. I feel like I'm looking down at myself from
eight miles above. Any kind of anti-disintegrating re-
integration program would work for me.

I feel rejection but somehow I don't feel like
destroying her office. Possibly because of the two dozen
orgasms I already had today. I'm okay with it.

†

S&M

Nat's too sweet to him. At this rate DJ is never going to change. I watch them walking back from the Fire House and she has her arm through his, laughing. He's higher than a kite and I'm pretty sure he's lost the plot. He's forgotten about prison and his mind is on … her. It's not what I want.

"Brandy, get her out of here, please." I say, "Nat, go. Leave him alone."

They go off quickly and quietly to the pool house. I get up from the sofa and wave DJ to sit down. I sit on the ground. I want the ground for this. I have all the time in the world but I don't want to waste it. I'm teaching here.

DJ sits on the sofa and pulls his legs up under him in lotus position. I feel a breath of relief just seeing that.

"What's going on with you, little brother?" I ask.

I can see his thoughts scatter from her to here and back to her.

"Uh," he says. He has no clue what's going on.

"Hmm. I don't want to say I told you so, or I know how you feel, but I'm trying here. Where are you going with this?"

He laughs. "I'm going nowhere fast," he says.

"Two weeks ago I was strung out, too. My brother didn't like to see me suffer. As long as you keep taking it, he'll help you out. Same as your smack house friends. You've got to get out of there.

"And FYI, Nat's off limits, baby. You can let her in, but you can't have her. Calm down. Get a little control. You know this has nothing to do with her, don't you? It's about you.

"Whatever is going down on the beach, the drugs, the violence, we're more powerful than that. Remember the jokers who used to show up during the big swells with baseball bats? As if you can beat the shit out of Mother Nature. Looking rough and acting tough isn't power. They were pretty pathetic, no?"

He laughs. He knows what I'm talking about. But he's only half here.

"Have some strength. What good is a baseball bat if you're not hitting a home run?"

"Smashing things!" he laughs.

"Yeah. Destruction. Are you into that? What you did in Mack's IC was really ugly."

"I'm sorry. You said it was two strikes against me."

"Yeah. Strike three will be if you keep molesting my assistant. You wouldn't last three minutes in bed with her. She's ten years older than you and you don't even know what you're doing. Could we concentrate on the drugs and the felony charges first and give your puppy love a rest?"

"She loves me, Sim," he whines. "My first."

"I love you, too, DJ, but that doesn't mean you can put your tongue in my mouth," I hit him in the shoulder just hard enough to shake him because he's not hearing me.

"Listen. Sean is going to try to get the narcotics charges reduced, drop the intent to sell charge because you weren't actually making the sales. Darrell told him that. And maybe they can drop resisting arrest because you were stupid enough to fall off the cliff. He can't do anything about possession of narcotics and being under the influence except to petition the judge to let you stay in rehab. For that we need to get some clean blood tests. I'm giving you until Sunday. Three days. Can you do that?"

"Can I use the pool?"

"How stoned are you, little brother? Are you even listening to me? You can use the pool, I'll teach you yoga, you can spend all day on Nat's massage table, watch surf movies, lift weights or sit in the sun all day having orgasms and drinking bourbon as far I'm concerned. Just *fucking* no more narcotics."

His eyes light on the water and the barbells, the lawn and then the Fire House and back to me. Something he sees makes him happy.

"Okay," he says. "Can Mack give me a full blood transfusion?"

"Oh, God, honey. Is that going to be necessary? Do you know how painful and expensive that's would be?" I'm shocked at how twisted he's thinking. And I'm kind of wishing I hadn't sent my assistant therapist away.

"Rock stars do it all the time," he whines.

"Little Dracula, where is your mind going? I'll give you a pint, Mack might give you a pint, but that's only about 15% of what you'd need. It's painful, and if you have another hit, you'll just pollute the clean blood and we have to start all over again. It sounds too bloody to me. You can't even donate blood you're so loaded."

"You can trade my blood to the hospital for people who need narcotics."

This time I pop him on the side of his head.

"Here's the deal, buddy," I say. "I'll give you a pint on Sunday. And if you put any drugs into *our* blood, I'll take it back the hard way."

This time he hears what I'm saying. He offers me a little bottle of oil from his pocket and says, "Sniff that, Sim. It smells like dreams. She gave it to me."

†

NAT

I'll regret this the rest of my life if I don't do something about it. Tantra teaches us to overcome sensual entanglements by enjoying them without becoming attached. I want to marry Jain, but right now I'm too attached.

I sit on the deck with Brandy drinking strong black tea and listening to the winds shift on the mountain. The jasmine is in full bloom and the scent weaves around us like a silk scarf.

Sim comes out the back door with DJ and they sit on the deck with us. He asks his wife to take a look at DJ's hand to see if there's any hope of swimming. Brandy unwraps it carefully and turns it over in her hands.

"Maybe Sunday," she says. "The stitches should stay in a few more days."

She kisses his hand and lets it go. He smashed it because he wanted to kiss me.

DJ laughs and points to his tattoo. "Look, I've only got a 3 now. The 6 is gone."

Sim takes his hand and inspects it. "That's a good omen. You've erased 36th Avenue and some really bad karma. Three is a yoga number. Three doshas, three gunas, three eyes of Shiva, and the three parts of Om, the beginning, the middle and the end.

"And probably three minutes." he snarls with a wicked laugh.

"Let me see it, DJ," I reach out to take his hand and hold it. There's a very small '3' tattoo right next to the scar where he split his knuckles open.

"You should tart this little thing up as an Omkara tattoo," I suggest. "Just add the tail and the cap and you'll have a beautiful little Om on your hand every day."

His eyes light up and he smiles at me with pure love and gratitude. "I will, Nat. I mean I would, but I'm under house arrest so I can't leave."

"No," Sim says to me. "That's good, Nat. We'll do it Sunday. Sunday's going to be the junkie's new birthday. I'll have Crys bring an inker up. I might even copy him. It'll take our minds off his pain."

I'm still holding DJ's hand so I volunteer to do some work on it while the bandages are off. I don't want to let him go. Brandy gets the helichrysum and birch bodybuilding blend. Sim just sits there staring at me. I've never been good at hiding my feelings and I know he can read me now. I'm going to regret this for the rest of my life if I don't let it go right here and now. It will haunt me.

"What's up, Nat?" he frowns. "Where do you think you're going with this?"

Brandy brings back a shot glass full of oil and hands it to me. I start rubbing it into DJ's hand, working very carefully around the stitches.

"Can I have a little time, boss?" I whisper to Sim. "I just want to say good-bye to him."

"Nat," he warns. "You shouldn't."

"Oh, but *I'm* sure I should, Steven," I say. I'm not speaking to him as my boss right now. I'm speaking to him as an equal, a yogi. He speaks my language.

"Ignorance causes a deeper attachment," I remind him. "It's what we teach. Enjoy but don't get attached. Would you please give me some time?"

He gets to his feet and smiles with amusement.

"Om Kali Devi, indiscriminate gourmet of all the world's flavors."

He takes Brandy's arm, then turns at the door to ask, "How much?"

"An hour?"

"With him? I'm betting three minutes max," he laughs and shuts the door.

I'm still massaging his hand. I want to do his feet but I don't have the patience now. He stopped breathing when the door closed. I put one finger up to my nose to remind him to breathe. We do ten slow rounds of nadi shodhana together, breathing the thick scent of jasmine slowly from left to right nostril and back slower and slower until it almost makes you high you become so balanced. When he's relaxed, I let it go.

"DJ, I'm going to marry Jain. But I want to say good-bye before I do. I'm not going to keep playing with you. I love you. But it's going to be like this."

I kiss him like I kiss Sim, very respectful and controlled, because if I kiss like this I can think straight. If I can kiss him like this, I won't have to give him up. He kisses back, very reserved, cool and serious now.

He winks at me. "Control," he smiles, proud of himself.

"I'm going to kiss you like that from now on, but right now this is a very special good-bye kiss that will never happen again. Just between us, you and me."

This time I kiss him like he kissed me before I taught him self-control. He can never taste so eager or inexperienced as the first kiss but this time it's better. This time he tastes of pure impermanence. Impermanence tastes even more delicious than inexperience.

I've never experienced a better teacher of Maya than the impermanence of a kiss. Maya is the illusion of a real world as everything passes by, turning into a memory and a dream as soon as it's over, rising and dissolving. There's nothing solid about a kiss.

Maybe Sim taught DJ about Maya, but not like I do. I give him a grand slam two course lesson in impermanence and experience that can never be repeated and never taken away. I ask him to remember it every time he looks at his new tattoo.

A kiss turns into a memory a second later. Experience turns into dream. The flames of fire transform matter into essence, from reality into smoke. Fire is the mouth of Shiva and its flames are his tongue. I die every day.

†

BRANDY

"Brandy, can you clean him up a little?" Sim begs me. "He was supposed to be under house arrest. Mack will kill me."

DJ looks wild and completely disheveled. He's a pretty messy boy right now. He's been sleeping in the same sweat pants for three days and probably hasn't combed his hair in a week. But he's got Nat's beautiful white silk scarf with Buddhist images around his bare shoulders.

They were out there nearly two hours, not three minutes.

When DJ follows her in dressed like that Sim looks worried.

"Gee, I don't you should advertise this by wearing the lady's scarf, DJ. You better lose that."

Nat puts her hand on the scarf and says, "Sim, it's no big deal. It's a common yogi blessing to give a scarf. This symbol," she points out, "represents healing and preserving beings from illness, harmful forces, obstacles and suffering. It's good for him."

"What else did you bless, Nat?" he sneers.

"Every last bit of divine perfection," she laughs. "Om Kamadevaya. I don't think I missed anything."

"Well shit. There's a board meeting in an hour and we're all supposed to prep for the press tomorrow. See if you can make him look nice, Brandy."

"What about my third strike, Sim?" DJ wonders, worried.

"Technically, buddy?" he says shaking his head, "You didn't strike out. Home run. You scored."

Sim walks Nat back to her office for abhyanga and I show DJ into the shower for a shampoo. He's in desperate need of a haircut and I'm inspired to tart him up. I lay out the mutilated blue jeans that I washed after he surfed them down the cliff. They're badly torn but beautifully frayed and immaculately clean. He laughs when he comes out of the shower in a towel and sees them.

I cut his hair wet, very short on top so that the crown chakra has a little Buddhist punk rock spike to it. I cut the front short enough that it's off his face and out of his eyes and above his ears. He's got the left ear pierced so I put one of my diamond earrings in it. I cut the back short enough that it doesn't hang over his silver chain.

He asks me for the abhyanga oil and while his hair dries he covers himself with sandalwood. I oil his back and then he pulls on the beautiful raggedy jeans. I put the blessing scarf back around his neck and arrange it neatly on both sides of his handcuff necklace.

Then I step back and admire him. He's a different person. He looks like Krishna's pimp. He's clean, peaceful and radiant. I'm amused that he's no longer bothered by me touching him, fussing with his hair, teasing him, watching him dress. It's as if he's not here anymore, he's so passive. He looks pretty high, but not like a junkie. He looks like an avatar.

"This will do for the photo shoot," I say. "You're a rock star now, baby."

We walk over the lawn to the Fire House arm in arm in the moonlight and I can see all our staff already gathered around the boardroom table. I pick a small sprig of jasmine from a pot by the door and tuck it behind his right ear. I wonder if Mack's been giving him lithium because he's so sedated he's floating above the Earth as he walks.

We're quite a bit late for the meeting but that just lets us make an entrance. Everyone in the room shuts up and stares at him when we come in.

Sim says, "Well you missed everything but I can fill Brandy in later. DJ, you just show up looking like that at 10am tomorrow. Don't talk to anyone. You won't be in the interview because of the felonies, but you'll be good in the photos. You look like a very expensive stripper."

Mack gets to his feet to shake DJ's hand and says, "Wow. What a difference a day makes! What have you been up to today?"

DJ looks happily around the room at everyone, smiles like an angel and says, "Yoga. Lots of yoga."

†

NAT

The moon is waning again and its quiet enough to hear its light falling on the grass on my way back to the Fire House. Jain is deep in sleep, beyond snoring. I put a bit more jatamansi on my crown chakra for sattvic dreams. I want to go so far down into sleep now that I hear the cosmic Om roar through the bedroom like a locomotive engine.

The last thing I do before I go to bed is look at the picture of my sweet guru. He is smiling so big I think he's laughing at me. My mind became so wild when I tried to control it, like a wild horse that doesn't rage until you show it a rope. I hear Sri Niranjan teaching, clearly, "You can hurt yourself trying to find Samadhi, you can fall down and break things and maybe even hurt other people around you." I'm carefully watching myself walking carelessly through all of this.

Om Kamadevaya vidmahe
Behold the God of Love
May this sweet flowering power direct us

You can never again be the person you were yesterday. We grow, stagnate and die each day in many ways. I know even stars, rocks and diamonds are impermanent. But consciousness may be the most impermanent of all. Today I saw a person disappear entirely. It was like seeing death and birth at once.

Maybe the narcotics destroyed him so completely that there was nothing left of him to bring back. Maybe his kundalini started such an intense fire that it incinerated every thought and desire he ever had. Maybe I broke his heart. Maybe I just blew his mind. Probably it was all those things happening at once.

But DJ is gone.

Gate, gate, paragate, parasamgate.
Gone, gone, long gone, gone far away

In my haste to quench the thirst of my desire, I blew his fuse.

Afterwards I massaged his feet and he just watched the moon steadily without a word. Finally, I asked, "What does DJ stand for?"

"David John," he sighed. "No one calls me that."

"I won't call you that, either, Kamadev," I whisper. "Om Namah Kamadevaya."

He laughed, "Kama Dave? What's that?"

"Kamadev. Yes, it's pronounced 'Kama Dave'. The God of Love." I touched his heart and put my white blessing scarf around his shoulders.

All the wildness was gone from his eyes, all the fear and desire and thirst. His face wore the peace of perfect composure and control. When I kissed him again, he kissed me like I was a child, with loving kindness. He was long gone over to the far away shore. I didn't mean good-bye to be that permanent.

†

MACK

Nat was up half the night studying and writing in my study, the only internet access on the property. I like it when she does that because she burns the midnight oil to a crisp and leaves it's ashes on my computer. The bookmark history in my browser is usually a treasure box of articles and resources for botanical medicine and Ayurveda the next day. I'm learning a lot by looking at her tracks.

While she studies, I sit with DJ. He tells me he's now Karma Dave before he dives off into the deep end of exhausted sleep. For some reason, he's not sick and he doesn't want me to give him any morphine tonight. The best way I can describe it is he's on another planet. But at least he's peaceful and his vitals are all pretty low key for a junkie. He's put so much oil on himself he glows.

In the morning I find an order on my desk for a couple thousand dollars, including four ounces of night blooming jasmine distillate, blue and white lotus attars, and a half liter of Sri Lankan sandalwood. She has a question mark next to mango flowers and has crossed out 'ashoka flower oil".

I'm a little curious about this huge shift in medicinal oils so I check out the websites she's been browsing. There's a wild array of botanical, medicinal and mythical information but the focus of her study is bizarre. She's researching the Ayurvedic use of the five flowers decorating the bow of Kamadev, a cupid-like deity who shoots Krishna up with so much love that he becomes adorable and venerable.

I went off morphine yesterday after Steven asked me to chill. Also working with a real junkie instead of a patient has opened my eyes. But my first thought is shooting the essence of Kama into my veins. I wouldn't mind that. I start to crave it. What is she going to do with this? Who would want morphine any more?

I check her list again and read her notes on the pad.

Ashoka - means without sorrow. Sacred ornamental flowering temple tree
White lotus – gives them strength and power
Blue lotus – mildly sedative
Mango flower ?
Jasmine - nervous system, psyche, emotions, confidence, optimism, euphoria - balances energy – increased passion, romance, peace and love! (Healing for sexual difficulties, impotence, premature ejaculation, and frigidity, hahaha).

Apparently she's not worried about sexual difficulties. The distilled Sri Lankan sandalwood, the thousand dollar order, isn't one of Kamadev's five favorite flowers but there's a note:

Vishnu bathes in jasmine and sandalwood - quiets mind & emotions, opens the heart and the third eye chakra, integrates body, mind & spirit, enhances romantic moods

Kamadev is apparently an incarnation of Vishnu, I read. It's sounds familiar somehow. And then it hits me. Karma Dave. Shit. I go back to IC to check on him and he's gone. It's 4am and still dark.

†

DJ

I'm asleep on the back of a serpent, floating in a lake of milk. There's a blue lotus flower blossoming from my belly and my body is humming with orgasms. Lakshmi sits at my feet and massages them with jasmine oil. She has a deep scar from behind her heart that cuts around her back all the way to her breast. It looks like Kali tried to rip her heart out through her back. She said Dr. Jain cut her to save her life.

I show her Tantric sex and then animal sex and then the way gods do it until sex becomes as essential as a glass of water. I show her control that makes her beg. When I stop for a minute to watch the moon move, she pleads for mercy. Sim pissed me off when he said three minutes. I'm stoned enough to control her for three days and nights if I want.

Afterwards she's rubbing my feet and I really don't want her anymore. I'm the god of love. She's just a mirror, Maya, the illusion of the world. She said good-bye to me. I'm experienced. I'm impermanent. I kiss her good-bye without any heat, without touching her, the way she said it's going to be.

So I'm sleeping here again, alone on the futon surrounded by sticky jasmine blossoms dripping in the air, night blooming jasmine arousing me with its scent then closing up at dawn so I can start to dream the world of Maya again.

I open my eyes and Maya is still there waiting for me, the illusion of a deck floating in space at the top of the world above the tree tops. If you have to be in a world, there is a very good view of it from here.

I hope Sim doesn't kill me for breaking in but he said as long as there's no fucking narcotics, I can do whatever the fuck I want to.

I'm just sleeping here, sated, dreaming I'm lying on a snake floating in the milk lake. It's from a myth I read at Sim's house. Vishnu dreams the world into existence while he's lying on the serpent of consciousness. He dreams one universe after another and this universe is just one of his many dreams. From what she taught me, I'll bet he's dreaming of sex and snoring very steadily.

Sim gave me the idea of sitting in the sun all day meditating on my orgasms. That's my plan for today. I'm going to ignore the entire illusion of a press conference and cover myself with that sandalwood oil and come all day. I'm Kamadev, god of love. And I'm not even going to talk to her, even if she wants to rub my feet. She can't touch me.

†

S&M

Bran gets up for water and whispers in my ear when she gets back in bed, "The beautiful crazy boy is sleeping on the deck, Sim. Naked."

"Shit, honey, how did he get in?" I know I locked the door. I've only been married a couple weeks and I need my privacy.

"Bathroom window," she whispers. "His jeans are in the kitchen. He's sucking on his knuckles like a baby.

"Should we call Mack? I don't want to wake him up, but if he's up he'll be missing a patient."

"Can you run over there and see? Ask him how much dope he gave him tonight please. Tell him he's safe here for now.

"And, baby, one more thing. When you get back can you make me more beautiful than him?"

When she leaves, I start nidra with my right thumb, index finger, middle finger, taking myself down to the bottom of my heart when I hear him calling from the kitchen.

"Sim, can I use the oil? I quit."

"You quit breaking into people's houses?"

"I quit dope. Can I use the oil?"

"You better talk to me first," I warn.

"Nah, I want to do this first so I can get dressed."

"Then no, you can't use the oil. Get dressed and come out here. You woke me up, fucker."

He comes out in his clean wrecked jeans looking mortally offended. "Excuse me," he says. "I thought you'd be proud of me. You told me I had to get out of there and I came over around 3am. I have been listening, teacher. I didn't want to wake you so I jimmied the window. I'm not under house arrest anymore because I quit using yesterday."

"That would be cool, but I'll believe it when Mack tells me. You look absolutely fucked up. Look at yourself."

He goes over to the mirror and puts his face up close to the glass and stares for a long time. Then he turns around and looks at me. His eyes are glazed and unfocused. He looks like a train wreck.

"I look fucking beautiful, Sim. What are you talking about? Brandy made me look like the god of love."

"Sit down," I say. "You quit? You didn't have any more dope last night?" He nods hard smiling.

"You did it for her? So you could move into her house?"

"Fuck her," he grins showing all his teeth. "I did it for you, Sim. And maybe for the pool and the surf movies." He laughs, a little crazy, amused by himself.

"I've got everything under complete control now. Everything. I just walked out of the Ice House when she was on the computer."

"You've got complete control? Because you lasted longer than three minutes?"

"Fuck," he hisses. "She was begging me, Sim. I made her cry. I may never let another woman touch me again. You were right. I can really hurt them.

"She called me Kamadev, the god of love. I'm killing her."

Brandy comes back into the house and looks at him curiously. Even though his eyes are blank, his hair is bed head perfect.

"Clean," she says. "Mack says he hasn't hit him since yesterday morning. So unless he has a hidden stash somewhere that he's shooting, he's clean."

DJ pulls his little bottle of spirit oil out and starts sniffing on it with deep breaths of nadi shodhana. He's smiling proudly and nodding slowly like a drunk.

"I'm betting on a stash of lithium somewhere. But maybe he's just really sick." I shake my head. "Okay. Here's what we're going to do, DJ."

"I'm Kamadev," he corrects me.

"Sri Kama Dave," I continue. "You're going to move into the Fire House. Get your oil from IC and take one of my bottles of sandalwood, too. You haven't got fuck all to pack. Take the room upstairs. It's got a private bath. It's fine to take towels or flowers out of the lab, but nothing else. Have fun with your oil over there and meet me out at the gym at 10. Got that?"

"Upstairs in the Fire House. Bath, towels, flowers, oil. Gym at 10."

"Keep the windows closed. Don't hurt yourself."

"Don't hurt myself. Got it."

He walks back to the shelf and touches the handcuffs.

"Can I have this?" he asks fingering the spare key on a chain.

"I need to have a spare key," I explain. "I'm playing with them."

He picks up his blessing scarf and puts it over his shoulders and heads for the door.

"Never mind. Take it," I say. "I'll tell you if I need it."

Brandy shuts and locks the door behind him and raises an eyebrow. "He looks wild. Is he okay?"

"No. He was stoned and she fucked his brains out. I don't think he's too focused."

I pick up the phone to warn Nat. I don't want to shock her.

"Sri Kamadeva is moving in upstairs. Just a fair warning. He's on his way over."

I put the phone down and reach for Brandy.

"Come back to bed, sugar. I want to be that crazy. Drive me wild and then see if you can make me look prettier than Kamadeva."

She curls next to me under the sheet and purrs.

"Prettier than Kama Dave? I'm not sure that's possible. What kind of god do you think you are, Sim?"

I'm surprised she hasn't figured that out yet. So I tell her. I'm the Nataraj.

Om Namah Shivaya. I'm Shiva. Then I show her how Shiva tears the world out of the cosmos and sets its rhythm with his dance.

†

BRANDY

At 10 I'm sitting on the sofa watching Shiva, Jain and Jake warming up on the bench press. It takes two to spot Jain with 275 pounds. He's a beautiful piece of machinery and the boys are out of his league as far as the weights go. He only works one day a week now at the hospital so he's replaced his pale complexion with radiance. As have I. Shiva no longer calls me his Ghost Girl.

As far as looks go, though, I've got to give it to Shiva. I cut his hair a lot longer than Kama Dave's. It's thicker so I could still get that live wire effect up top without going so short. I'm thinking of burning his cop hat so he can never cover his head up again. Maybe I should burn his clothes, too. He looks like a dark star going supernova. I wish I could have put some red tips on the ends of his beautiful black hair, but I settled for putting a big red ruby earring is his left ear instead.

I smell Dave on the breeze before I see him coming on the path from the Fire House. Nat's walking a few steps behind, but he's not looking at her or talking to her. Yesterday they couldn't keep their hands off each other. Today, it's like he's walking all alone on his own planet.

He's got white jasmine buds tied in a long twist through his hair that make my hair cut proud. There's a big bunch of loose jasmine tucked in the waist of his jeans. The white scarf, handcuff key and the little silver necklace adorn his bare chest and back, and he shines with sandalwood oil. Even his bare feet are glowing.

Jain stands up from the bench, sees Dave, frowns and flexes his chest. Kamadev holds up his hand in the universal mudra of peace, an open empty hand: I don't have a rock or a gun in my hand. Ahimsa. No harm.

Mack calls him over to the table where he's entertaining Chris Croft and I follow him. I'm supposed to escort him out of here in case anything happens. Sunny is telling Chris about the corporate mission. She stops so Mack can introduce the god of love.

"Chris, this is Kama Dave, a patient. No interview with him yet. He's going through an enlightenment phase right now. He's not talking to any one. Just photos."

Dave puts his fist out so Chris can bump it. He's not talking, just like Shiva told him. I put my arm around him and walk him back to the sofa, but Nat's sitting there and he won't go near it. He takes my hand off him and sits down on the grass in the sun, eyes half closed.

The photographer who came up with Chris is focusing hard on the workout shots. She's a beautiful young woman and she is obviously relishing shooting the boys.

Between sets, she turns around and notices Kamadev stretched out on his side sniffing his bottle on the left of his nose and then the right; her smile explodes. She knows him.

"DJ! Remember me? Amber, from the Point. Look at you, gorgeous boy. I thought you were in jail."

He shakes his head at her. He's not talking to anyone.

"Amber," I say. "Hi, I'm Brandy. I'm his nurse. He doesn't want to talk. But he likes to be called Kama Dave now. Make sure you get that if you run any photos of him. DJ is history."

She asks if she can take a few pictures of him on the sofa with us. I don't think he'll do it, but he shrugs and sits between us, detached and cool. She shoots us, then he leans back against my shoulder and kicks his feet up in Nat's lap. He crosses his arms over his head and smiles like a god coming. I put my hand on his heart and she puts her hands on his feet for the photo. It's going to be a centerfold pin up.

"Front page, Dave baby," Amber laughs.

†

NAT

I'm afraid I hurt him. He let me fix his hair and tie flowers in it and asked me to oil his back but otherwise, he's staying as far away as me as possible, as if I were poison. He came into the lab and took a stack of towels and a fistful of jasmine. He has his own oils and he puts them on himself in his room. He uses much more than necessary, but it calms him down. When we left the house it reeked of sticky white buds and sandalwood oil.

He's maintaining silence now. Sim is wrapping up the interview with Chris while Amber takes a few more gratuitous portraits of Kamadev. I want to put ten more silk scarves on him. I'll bet she feels the same way.

She packs her camera and Chris shakes hands all around. "We'll be at the point tomorrow when you get there. Go hard, boys! I like what you're doing, integrating yoga, Ayurveda, bodybuilding and medicine. It's an interesting mix."

"As the President and original patient, I can assure you it's pretty mixed up," Sim says. "It's a twist on the Garden of Eden and a mad house."

"Then you must love it here," Chris laughs.

"Absolutely crazy for it."

When Chris is gone, Sim walks over to the sofa and smirks at me. His hair is pretty and he has a big ruby in his ear like a pirate who's robbed the queen. He curls his lip and shows me his right canine tooth in a snarl.

"Oh, payback time, honey," he hisses. "I need to have a few private words with you in my office. How much do you owe me now? *'Please, boss! With sugar on it! Please, boss!'* We have a deal."

I remember the promise and where this started two days ago when Kamadev wouldn't let me touch him or talk to him. Here we are again. He won't talk to me, but I made a deal. I follow Sim to his house and out back to the deck.

"Sit down. The futon is pretty comfortable isn't it?" he smirks. He knows I know.

He sits next to me. He smells like frankincense and sandalwood with a lot of sticky sweet helichrysum.

"So this is not about playing or pain, Nat. It's just going to be cosmetic. This is just for the beach tomorrow. It's going to be a message."

I'm a little worried to tell the truth.

He stands up and pulls his belt out, not sexy, but very businesslike. Is that what he wants me to do again? Beat him with mindfulness, precision and intention? I'm actually in the mood for it. I'm ready to kill him. I stand up and take the belt from him.

"Like I was saying, this isn't just for fun today, Nat. I want to wear it. Six serious welts. Take the paint off the walls this time, honey."

Now *that's* a different story and not where I thought he was going at all. But I'm still interested.

"How about three, Sim?" I suggest. "I can do three neatly but with six I might cross over and tear some flesh. It could be uglier than you planned."

I run my hand over his upper back and shoulders, the part without any scars like a blank canvas. His skin is still warm from sitting in the sun. I want to hurt him because he let me hurt Kamadev.

"Three," I repeat. "I might get five if your back was as big as Jain's."

"Deal," he says. "Then we'll see how three looks."

"Sim," I add with a little anger. "I think I hurt him. Maybe you should have stopped me."

"Nat? What's the job of the goddess Parvati?"

"She aborbs the energy of Shiva and releases it into the world for the benefit of all mankind."

"Right. You're just doing her job for me. Now release some of that energy on me, honey."

He turns his back and leans into the wall for an easy target. I feel the prana burning in my feet and I let it run hot. I want to hurt him. But I want it to be cosmetically aesthetic. Three beautiful forks of the same river rising up his spine like snakes flowing from the same source at manipura chakra. I'm just doing my job.

The left hand snake surprises me with its dark venom. I watch for about a half minute while he tries to slow down his breath. It worked. I see a wide burn rising and already it has the halo of a bruise. Strike one. I put another beautiful snake on his right shoulder and don't even wait to see if it worked. I can feel it.

I put the last one right down the center behind his heart.

"You'll like this, boss," I say. "I did it nice."

He sits down on the futon with his eyes closed breathing hard. "Oh fucking Nick."

"I'm Nat," I remind him.

"You're fucking Kali biting the heads off men, Nat. How does it look? Is it nice?"

"It's much better. I know what I'm doing now. It looks very professional. Scary. Precise and premeditated. Oh, you'll like it."

I take his arm and help him back to his feet and back into the bedroom. He looks over his shoulder in the mirror and whistles, "Yes!"

"No," I say. "You can't even see it. Do you have another mirror, a hand mirror?"

He gets one from the bathroom and holds it so he can see his back without twisting. Now he can see the perfection, the three purple snakes in parallel just short of bleeding. I hope it hurts as bad as it looks.

"You know what you're doing, don't you? We're even now, Kali baby."

He recites proudly for me,

"O Kali, raimented with space,

three-eyed creatrix of the three worlds,
  whose waist is beautiful with a girdle
  made of dead men's arms.
"Kali means time. She's one of my favorites.

"I know you're mad at me, Nat, but Kamadev threw himself under your feet. As the story goes, Shiva threw himself under the feet of Kali to stop her from killing everything in sight. Some say he threw himself under her feet because he was so turned on by all her destruction. Probably both. Disintegration is very seductive.

"That's all Kamadev is doing at the moment. Disintegrating. He threw himself down. I'm sure you didn't hurt him. Maybe you scared the living shit out of him, but he'll be fine when he remembers where he put all the pieces."

I look in the closet and find one of Brandy's shawls, the color of blood. Good choice I think. I cover his shoulders and tell him to try to keep it protected so it doesn't bleed and scar. Good luck sleeping with that but you asked for it, honey. No medicine till the show's over so it will look its horrible best. And then I'll make it disappear.

†

DJ

I've been meditating in the sun a long time. I watch her walk away with Sim to his house. Then he comes back with a big red shawl around him like a bullfighter and she has her arm around his waist. He looks a little sick and I wonder what she did to him. She knows how to do a lot of stuff.

I'm thinking about the deep dark scar she has around her back that cuts right below her breast. I'm thinking of her breasts white as jasmine, white as the evening moon. Then suddenly I see it and wonder how I missed it yesterday. I had sex with her and didn't recognize her. But now I see her clearly, as if she stuck her tongue out at me to prove it, walking with Shiva subdued. She's Kali, mother goddess of time, biting the heads off men.

In the legend Shiva subdues her anger by lying at her feet letting her trample him. I can see she's trampled him and I can guess the rest. She has four arms, with a sword in one hand, a severed head in another, and two more hands held up in ahimsa, 'No Fear'. Real skull jewelry, her skirt made from dead men's arms, breasts covered with blood from killing everybody.

I jump up to my feet to get the fuck out of here, but my legs are dead from sitting on the grass so long. Dr. Jain stops me. He says he's Sim's personal trainer and it was tough stitching him up because he knew him since he was 12. It took two doctors eleven hours to sew Sim up. He apologizes for joking about my stitches.

He shows me some easy wrist curls to start rebuilding my hand. I tell him I have to go, but he says, no. Calm down. Work on your hand. I want to ask him about the scar he cut on her back, but I'm not supposed to know she has a scar around her breast. I'm careful what I say to him. If he's going to marry Kali, I'm worried about him.

So I tell him about this beautiful woman I knew who floated in a bed of seaweed and sparkled like the sea. She was a body builder like him and she was as strong as she was beautiful.

"Do you mean Sim's friend, Nick?" he laughs.

"How do you know her?" I sniff my bottle hard. I'm disintegrating. I'm jealous.

"How could I forget her? She had a barbell in her living room. Sean took me to her house to hire Brandy.

"Nick was a beautiful woman," he says. "A little bit rough. Maybe a little too old for you?"

I think that's a good question to meditate on and I start wondering if I'm too young or old for anything. Then I remember the sun in her eyes, green like sea glass. Numbers have nothing to do with her green eyes.

Sim sits down on the sofa with Nat to watch us. "No girls tomorrow, right?" Jain asks.

"Yes, I changed my mind. There was enough of that today. This is just going to be quick and dirty. You, me, Sean and a lot of cops. It's not a day at the beach, it's just press. I'm dressing up. Anything you want to wear is fine as long as there's no shirt involved. I want you to scare them, Jain," he laughs.

"Kama Dave was just telling me about Nick. I was at her house when you were in the hospital."

"Oh, Jain! She has a body that could cause a car wreck. Literally. She caused regular smashups at the Point just walking across the street. He has impossible taste."

He winks at Nat.

"Speaking of bodies, Sim," Jain says, "Nat needs rehab on her back. The scar is getting better but I had to cut through the lat muscle and it's not firing right. I thought you could help her since you're doing a lot of back work. She doesn't need to do power lifts; she just needs therapy. Can you help me with that?"

"Sure, Nat. Let's see what you can do for a single with 10 pounds."

Nat takes her shirt off and she's wearing a little yoga top underneath. I can see the scar when she sits down and reaches for the bar. I get a sudden orgasm when I see that scar again and I stop breathing while I watch her. She pulls the bar down unevenly and slowly. I can see the left muscle working but the right muscle fires all at once and seizes. Off then on. It's not smooth.

"Gee, that's not firing right, Nat," Sim says. "You should do very light weights and easy Vinyasa. I'll work with you. Lots of massages, too. Is anyone here as good as you?"

"Brandy and Sunny both."

"Cool, we'll turn you into Ms. Kalifornia in no time. I'm going to need some help prettying up, too.

He's standing behind her inspecting her lat muscle. He has her stand up and do some range of motion checks while Dr. Jain and I watch. Then he puts the pin on 50 pounds, hands her the shawl and starts doing a set.

"Just one rep," she says. "I need to see if the skin is going to crack."

Sim pulls the bar down slowly.

"What the fuck!" Dr. Jain swears.

I knew it. Fuck it's massive. There are two snakes on either side of his back ripped into his skin and a very bruised third snake down his spine right on the bone.

I can see her with a belt in one hand, a mirror in another and two more hands held up in ahimsa to promise she won't really hurt him. Four hands and she knows how to use them all at once.

I remember him saying, you ain't seen nothing yet, honey. He asked her to do that. She trampled him.

Nat looks at the snakes and tells his it's fine. Try a couple more reps. It's not bleeding.

"It's just cosmetic, Jain," she says. "It won't even scar. We're being careful."

"That's careful?" he gasps. "How'd that happen?"

"A belt works really well," Sim laughs. "It's just for publicity. It's a message. The right people will know what it means. The fucking Kings of 36th Avenue will understand.

"Even Sri Kama Dave knows what it means."

Jain looks at me and waits. Kali turns around, too and waits for my answer. She hasn't even got a clue why he asked her to do that to him.

"It means he'd take a hit for his brothers," I explain. "Except it's never been that bloody before."

†

S&M

Kamadeva follows me home like a lost dog. I can tell Jain makes him nervous and Nat completely freaks him out. He doesn't want to go back to his room. I wonder how stoned he's getting off all the botanicals. It's working for me, really sedative and lighting up my high perception. It's smooth as glass. But he was also meditating in direct sunlight and that's a good recipe for derailing a train.

"Fucking Kali," he warns me. "She's been fucking Kali all the time. Be careful with her, Sim."

I stop on the grass and look in his eyes. "Of course she is, Sri Kama Dave. I knew that when I hired her as my assistant therapist. I warned you, buddy. But don't be afraid of her. Kali is one of my favorites. She's my pet. I have complete control over her. She loves you. She'd cut her hair off before she'd hurt you."

"But she hurt *you*. She *trampled* you," he whines.

"It just looks like it hurts. Actually it just fucking itches."

Brandy is in the shower so I take advantage of her closet. The only thing on my mind now is her pink silk kimono. I can't bear the itch of the shawl on the welts. It's like fingernails on a burn.

The kimono feels like a cool breeze on my skin. Brandy comes out of the shower in a towel looking for it.

"Sorry, honey," I say. "I need to borrow this. Please."

She doesn't argue but gives me a curious look and smiles at Sri Kamadeva.

"How about giving Sri Dave abhyanga before I take him home? He's still worried about Nat."

Kamadev and I sit on the futon and wait while she gets dressed. He's definitely calmer around the jasmine and wants to bring some home. I remind him that Nat has bucket loads of it already in the lab.

"You need to try one of these, Kamadev," I say, letting him feel the arm of the kimono. "It's silk. I think gods are supposed to wear this kind of stuff."

When Brandy comes out in her white sweats, I tell her I'm going to order more of these for patients. Silk.

"It's therapeutic, Bran," I tell her, "The shawl sucked."

"Got a sunburn, Sim?" she teases. "I've never seen you wear so much clothing."

"No, I'm just in Hollywood with Kama Dave," I smirk. Then I remember she's only known me for a couple weeks now. I wonder if you need to be crazy to be a nurse. She should be scared to death.

I feel my feet boiling up again and look around for something to smash. There's nothing around me, only space. I take a deep breathe and taste the jasmine. I smell the oils Brandy is pouring in the glass and I want to push the futon off the side. I taste honey in my throat from the sticky resin. I want to hurl Dave over the edge of the world into the abyss to hide him. I want to see the sea blotted out for its own protection. I want to burn everything.

I try to breathe all of that out through my left nostril and its getting fucking dangerous. I'm afraid all the demons from the beach are going to come up the mountain and find me, one by one, and destroy my office at the top of the world and kill all my friends.

"Hey, Kama Dave," she purrs in his ear, "how beautiful you look today. Amber melted at your feet."

"Local girls," he recites, "we don't look at them or talk to them."

"Poor local girls," she says. "You've been teasing them for years."

"I'm not teasing," he says. "I don't want to hurt them."

God, I'm good. He knows the important stuff on a cellular level. I remind myself to thank Mack again for teaching me to be such a good teacher. If I taught him nothing more enlightening than 'don't fuck with the local girls', my life has purpose.

"Sri Dave, why aren't you sick?" I ask. I'm feeling pretty sick myself. "When was your last hit? Thursday morning? Wednesday night?"

"Right. 2am. Mack hit himself, too. I *am* sick. I haven't seen you stop spinning in front of my eyes. I'm just like very, very inside myself sick. I look fucking good outside but inside sick. Have you ever been that ruined?"

I could remind him that I was shot twice, in surgery for half a day, that I was strung out to dry on narcotics for weeks, that none of my friends knew where I was or what happened to me, that my house was full of dope dealers when I was unconscious, but I've only got so much air to breathe and he should know that if he were really here. He's right. He's sick.

So I give him a prescription while Brandy massages him. I tell him to do at least four therapies a day, meditation, nidra, sunbathe, abhyanga, yoga asana, weights or swim. It's okay to do meditation or sunbathe on his own, but get someone to work with him on the rest or it doesn't count. You've got two nurses, two doctors and two therapists. Use them.

When Brandy has finished, I put the red shawl around him and he growls, "I'm killing her, Sim. Kali is my pet."

"You have no idea how right you are, little brother," I say. "And she works for me so let her help you."

"I made her cry," he brags.

"It's not something to brag about. You're not supposed to hurt her. Be a little bit nicer if you can. Polite. Do you know how to do that? Pretending you care even if you don't?"

I walk him back to the Fire House and try to sneak him in the back door by the stairs so he can escape to his room without running into Kali. But she hears us come in.

"Hey," she calls. "I've got some really good new stuff." She could be a hooker or a dealer if I didn't know better. She's got a little package Sage delivered this afternoon.

We go into the lab and she's got two small bottles of oil and four bottles the size of my little finger, two drams each of blue and white Lotus attar. She pours half an ounce of sandalwood and a teaspoon of jasmine into a glass, then adds a few drops of distilled lotus. It smells like a bed on a cloud above the rising sun. I want to drink it.

She pours the mix into two amber bottles and gives one to Kamadev and one to me. Then she gives him a dram bottle of blue lotus to keep and sniff. It's a sedative and an aphrodisiac. She winks at Kamadev and says, "Any time. I've got a lot of it."

I wonder whether she means a lot of lotus oil or a lot of time. Probably he thinks she means both because he backs up so fast he hits the wall.

"I like the silk, Sim," she says fingering my sleeve.

"I couldn't stand that shawl," I frown. "It itched like hell. But this makes me feel like a fighter. Bring on the next contender!" The silk excites me. It kisses my pain.

"Do you think Jain would wear one? It would be a good uniform for the staff and the patients."

"Probably more professional than running around without a shirt, boss. It's a nice look, very serene. I'd wear one for work and Jain will dress however I ask. So, yes."

She's looking at Kamadev with a smile and I can read her mind. She's imagining Dave in a silk kimono with that blessing scarf and a bunch of jasmine in his hair. She's thinking she loves her job. Then she turns me around and slides the kimono gently off my shoulders to inspect her artwork.

"Very beautiful, Steven. You look very serious. Do you know how much this would cost if it was a tattoo? Thousands. It's a bit uglier than earlier, kind of blistery. Have fun sleeping on that tonight, boss. Call me when you get back from the beach tomorrow and I'll see if I can make it disappear."

"Will you ask Sage to get the silk kimonos? White or saffron would be good colors. Saffron's better. For Sunrise. Maybe both. Lots of kimonos. Do you think Mack will approve it?"

"I just spent $2,500 on those oils this morning. He didn't scream or anything. I'll do my best."

I take the kimono from her and put it on Kama Dave, then I put a little piece of jasmine behind his ear. He stares at me smiling at the nice feel of silk on his skin. He likes it very much. Nat starts laughing and shakes her head. She knows I read her mind. She can't get her mind off him.

"Let go of your attachment, Kali baby," I warn her. "Don't hurt him while I'm gone."

†

NAT

The boss laid down a new set of rules last night. I'm not allowed upstairs in the Fire House unless Kamadev asks. Early this morning Sim, Jain and Sean set off for dawn patrol with the media. They left me in charge but I'm not allowed to go up to his room. It's his private space. I'm grounded. I think that's pretty funny since I was his kundalini teacher and I taught him his root and his ground.

Sim sent Brandy over around midnight last night to take care of him. She slept on the sofa bed near the foot of the stairs so she can hear him if he cries. And that boy can cry! It's hard to tell if he's crying out in pleasure or terror but he wakes the house up all night with sudden yells. He's sick and he seems to be enjoying it.

I'm not allowed to touch him, talk to him or look at him unless he needs or asks for help. And he's not allowed to shut or lock his bedroom door so Brandy and Jain can check on him. Sim told Kamadev that Jain is his personal bodyguard, so Dev trusts him now.

I'd like to feel his pulse and sing mantras to him to calm him down and bathe him with sandalwood and frankincense and take him deep into yoga nidra. It worked so well with Sim. But I screwed up my relationship with the patient. I fucked him. I had a thousand good reasons for doing it but no matter how good they are, he won't forget.

I thought I was starting to understand the boss, too. He has some kind of organic divinity complex, as if he were the tortoise bearing the weight of the world across the cosmos. But I don't really know him at all. Brandy thinks he's mad. At least right now, she says, he's potentially violent. He told her to leave last night and sleep here so he couldn't hurt her, then locked himself out on the yoga deck for the night.

I walked over around 1am to see if he wanted to talk, but he wouldn't open the door. He just yelled, "Fuck off, Nat!" and then I heard something big crash from the deck to the trees below. I wondered if he jumped so I knocked again.

This time he growled. "Get the fuck home."

So at least he was alive. Maybe not well.

At six am, Brandy and I are having coffee with Jain and Sean in the Fire House kitchen when Sim comes in the kitchen door. He looks worried. Maybe disturbed is a better word. He's wearing jeans with a belt, his cop hat, Brandy's pink kimono and all his favorite hardware.

"How's Dave?" he asks.

"Sleeping now," Brandy says. "He was a noisy boy screaming all night. Next time *you* sleep with him."

"Morning, S&M," Sean says. "Are you going to the beach dressed like a girl? Pretty sexy lingerie even for you, don't you think?"

"Beautiful, aren't I?" he laughs. "Actually, Sean, it's just for the ride down there to keep me from sticking to the squad car seats. You get some pretty dirty people in the back."

Then he turns around and drops the silk like a stripper so Sean can see his back. Jain and I have seen it. Brandy cries out, but Sean doesn't seem surprised in the least.

"Nice job, S&M," he says. "Don't bleed on my seats."

Sim picks up the kimono and smiles at me.

"Nat, do you think you could fix up my office while I'm gone. There's been some damage. And get these." He shakes the silk robe at me and puts it back on. Then he whispers to me, "No, I didn't sleep at all last night, thank you."

After they're gone, I walk over to pool house to check on the damage. The front door is unlocked and wide open. So is the kitchen door.

Things are re-arranged on the yoga deck and a lot of things are missing. I can see the massage table far below me in the tree tops. I wonder if it's okay, if someone can retrieve it. The futon met a better fate. It was too bulky to fall far so it's caught on one of the deck supports.

The Medicine Buddha is still sitting safely on the edge wrapped in gratuitous fistfuls of jasmine. But most of the potted herbs and other flowers are simply missing, probably smashed on the canyon floor below. The yoga mats are really the only furniture left.

It's nice to have some work to do. I sit down on his bed and call Sage. One dozen saffron silk kimonos, two XL, four L, six M, another massage table, a half ounce of wild French lavender for his scars and an ounce of helichrysum for the internal bruising.

Sage is curious about Sim so I tell her he's at the beach. She can just read all about it tomorrow in the Sunday paper. The story is already written.

†

SEAN

S&M is riding in the back playing with his handcuffs. Jain is sitting in front with me and we've got four other police cars caravanning with us to the Point. It's a beautiful beach day with a building south swell but the streets are eerily quiet for a Saturday morning. Last night we had three rapes, two stabbings, four narcotics possessions and six driving under the influence. A pretty normal Friday night in the neighborhood lately.

No one's been shot this week, not since Darrell was murdered four days ago. At least that's solved. Most of the ones who get locked up are just fucked up locals. The violent ones don't get caught and they just keep going.

When we pull up en masse with five patrol cars and park in the no parking zone, the population shifts. I see a few guys leaving in a hurry. We just sit there in the cars, watching the surf, not harassing anyone. S&M takes off his silk robe and stuffs it under the car seat and steps out of the car to watch the clean south swell rolling like a crystal snake across the reef.

There are only three guys surfing out in the morning glass. S&M stands there for a few minutes enjoying the sun on his back, then he walks around to my side of the car. I roll down the window and he says,

"You know, Sean. Maybe it's not such a problem after all. Maybe it's good that drugs and murders have become so popular here. There're only three guys out surfing on a Saturday morning with a shoulder-high swell. I can live with this."

"No women or children?" I laugh. "Only the tough guys get to surf?"

"I'll have to think about that," he smiles and walks back over to the cliff to watch.

Chris and Amber walk over from the news van across the street.

"And that," Chris says waving with a flourish at the empty point, "is the story. It's not safe to come down here. Unless you've got 5 cop cars," he laughs.

Amber asks S&M to do some photos leaning on the patrol car like he owns it. He leans back and holds both his arms over his head like he's under arrest and shows her the patented lady killer smirk. He makes Kama Dave look like an altar boy. Then he asks me and Jain to get in the photos with him. We're the cleanup committee, he says.

Amber's excited about the shots yesterday and says the bodybuilding pictures are beautiful. She says her favorite, beside the Kama Dave centerfold of course, is S&M working his back.

"You have a beautiful back, Sim," she smiles and tries to put a hand around him. He grabs her wrist, twists it and laughs at her.

"If you touch me, honey, I will be forced to use these," he smiles showing her the handcuffs. "Hands off. I'm not available."

"Ouch," she says.

"Oh, yeah, ouch," he says sweetly. "It hurts me more than it hurts you."

Then he turns around and shows her how much more beautiful his back is today than it was for the photos yesterday.

"Don't put any of that in the paper, honey," he whispers seriously. "It's personal."

While S&M is busy teaching the photographer restraint, a little crowd starts gathering, not a lot of people, but neighbors. Most of them are really pleased to see him alive. The heroin dealer rumor gets tripped up immediately by his police escort and people are curious what's up.

S&M recognizes a lot of neighbors, shakes hands with the guys and just smiles politely at the ladies.

"Good morning," he says. "We just wanted to come down and throw down a gauntlet. The Point Guard is sponsoring a fund raiser to support our new community clean up project.

"It's been a long time since it was dangerous for a girl to come down to the Point and we want it to be nice again. I've got a lot of personal karma here, so we're launching a community challenge tomorrow in partnership with the police department. Check the Sunday paper. Chris has the whole story. Nice to see everybody."

He turns around and starts talking to me about swimming. He just wants to jump back in the ocean and pretend this never happened. A guy a little shorter than him comes up from behind and leans into his ear.

"They should have shot you in the *head*, fucker," he hisses. "That was a rookie mistake shooting you in the body."

S&M wheels around and punches the guy in the face, but I pull him back and Jain holds his arm. I help the poor victim to his feet and ask him nicely for his identification so we can keep an eye on him. When he refuses, I wave one of the other officers over and ask him to take the gentleman to the station to identify him. Go ahead and hold him on a murder threat charge, I add.

"Let me do what I do best, S&M," I tell him. "And you do what you do. No guns or knives. If you want to swim out to the reef and back, fine, we'll cover you. Just stay off the beach and get right back in the car."

S&M unlocks the handcuffs on his left wrist and hands them to Amber. Then he pulls his belt out slowly winking at her and chewing on his lip in a wicked tease. He slaps his palm twice with the end of the belt, then hands it to her, puts his cop hat on her head and says, "Don't go away, sugar."

Then he goes straight down the cliff and runs into the ocean in his jeans. I can hear him howl when he hits the cold water and a surfer taking off on the wave howls back in recognition. He swims out, treading water on the reef. It's shallow enough that he finds an occasional foothold to stand on before the swell knocks him off.

The surfers circle around him and I can hear the hoots and laughter. Then one of them gets off his board, shoots it to S&M and swims in. I hear S&M yelling Sanskrit blessings after him the whole way. He takes off deep on the next set and surfs into the beach.

When he climbs back up the cliff, he yells loud enough to wake up the rest of the neighborhood, "That's one for Darrell!!!"

Amber puts his stuff back on him, being careful not to touch him. He's freezing cold and the snakes on his back are nearly black against his blue skin. She puts the cuffs on his left wrist and puts his hat on backwards. Then she makes a NASA mission out of rethreading his belt through the wet jean loops.

"I got a beautiful shot of you surfing, S&M," she purrs. "Of course it's Chris' story but I'll bet he leads with that. One for Darrell."

†

DJ

It's a bad night. I can hear things through the open window. Sim said keep the window closed but I hear things out there. I hear him singing. Nice blues. I hear a few crashes then he sings some more. I hear the wind kiss the trees and then I hear moonlight falling on the floor of my room.

Brandy comes up the stairs to check my pulse but I pretend I'm sleeping. When I really sleep I wake myself up screaming. I'm dreaming of the other one. I see her tearing my flesh open, three snakes across my chest and her breasts are covered with my blood.

She has four hands and she knows how to use them. She puts one of them around my neck and one in my hair, one on my heart and with the fourth hand she's shifting my gears. I've only got two hands so I keep them mostly on her ass for control. She's only got two legs but they're wrapped around me like ropes.

My dreams are wild but in the end I sleep late. The sun is as high as I am when I open my eyes. I'm alone and I'm nervous, the first time I've slept up here. I shower and then cover myself with lotus and sandalwood and jasmine while my skin is still wet, put on my jeans and scarf and sneak down the stairs.

There's no one in the house. I check the lab. No one's home. In the kitchen there's juice and croissants, tea, jam and honey. There's a note:

Kama Dave, we're working in Sim's office. Dial '5' if you need us. – Bran & Nat

I don't see why I'd need them. I pour a half glass of orange juice and cover the croissant with honey and take it into the boardroom. I fill the rest of the glass with bourbon and put my feet up on the table.

On the second whiskey sour, I put the honey in the glass with lemon, cherry jam and bourbon. Fuck the orange juice. As long as there's no narcotics, I think. I've got my feet on the boardroom table, a cherry jam bourbon sour and I'm sniffing my blue lotus "quiet time" oil, when I hear a knock on the front door.

I can't be fucked getting up and anyway, I think, I'm not technically here running the board. But I hear a girl's voice, "Nat, it's Sage. Open sesame."

"Oh, Sage," I open the door and lean across its full width so she can't come in. "What do you want? I'm very busy right now."

"I'm delivering this order personally. She wanted it this morning. I was hoping to talk to S&M."

"Oh, well. Then talk to me, honey. He's out. She's out. I'm in charge. Would you like a drink?"

She comes in cautiously with a few boxes and sets them on the boardroom table. "Just tea," she says looking at me curiously. I put the kettle on and make another lemon cherry jam whiskey sour.

"What's in the boxes?" I ask. I recognize the labels but these boxes are huge. Usually the stuff comes in little tiny boxes.

"Silk kimonos," she says. "There's another big box in the car, a massage table. The herbs are in my pocket." She pulls out two little bottles and lets me smell the lavender.

"That helps with scars. Nat says he needs this today. Could you help me with the massage table?"

"Sure. When I'm done with breakfast," I say. "But we already have two of them, one in Sim's office and one in Nat's. There's no more space."

I hand her my blue lotus bottle and wink at her.

"This is good, Sage."

"Then you must be Kamadev," she muses. "I thought so. You're the reason she's buying all the jasmine, sandalwood, and lotus attars all of a sudden. After weeks of painkillers, sedatives and detox oils for S&M's wounds.

"She told me she had the God of Love as a patient. Gosh, honey, what is she treating you for? A broken heart?"

"My heart's fine," I say taking her arm and putting her hand on my chest. I can feel the heat of her palm on my heart. "She's just treating me for heroin. This blue lotus is really nice. It helps me stay calm."

I take the bottle back from her and look around. Do I still have a drink somewhere or was that the last one?

I put some honey in the bourbon. I sniff the blue lotus and then put a drop of it into a smear of honey on my finger and rub it into my forehead. Then I put a few drops of blue lotus into the bourbon. Oh, the silk!

"Sage. Fuck. You got the silk? Open the boxes. Open sesame. Sim said gods are supposed to wear this kind of stuff."

I'm feeling naked since Sim took the kimono back. She opens one of the boxes and hands me a saffron gold silk kimono. I let it sit in front of me and just stare at her. Then I get up and go back to the kitchen for some more cherry jam and lemon and this time I put a big dash of bitters in it. I'm hungry. I pour her some dark black tea.

I take it back into the boardroom and fill the rest of the glass with bourbon. It's delicious. I sit back down at the table and stare at her. Don't look at them or touch them or talk. I'm just looking. I'm not talking much.

"Fuck, Sage," I say finally. "Do you want to see me in this or not?"

I want her to put the silk on me and I'm waiting. Her eyes light up as she gets my drift. She picks it up and walks around behind my chair and dresses me like I'm her toy boy. The beautiful golden silk feels like a massage kissing my skin. Then she steps over me and sits on my lap. She pulls her top over her head and she has no bra on. She puts four hands all over my shoulders and neck and presses her breasts against my heart. Her mouth is on my neck then she's blowing in my ear, saying I smell like the garden of paradise. I feel her teeth on my skin as she sucks a deep kiss on my neck.

I don't even need to take her hand to show her where I'm coming from because she's sitting right on top of it.

As she's going south, I hear Sim coming in the back door with Jain, calling for Nat. He takes one look and says, "Nice kimono, Sage. Good to see you but get the fuck off him. You can't afford him. He's on $500,000 bail. Where the hell is Nat?"

"Line 5," I say.

He picks up the phone and points at my drink. Sage gets off me and I go into the kitchen to make two more.

"Do you know what's going on over here?" he hisses into the phone. I hand him a cherry jam bourbon and he polishes half of it off.

"You've got a delivery, Nat. And Kama Dave has gone through half a bottle of bourbon and half of Sage's clothing...and oh yes, you *can* believe it," he laughs.

"I can have Jain watch him, but you need to get over here right now. I need you to fix me. Do you know how bad salt water fucking hurts on welts?"

He hangs up and watches Sage putting her top back on. Then he fishes through the box and finds an XL kimono and tosses it to Jain.

"Jain?" he says, "Nat says you'll wear one to work. Good for bodybuilding I think. It makes me feel like a boxer."

Jain tries it on and leaves the front draped open so his pecs and abs are framed in saffron silk. Sage watches him and smiles as he flexes for her. He's my bodyguard now. No one can touch me anymore unless I ask.

Sim takes another kimono out of the box and hands it to Sage, turning his back so she can put it on him. She stares at the scars on his back, the old surgery scars and the fresh black and blue belt welts.

"Nat said lavender and helichrysum would take the snakes off, what do you think, Sage?" he asks as she covers him up with silk.

She's speechless. I pour her some more tea and put my hand on her ass while Sim's not looking.

Nat comes in the kitchen door and sees all the saffron silk.

"Oh, beautiful, Sage! Nice choice. Oh my god, Jain!"

Sim hands her a kimono and points to the lab, "You need to get to work, Nat. Now."

Then he turns to me and says, "Kamadev, man, you should have seen my wave, brother!"

Nat takes the little bottles, asks Jain to get the massage table, and then follows Sim into the lab.

"You're probably not on his list of prescribed therapies, Sage," Jain says, showing her out, "but you're welcome to come back for the party tomorrow. We'll be on the front page announcing our community challenge. You might be interested in it. I'll warn you though, it's a $20,000 buy in. Sunrise Wellbeing has already committed."

"Sunrise buys that much from me in a month. You have some very expensive patients here," she laughs. "I'll think about it."

She puts her arms around me again, but this time she only uses two hands. She's on good behavior now in front of Jain. I kiss her with complete cool, no hands, no heat, controlled just like S&M. She puts a hand under my scarf and pulls it back a little to look at my neck.

"Nice hickey, Sri Kamadeva. Something to remind you of me."

†

S&M

"I may never let another woman hit me again," I sulk. "What would be the point? It doesn't get worse than this. Fucking salt water. The wave was worth it but I'm paying for it over and over. Get the snakes off me, Nat."

She says Sage brought some high altitude French lavender especially for the scars. She mixes it up with helichrysum and birch oil and works it very gently and slowly into the snakes. I want to rush her but she takes all the time in the world. An inch a minute, the pain dissolves under her fingers.

When she's done, I tell her to lie down so I can put the oil on her scar. It's a really nice recipe and I want to share.

"Does it hurt?" I ask.

"Mmm, yes," she says. "It hurts on the surface of the scar and it hurts deep in the muscle and in my ribs. It hurts all the time. You know I can get Norco any time if I wanted it. I've got scripts. But like you said, pain is just weakness leaving the body. It's amusing."

"Fucking Sage," I say. "How amusing was that? On the furniture in the boardroom."

She doesn't answer.

"Jealous, baby?" I offer.

"I left my attachment on the deck, boss. Yes, that was very amusing. Sorry I missed it. Do you think he threw   himself   under   her   feet,   too?"

"No. From what I saw it was the opposite. He was going along for the ride, but she was definitely driving. She was pretty experienced ten years ago from what I remember, and I remember a lot."

"It was my mistake telling Dev the boardroom was 'party central'," she moans. "He's too suggestible. I neglected to say it was for house parties, not private entertainment. Is there a rule about no girls in his room other than staff?"

"There's a hard limit rule against his having any guests period. If he walks out the front door, he violates his custody. Narcotics aren't his problem now. He's going to prison just as fast if he follows her out to her car and goes for a ride. If she wants him, she can put up his bail.

"And fuck if she can't afford that. But I don't think the judge would consider her to be a rehabilitation provider. She'll tear his head off and then he'll have a lot of time in jail to think about her. Tell her to back off, Nat, or I'll hammer her."

Her back has a nice shimmer to it and I remember my promise to help with her therapy. Like me, she works here but she's also a patient. One of the edges most therapists come up against is self-care. Healing other people is therapeutic, but therapists need to heal themselves first. Like they say before the plane takes off, in case of an emergency put the oxygen mask on yourself first so you can help others.

"Let's work at my place," I say. "Vinyasa and some weights. We'll take Dev swimming afterwards to sober him up. He hasn't done shit for therapy all day. I don't think alcohol and sex count."

Kama Dave is sitting at the boardroom table with Jain when we come out of the lab, but now he's drinking black tea instead of bourbon. Jain is showing him all the bodybuilding pills and powders, DHEA and crystal amino acids, ashwanganda, ginseng, guggulu and triphala. He's filling little paper cups with the right daily doses.

"How's the hand, Jain?" I ask. "Can you take the stitches out? I want to take him swimming. I also want blood samples for court."

Jain takes him into the lab, snips the stitches and draws some blood. I wave Nat to follow us in and hand her the rest of the scar oil. The last time he trusted her, she was massaging the scars on his hand. I figure that's a good place to start picking up his pieces.

I don't even wait for him to say yes, I just take his wrist and hold his hand flat out on the table for her. His eyes widen but he doesn't say anything. She pours a little oil on his hand and rubs it in slowly looking in his eyes. I know the oil takes the pain away. But the way she's looking at him is even stronger than the oil.

She's looking at him with pure adoration, love that has nothing to do with sex. I feel his hand relax and then I let his wrist go. He's smiling at her again. He knows how beautiful he looks in his gold silk with the white blessing scarf around his neck.

†

DJ

Sim takes us to his house for yoga. He can't stop talking about his wave.

"Kamadev, man! I didn't even have a surfboard or a wetsuit! I just swam out and Billy Lee let me use his board. It was epic.

"But fuck the pain shocked me. I forgot about salt water. Shit, Nat, do you believe that pain can erase karma?"

He stops and turns back to see if she's listening. She's walking behind us because I'm still a little nervous with her.

"Some kinds of pain might," she says thoughtfully. "Personally I thing meditation and service is a much better way to release bad karma than thrashing yourself. You know, if you really hurt yourself, you just plant more bad karmic seeds." Then she laughs and adds, "You must have been a very bad boy, boss."

"You know it. I've been trying to erase it for ten years," he sighs.

"Billy's suspended," I volunteer. "He was kicked off the tour for junk."

"Yeah, Sean told me, but he wasn't arrested, it was just a disciplinary warning."

"Not as bad as me," I laugh. "I take the cake. Everything all the time."

Sim puts his arm around me and says, "No, baby, you're doing fine right now. Just don't replace your cake with a different flavor. Don't jump off dope and dive into sex."

I can feel my face flush.

"I didn't dive into anything. I didn't touch her," I squirm.

"You didn't have both hands on her ass?"

"For my own protection, Sim. I was trying to slow her down."

Sim falls down on the lawn he's laughing so hard. Nat and I have to stop until he gets over it. Then he gets back to his feet and looks at her.

"You see where this in going, Kali baby?" he smirks. "You've created a monster."

Then he turns back to me and says, "Dave, I'm going to make you a list. If you have any questions about it, ask me. It's going to be very simple.

"First, Brandy. You're safe with her. My wife treats you like a little brother.

"Second, Nat. You're absolutely safe with her. Get over it. She loves you too much to see Jain kill you."

Nat laughs a little and shakes her head, "True. True."

"Third, Sunny. Safe. Everybody's safe with that mean little red head.

"Fourth, Amber. You did a beautiful job not talking to her yesterday. Keep it up, she's extremely dangerous for you. She tried to hit on me, too, this morning. Talk to me or Jain if she comes near you.

"Fifth, Sage. Time bomb. No good for you. Nat has already told her to leave you alone. Both Amber and Sage will be at the party tomorrow because we're working with them. Just let me know if they bother you."

"Got it," I say. "Brandy, Nat, Sunny, they work here. All safe for me. Amber and Sage are trouble. Don't look at them or talk to them."

"Mack knows what he is talking about," he says to Nat. "Sometimes it's just better to keep them off the starting line."

The yoga deck looks funny. It's empty except the mats and the Buddha so there's a lot of room to move. The futon is stuck below the deck on one side. Sim points down the mountain at a massage table stuck on a treetop.

"You're not the only one with a cake problem," he laughs. "That's why we're here."

Then he does something I haven't seen him do in a long time. He pulls one of the yoga mats to the edge of the deck and turns it perpendicular to the other mats, then sits sideways on it facing us. And he starts to teach.

"Today we'll focus on the dharma and ajna chakra. Ajna is the third eye, the door of perception. A really nice way to open the door is through balancing asanas. Man, I so need this."

†

S&M

For the second night in a row, I'm not getting any sleep, but at least I'm not feeling terribly violent this morning. The wave smoothed me out like a sheet of glass and then the yoga polished me off like a mirror. Nat still can't touch her palms together overhead, but I've nearly got full range of motion now. Dave's poses are textbook perfect, but his mental state isn't sharp enough to cut paper.

After class, Jain brought the new massage table over and helped me pull the futon back on the deck so it's beautiful for the house party. He took one look at the massage table in the tree and said, "Christmas! That's down there permanently, Sim. Maybe it's something you should meditate on for a while."

We take Dave for a swim but I don't care to find out how chlorine feels on my back, so I sit it out and Nat works on my scars. Dave goes nuts over the pool and swims enough laps that I know he'll sleep deep. After dinner everyone turns in early. I'm really happy to be back in my own room, but the bed still feels like hell, so I show Brandy how to do it on a chair. I taught Sage the furniture move when she was seventeen.

At four am the phone rings. I pick it up on the first ring so it doesn't wake Brandy. There's only a couple people who would disturb me at 4am. Either Kamadev has escaped or it's Sean finishing his shift. Either way it's trouble.

"Got a spare bed, S&M? I've got a little trouble for you," Sean warns. "Not as bad as Tuesday though. Can you meet me in ten minutes?"

"Please not another junkie, Sean," I beg. He assures me there's no drugs or criminals involved this time so I tell him to come around the front of the Fire House. I'm pretty sure Nat's bed hasn't been slept in since she's been here.

I'm sitting on the front steps of the house when he pulls up and it looks like he's alone. He gets out without his jacket and says, "Good morning, I guess."

"Is this a joke?" I ask.

"Nothing funny about it." He opens the back door of the patrol car and there's a body on the back seat wrapped in his jacket, curled up in a little ball. He reaches in and helps her sit up and her beautiful green eyes open and then roll back. That's all I really recognize.

Her face is dripping with blood, her nose is smashed open just below her third eye. The tip of her nose is scraped and bleeding and her lower lip is split open. Both eyes are black and blue and starting to swell shut.

She looks like she stepped out of a fight club or maybe a concentration camp. She looks like every last drop of life has been beaten out of her and there's just this skinny skeleton left of her. I take one of her hands and squeeze it and hold her chin up.

"Nicky," I groan. "Shit, honey."

She opens her eyes and recognizes me. "S&M, baby, I thought you were dead."

"Who did this to you, baby?" I ask.

"The fucking sidewalk," she swears. "The more I kiss it, the harder it kisses me back."

"Crys found her in the parking lot behind the bar when she closed tonight and asked me to help," Sean explains. "I didn't want to take her to jail again or the hospital either. I'm not sure if she has a concussion or if she's just drunk."

"So you thought of me," I say. "What are friends for?"

"There's no charges or warrants on her, Sim. I'm just cleaning up the street."

I get the front door and he gets the body. Nat's bedroom is empty, so I pull back the covers and stack some pillows to sit her up in bed.

"What do mean 'jail again'?" I ask Sean.

"She can tell you all about it, buddy. I need to get some sleep and I'll be back later with Crys for the party."

Then he remembers something and says, "Oh, wait a second."

He goes back out and comes in with a stack of Sunday papers hot off the press.

"It's nice, Sim," he says. "Have the doc take a look at her. We'll see you later."

On the front page there's a photo of me surfing in my jeans on a beautiful head high wave. The headline says, "ONE FOR DARRELL!" and then in smaller print, "Steven Mack Attacks the Point".

Nick groans a little so I show it to her.

"Yesterday morning. Perfect sets, only three guys out."

She smiles in a little bloody grimace and says, "Good job, baby."

"Yeah, big fun," I say. "I had five police cars with me and some creep offered to shoot me in the head next time."

†

JAIN

"Jain," Sim shakes me awake and holds his finger up to his lips. Nat's asleep naked in my bed. He gives her a little lecherous leer so I pull the sheet up quickly to cover her and follow him out. The lights are on in Nat's bedroom and he just points the way. There's a girl in the bed groaning with a broken nose and split lip and a lot of blood on her.

"Special delivery from Sean," he says. "He thinks maybe a concussion or drunk. They found her behind the Nest face down on the asphalt."

I sit down on the edge of the bed and take a look and then do a double take when I recognize her. She doesn't so look rough any more. She just looks beaten. I take her hand.

"The beautiful woman who floats in a bed of seaweed sparkling like the ocean and causes cars to crash," I say. "How are you doing, Nicky?"

She looks surprised to see me. Maybe she recognizes me, maybe not.

"Stupid," she says. "I'm feeling stupid."

Sim is leafing through the paper and opens it to a shot of me bench pressing. He shows it to me and then to her. He turns another page, then folds it up quickly and sets it aside.

"She doesn't need to see that one," he laughs.

"Is this it?" I ask, "Just your face? Or is there more?"

"There's weeks worth of more," she says. "I wouldn't have smashed my face if I could walk right. I think I broke my foot or my toes last week. The more you fall the more you fall."

"What are you doing in the bar, Nico?" Sim asks. "You don't even drink."

"I don't want to get shot in the head either, S&M," she whines. "The bar is safer than the beach. They don't let the dealers in there and the boys take care of me buying me drinks. I haven't been home since Tuesday."

I get up and go into the lab for antiseptic and towels and start cleaning up her face.

"It looks like the boys aren't really taking very good care of you in there, Nick," I say. "You've been in the bar for five days? Come on."

"More like 3 weeks, but I quit going home Tuesday. It opens at 10, safe and warm and closes at 2. I slept in my car and used the shower at the gym. But I missed my car last night. The fucking sidewalk rushed me."

"Does this hurt?" I ask. "Do you want something for pain?"

She shakes her head. "I don't feel anything. They shot Darrell right there on the beach Tuesday. Right where they shot you, S&M. The morning after the police took the little fucker to jail."

"Keep your voice down, Nicky," Sim laughs, "or you'll wake the little fucker up."

"Yeah, this is the first night he hasn't woke us up crying," I say. "I gave him a really good mix of bodybuilding aminos to help him sleep. Arginine, ornithine and theanine. I'll get some for you with a little triphala tea so you can get some sleep. Nat will take care of your foot when she wakes up."

"Hang on," she says desperately. "How can I wake him up? He went to jail."

"Oops, surprise," Sim says. "He's upstairs. But don't worry about him, baby. He's really not here at all. He's kind of on a leave of absence."

He opens the paper to the center and shows me the shot of Dave with his feet up on Nat's lap and his head on Brandy's shoulder. He doesn't show it to Nick. He just whistles and says, "Every girl in town is going to have this up on her bedroom wall today. I'm going to have to make him a longer list."

†

S&M

Mack is in a bloody good mood this morning. The phone isn't ringing off the wall because we didn't give the number out, but he's already got a ton of emails from the website about the challenge. There's already 12 potential teams applying and counting our team that's $260,000. With matching funds, that's more than a cool half million. We've got at least 40 surfers applying to train with us or be on the Sunrise team and its still Sunday morning. We're going to have to shut applications down before the day is done.

There's also 187 love letters addressed to Kama Dave and 96 for me. Dave's got some out and out marriage proposals. I guess there's no one sexier than a man who's already got his hands full.

I'm kicking back with Mack in his office, drinking the hot black stuff and grinning.

"Cool, Steven," he smiles. "This makes up for all the thousands we spent on the exotic oils and the silks, the massage table in the tree and your very expensive junkie friends. This makes up for all of it. You rock, baby brother."

"I'm just the front of house, Mack. This was Sean's idea. I would have happily Om'd you into bankruptcy with my expensive friends," I laugh. "Nice that Brandy worked out the non-profit and the financials. Did you give her a raise? Executive Assistant to the CFO? Have you kissed her yet, my brother?"

Mack goes red then white. Oh, yeah, he's sleeping with her for sure. She got a raise. All alone in that big Ice House with no patients, working all day on corporate finance, it's the perfect recipe for perversion.

"You know," I suggest, "we're going to need more room for clients. It just makes sense to share bedrooms."

He hates it when I pull rank on him with sex. He's got eight years on me but I've got the equivalent of twenty in that department. I put my feet up on his desk and suck on the pu-erh tea. I'm thinking, I've got seven years on Kama Dave but he's catching up to me fast. With sex, it's not quantity that counts. It's depth. It's karma.

This morning I ended up in bed with Nicky. Not sexual, just holding onto her and sleeping for a few hours. She's a bloody mess and she's hurt. Around 6am I wake up to see Dave standing in the doorway, watching.

"Nicky!" he whispers. "How did she find me?"

"Oh, buddy," I lie, "she's been looking all over for you."

He comes in the room and looks at the mess on her face and laughs.

"She hit the reef, Sim. She planted her face on the reef."

"Yeah, bud. She hit the reef really good. We're going to fix her."

Then I'm hit by divine inspiration. There is no better plan for a person who needs supervision than to give them someone else to supervise. It occurs to me that all the guardian angels in the cosmos are probably celestial derelicts assigned to watch over errant humans. At the end of the day, minding someone else's business can keep you out of the deep end of trouble.

I can't say there isn't a certain amount of amusement in it for me, knowing how much she considers him to be an intolerable pest.

"Kamadev," I whisper, "she needs help. Do you think you could watch her for me for a while? You're not allowed in her room, but if she needs anything, you can help. If she needs anything more than tea or toast, get Nat or Jain. Are you talking to Nat yet?"

"I can talk to Nat, Brandy and Sunny," he smiles. "Where is Nicky on my list?"

"She's not on your list yet, honey. Let's see how you go first."

I pull up a chair for him outside her door and give him a copy of the paper. I'm not worried anymore about the hundred and eighty-seven women coming after him. He'll never even notice them as long as he's watching Nick.

†

NICK

When I wake up, I feel the ache. My face hurts worse than my head. I'm not really sure where I am. I just hurt. I rub my eyes and feel a thick crust of bloody scar on my nose. My nose is numb but it tingles where I touch it. It throbs. I can take my own pulse just by concentrating on my nose. I lick my lips and taste dry blood. But I'm dressed and in a clean bed. It doesn't look like the hospital or jail. It looks like a nice house.

I hear a whisper, "Are you okay?"

There's no one in the room but me. I roll over and look at the door. Now I'm starting to wonder if I died or if I'm dreaming. He's standing with one arm overhead leaning against the door frame like an expensive model, barely dressed in a silk kimono with a scarf around his neck. His hair is perfect and his body is tan and oiled. He's standing in the doorway barefoot in lacerated jeans.

"I'm not allowed to come in," he says, "unless you need something. But Sim said I can watch you. You're not on my list."

Suddenly I'm extremely worried.

"What do mean watch me? You little pervert. Are you a voyeur now? What list?"

I want to run but I can't even walk.

"Not like that, Nicky," he says softly. "Jain's my bodyguard. He watches me. Sim says I can watch you to see if you need anything. I can make tea or breakfast for you or get the wheelchair if you want to get up. I'll just sit out here. I can get the paper for you. We're all in the paper today. Our whole house."

There's something in his tone that calms me down a little. He's not the same person I knew. He looks much, much older and much younger at the same time, experienced and innocent. His eyes look sedated and vacant, harmless and lost.

"Fine," I say. "Black tea. And the paper. But don't come in. I mean, it's okay to bring it in but otherwise stay out there."

He smiles like an angel and picks up the paper from a chair by the door. I wonder how long he's been watching me. He hands me the paper and gets extra pillows so I can sit up and says, "Your tea is on the way, Nick." Then he disappears.

I look at the front page and there's S&M surfing. Now I remember he was here in the middle of the night. They want to shoot him in the head. I wonder whether they can find us, where we are. There's a very long feature article about him and as I read it the pieces start falling into place, why they kept the story of his shooting out of the paper until now, how they caught the guys who shot Darrell, how they plan to fight back.

There's a very sexy shot of S&M with handcuffs and a cop hat and then another one of him shaking hands with Sean and Jain, the "cleanup committee". Jain has no shirt on and he looks like a terminator; his chest and arms are epic. There are five police cars lined up behind them on the cliff. No wonder they want to shoot him in the head this time.

The most interesting part is the community challenge. Steven Mack is now the president of Sunrise Wellbeing Corporation, working with his brother Dr. Mack and business partner Dr. Jain at a private facility for injury and drug rehabilitation. Sunrise has set up a non-profit for the Point Guard and pledged $20,000 for a fund-raising surf contest.

They're challenging the community to participate with a $20,000 entry fee per four-man team. All proceeds are going to make the beach safe again and fund rehabilitation and law enforcement. First prize is simply bragging rights and a perpetual trophy. They have matching funds from the county so in effect every dollar they invest is doubled and goes right back into protection and rehabilitation.

When DJ brings my tea I'm so absorbed in the paper I don't even notice him. He sits back down in the chair outside the door. I'm looking at the bodybuilding pictures of Dr. Jain bench pressing some serious weights and Sim working on the damage to his back. Dr. Jain is the team trainer it says. I remember him now, too. He was at my house and he washed my face this morning. I recognize Jake, the EMT spotting Jain on the bench press. I want to play with them!

"Are you okay?" he checks again a few minutes later. "More tea? We've got croissants and some really nice cherry jam," he suggests so politely I have to take a second look to see if it's really DJ.

"Sure. Sure," I answer automatically. I'm starting to feel hunger again. I can't remember eating all week.

So this is where I am. Sunrise. Wherever it is, there's no mention of the location or phone number in the paper, just a website contact form. "By application only." Sean is on the screening committee. I give a little sigh of relief. I think I'm safe.

DJ comes back with a croissant and jam and refills my tea, then sits down on the chair outside the room again. I can smell the scent of jasmine and sandalwood in his wake. I turn the page. There's a gratuitous centerfold of him kicked back on a sofa on the lawn with two women, looking like he's just come hard. The caption says simply, '*Kama Dave with Sunrise staff Brandy and Nat.*'

"Dave?" I try. "Kama Dave?"

"Yes, Nicky? I'm here. What do you need?"

†

NAT

Jain wakes me up with a cup of coffee and a smile.

"We need you, witch doctor," he whispers. "Little broken bones are too tiny to set. The doctor of the house is helpless, Nat. I didn't wrap it or anything so you could do your magic."

"Oh? Who's hurt?" I yawn.

"We gave your room to the new patient Nicky. We didn't think you'd miss it."

"I won't," I laugh. "I'm sleeping with you forever, Dr. Jain."

"Is that yes then?" he smiles.

"It's always been yes. Is this an emergency or can I have coffee first?"

"No, she's in Dave's hands. Take your time."

"Dave? That sounds like a potential emergency," I laugh.

I sip on the coffee then I remember the first time with Sim, what he said when he was frustrated, not with sex but with desire: 'Where is Nicky when I fucking need her?'

"I'm up," I say. "Enough coffee for now."

Kamadev is sitting on one of the boardroom chairs outside her bedroom drinking tea. He gives me a strange little smile and says, "I'm watching her, Nat. I gave her breakfast."

I'm not prepared for the shock when I see her. Her face is bruised and bloody and she looks very depressed.

"Hi, Nicky," I say. "I'm Nat, Sim's assistant therapist. Dr. Jain asked me to look at some breaks or fractures. Ouch. Not much I can do with a broken nose, but I can get rid of those scars in a few days. Can you walk?"

"My foot's broken," she says. "First I broke my heart, then my foot, then my face," she laughs like it's a cruel joke. "No, I can't walk."

"Kamadev, honey, can you get Jain to carry her to the lab? Thanks. And don't leave the house, baby."

"You weigh nothing, Nicky," Jain teases her. "What happened to those muscles, honey? Don't you want to be on our team?"

He sets her down on the massage table and I look at her right foot.

"It looks like all five toes are fractured," he says. "Rest and massage should fix it. She probably needs some help with detox, too."

I pull the hem of her pant leg up a little and see more scrapes and bruises on her shin.

"Okay, I got it, Jain," I say. "I'll yell when I need you."

When he leaves I look at her carefully.

"It's not just your foot, is it, honey? I think you should take you clothes off and let me look."

She lets me help her undress and then I cover her with a sheet. I see enough. There are big finger mark bruises on her arms where she's been picked up and hauled to her feet and black bruises on her ass where she's fallen. Her elbows and knees have scabs on the joints and her ribs are discolored. The whole right side of her hip and thigh is red and blue and purple with old marks and fresh injuries.

I mix up some of Sim's trauma blend and start with her hand.

"I'm going to do your whole body, Nick," I tell her. "It's all connected. Tell me if anything hurts when I touch you."

"It smells nice in here, Nat," she sighs. "Thanks for helping me. I'm just smashed everywhere. I thought S&M was dead. Darrell's dead. Everyone ran away. The dealers tried to rape me."

"Sim talked about you, Nicky. He said he missed you. And he, um, asked me to do some unusual stuff for him. You're part of the reason we've got the new silk uniforms. It doesn't hurt on scars and bruises."

She looks at me curiously but doesn't answer.

"You know yoga?" I ask.

"I studied tantra with him," she nods. "For many years."

"Cool. Then you might want to take this to heart, something my tantra teacher told me about staying steady in your practice and not going too fast. It helps me whenever I crash and burn. We all find the ragged edge at some point.

"'You can hurt yourself trying to find Samadhi, you can fall down and break things and maybe even hurt other people around you.'

"Our official corporate mission is to provide integrative health and community service. But really, we're all just trying to help each other find Samadhi without hurting anybody or breaking things. It's a little crazy sometimes but we're just humans doing our best."

†

DJ

Nicky is more beautiful than ever with blood on her nose. She looks like she's been fighting and I think she's been fighting to get back to me. She went hard. She finally found me.

I go over to Mack's house and get the wheelchair for her. She can't walk. She can't go up the stairs, so I can't show her my room. Maybe I'll move out of my room. I could move the sofa outside her door and sleep there. Maybe I can sleep with her and hold her like Sim was doing if I behave myself. I've got control. I could sleep next to her and never hurt her.

I ask Jain to help me get her in the chair so I can show her around. He says fine but I'm going to help you watch her if you want to take her outside. He lifts her out of bed and we put one of the silk kimonos around her. I take my blessing scarf off and put it around her neck and she smiles at me, a crooked fangy little smile with lots of teeth. Then she laughs at me.

"DJ! I mean Kama Dave. Your neck!"

Oh fucking Sage put a hickey on me. I'm ashamed. I'm trying to think of a good story to tell her, but I can't think of a proper lie. All I can think of is half-assed.

"I swear I didn't touch her," I say. "Much." I correct myself. I can't erase a hickey. She giggles.

I push her out through the kitchen door and Jain walks beside us. We're walking up the path and the sun is sparkling in her hair. When she sees the gym, she nearly starts crying.

"Oh!" she gasps. "I saw the photos but I didn't connect the dots. The gym, the pool, the lawn. Dr. Jain, don't tell me you have a putting green. This is like a resort."

"More like a retreat. Maybe a last resort," he says. "And no. No putting green. Take a rest today. There's going to be a big party out here in a couple hours, media and friends. If you want to start training Monday, I'll help you get back into upper body workouts. When the toes are a little better, Sim can help you with some standing poses."

"Nicky," I break in, "Sim has a yoga shala on the edge of the world. Over there, behind the pool house. That's his house. There's a massage table on the top of a tree and a medicine Buddha."

Just then, Brandy comes out of the pool house and sees us.

"Nicky!" she screams and comes running. When she gets closer she sees the blood.

"Are you okay?"

"Good enough now," Nick says. "Just a little smashed up. I can't wait to try the gym! Good to see you again, Brandy. So you've been working here since you left my place?"

"Uh, yeah. Crazy. I'm married. I'm actually looking for him. He disappeared in the middle of the night but that's more or less normal for Sim."

"You married S&M?" she says shocked. "I didn't think he – "

"Mmmm. I'm still shocked, but he was very, very stoned that day. Pretty sick, too. My good fortune that he needed a nurse."

She winks at Nicky.

"Nicky hit the reef, Brandy," I say. "Nick nicked herself this time."

Brandy turns to look at me and puts her hand on my neck.

"Oh, baby Dave!" she laughs at my hickey. "Nice work. She just got here."

"No! It wasn't me," Nicky moans. "I haven't touched him."

But I hope it puts seeds in her mind. I hope the thought makes her wonder what my neck tastes like. Sage said I taste like milk and honey.

"How about the team?" Nick says. "Who's on S&M's team?"

I haven't got a clue, but Jain says, "We invited Billy up today to talk about it. Sim is team captain of course. Jake is our caddy. Maybe Dave."

"Maybe me? Maybe I'm on the team?" I'm getting hot and excited now.

Jain points to my hand and says I need to start training. He says it depends on if I have to go to prison and it depends on how hard I can go with my hand smashed. I will tear the paint off the house. I'll show him how hard hard is.

Sim comes out of the Ice House, walking as slow and cool as a drink of water. He doesn't even smile at us. He sneers.

"Oh, Kama David baby," he says, "I've got about forty seven women lined up wanting to marry you. Are you looking, honey?"

"I'm not available, Sim. I'm a very busy man," I say with all sincerity. "I'm training for the team."

"Oh? Did I invite you to be on the team?" he smirks.

"Oh, you will when I burn your gym down."

"Fair game," he says and puts his hand out to shake mine. When we shake he squeezes it hard enough to break every bone in my hand that isn't already smashed. It's only physical pain so I laugh at him.

"Game on, teacher. Go hard or go home."

†

S&M

I'm so ready for this party. This time I'm drinking because tomorrow the gauntlet drops in the gym. I've got my team picked. Me, Billy, Kamadev and Nicky. Nice that Billy got kicked off the pro tour because now he can compete in an amateur contest. When we win this, he'll get right back in the pros. And honey, there is no doubt that we'll win. We own the ocean. We own the mountain. We own space.

Nicky doesn't want to come to the party looking like the Bride of Frankenstein and I don't blame her. She's a horror show. Nat's working on the face scars but says it will take about five days. My back doesn't hurt much now and Nat says the snakes will fade completely. This time, I'm happy to see them go.

The Queen of Finance, Sunny has arranged an extravagant feast of lamb tacos with every grain and vegetable known to mankind, a filthy sweet carrot cake and bowls of berries with whipped cream. She knows I don't much like meat, but I'll eat lamb anytime for the high levels of carnitine. Carnitine builds strong bodies. I've never seen it done with Wonder Bread.

Billy shows up earlier than the rest so I give him a private tour.

"Man, Sam," he swears, "You've got it going on. I'm in. I'm in 110%."

I love this guy. I haven't been called Sam in five years. I ask him about the suspension. Mostly I want to know how much junk was involved and how he stands with it now.

"I never liked it, Sammy. I don't like to give my control away. It was just a nightmare and a horrible mistake. All the guys were doing it and that's as stupid a reason as it gets. I miss the tour. I can't tell you how stoked I was to see you swim out at the Point. God fucking bless you, S&M."

"She does, Billy. So here's the deal. We train with Jain at 10. I'll teach yoga starting Tuesday. Monday's a religious holiday for me."

"What kind of religion have you got that takes Mondays off?" he laughs.

"My kind. It's a medical fact that more people drop dead on Monday morning at 9am than any of other time during the week. My religion teaches it's better to murder time on Mondays than die.

"Of course all the training is optional for you, I know you've already got the works. But come up and train with us and we'll feed you. Anytime you want to stay, you can share a room with Dave or camp out. We've got nothing but options. Good to have you on the Sunrise team."

Chris and Amber are the next to show. Chris says the newspaper wants to sponsor a team. Then Sage comes around the back and hands me a little package.

"I'm in for the 20 grand," she says. "This is just a little peace offering."

I unwrap the package and there are two little bottles of exquisite saffron attar.

"Traditionally used for heart-opening and compassion," she smiles. "One for you and one for Kamadev."

I open one and the stuff smells like golden sunshine.

"Very potent aphrodisiac, too, isn't it?" I leer at her. She never gives up. I'm thinking about taking her on one of the boardroom chairs and finishing what we started ten years ago.

I have to slap myself mentally to let go of the thought. Thoughts are memories and desires arising from karma sprouting on their own, spontaneously. They're not stored in the brain, they're called up from the soul from the unmanifest cradle of creation.

"Anytime, baby," she says. Anywhere, too, I think. Beach caves, furniture, back seats, shit I've got to get my mind back on track. There's no such thing as casual sex. Everything you do remains forever like an autograph on your heart.

I haven't eaten lunch yet but I go straight for the carrot cake and a half glass of bourbon. Where's the cherry jam when I need it?

I'm thinking Dave's as crazy as a fox. I haven't seen him all morning but Nat says he's diligently guarding Nicky. He's talking to Nat again, too, and she's filled with light-heartedness, laughter and love. She looks impervious to hurting or being hurt by anyone.

Sean drags in with Crystal holding him up. He looks like shit. I shake his hand and whisper in his ear. Half a million dollars, baby, so far so good. All the shit disappears from his face like a magic slate. Crys introduces Beau, an ethereal tattoo artist with dark skin, copper hair and golden eyes.

Halfway between the lamb tacos and the whipped cream, I'm sitting on one of the deck chairs next to Chris, talking story. I don't see him much, but he's a legend and I suspect he's going to be my toughest competitor. I'm right in the middle of a sentence when Brandy comes over and sits on my lap. She doesn't just sit. She squirms. She can't get into that patented Sage position because of the chair arms but she's making herself loud and clear.

"Good God, woman," I swear. "Get off me. We've got company."

She bites my ear and persists, "I love a man in a chair."

"Keep it up," I warn. "Keep it up."

"Oh, sweet baby, you keep it up," she sighs. "All the way up."

"Seriously. Brandy. I'll lock you up and throw the key away if you don't get off me NOW, woman. I have company."

"I like that. Lock me up, honey. Throw the key away."

Instead of behaving, she gets more provocative, squirming like a wrestler in heat. I pick her up and set her on her feet. She wobbles like she's a little drunk. I look around for help and my eyes land on the vicious red head.

"Sunny, please," I beg. "Get her out of here. Chain her up if you have to. On second thought, take her over to relieve Kama Dave. I need to see him out here. And bring Nicky a plate of food. She looks like a skeleton."

Sunny takes her arm and walks her over to the Fire House for a timeout. Now I've got Nicky supervising my wife. It works for me. I'd pay to be a fly on the wall when those two start trading notes. Man, my ears are already on fire. Brandy doesn't even know me.

Dave comes out walking on sunshine with the same impervious air as Nat, bulletproof, inviolable. I want whatever he's on. I introduce him to Beau and explain our ink project, turning the stupid little '3' tattoo on Dave's hand into a beautiful omkara. I draw the Om out for him with exquisite flourishes the way I like to write it, with a curvaceous tail and the crescent moon cap separating the unmanifest dot of creation from the world of Maya.

"Piece of cake, mate," Beau says. "The '3' just needs a little embellishment. What was the '3' for?"

"Long story, buddy," I say. "Long and ugly. We want to forget it ever happened. I want you to do one just like it from scratch on my hand. Might as well do mine first so Dave can eat."

While Beau's setting up, Nat says, "Show him the snakes, Sim. Get an estimate of how much my artwork would go for in a permanent version."

"I'm really not interested in doing that, Nat. I've got enough scars on me to open my own art gallery."

But she's peaked Beau's curiosity. "What art? I love art. Let me see."

"Nah," I say. "It's nothing."

Nat puts her big eyes right in front of my nose and starts pushing my buttons as only she knows how.

"Please, boss. With sugar on it," she begs. "I want to know how much to charge you next time. I'll bet Nicky's never done anything quite as kinky as that."

"Shit," I say, just for the peace of the house. I don't want Mack to see this. Mack would kill me, but he's busy drinking and whispering with Sunny now. I get up and take off my silk.

"Oh, man," Beau whistles. "Do you know how hard it would be to do a tatt like that with all the, um, coloration? I'd have to charge you a couple G's and it would take a few sittings to get all the gory detail. Can I get a photo of that for my files? You might start a fad."

Nat swells with pride. "It took me a little over a minute to do that."

"Ouch," says Beau. "Triple ouch. Hurt much?"

"Only when I surf," I laugh. "Or try to sleep. I threatened to kill my wife if she touches me again. I can think of a lot more enjoyable things to do with a belt."

"It'll be gone in a couple days," Nat brags. "I'm saturating the scars with lavender and helichrysum."

She gets into a long discourse with Beau about the effects of botanical oils on skin, scars and bruises and introduces him to Sage, purveyor of exotic erotic and medicinal treasures. Before long, I've got a beautiful little Om tattoo below my right knuckles just beneath the face smashing section of my fist. It's sweet. I flash it at Kama Dave and he explodes with excitement and trades places with me for his turn.

"Nice job, Beau," I thank him. "I'm going to treasure this. The Vedas teach 'Whoever knows this one syllable obtains all that he desires and is adored by the gods.' It's probably a better fad than bloody snakes."

"Yeah, mate," he laughs. "It's going to be a whole lot cheaper for you, too."

"The real meat of Om," I explain for Dave's benefit, so he doesn't just think about sex when he looks at it, "is that it represents the separation of Maya from the true nature of infinity. Maya is the dance of existence but creative consciousness is the supreme 'dot' behind the curtain.

"If you achieve Samadhi, you not only know the truth, you become knowledge itself. Om signifies the ultimate truth."

While Beau polishes off the embellishments though, I can see Dave isn't so much listening to me as looking at Nat. He's dreaming no doubt of the jasmine scented futon on the top of the world, of losing his inexperience while floating on the back of a snake in a lake of milk.

Nat catches his drift and winks at him. "Om Kamadevaya Vidmahe," she whispers. There's a strange peace between them now, as if they're complicit in some crime, but there's nothing criminal about it. She's just a good teacher.

I give him one of the little bottles of saffron attar from Sage and warn him to be careful with it. He lets Nat have a sniff and she grins.

"Yeah, take it easy with that stuff, Kamadev. It's a very powerful love potion."

"Can I drink it?" he smiles with mischief.

"No," she laughs. "Use it like the Blue Lotus. Sniff it or add it to your massage oil. Or mix the saffron and lotus both together if you want to destroy all the women on the planet."

Oh, the body language written all over that boy. He puts his head down on his arm on the table as Beau works on his tattoo and turns his face up to gaze at her like a pet at her heels. He's catching up to me so fast now he's dangerous. I won't ever be able to look at that little tattoo on my hand again without thinking of sex and blood and snakes and jasmine milk.

†

BRANDY

I miss him. I'm hurt. He kicked me out of the pool house Friday night and last night he spent with Nick. Amber, Sage and Nat have all been groveling at his feet this afternoon as if he walks on water, which he apparently does judging from the Sunday paper. I can't get his attention. I have a few drinks and watch him laughing with his friends. He's drinking pretty hard so I give him time to loosen up.

When I saw my gorgeous husband's photo on the front page this morning and all the beautiful sexy shots at the Point, I couldn't wait to get my hands on him. The centerfold of Kama Dave doesn't hold a candle to him. Sim is divine perfection. I've loved him since the first time I laid eyes on him and I'd do anything for him.

So I try to let him know, I'm here, baby, I want you. I sit on his lap and cuddle and whisper in his ear but it just makes him mad. He's too busy for me. He picks me up and removes me from his lap and tells Sunny to get me away from him. I'm devastated.

We bring a plate of food to Nick's room. Dave is sitting outside the door patiently waiting. I give his hair a little tousle and kiss him softly. He looks at me with pure love and light and it cuts my heart further. Why won't Sim look at me like that today? What have I done wrong?

Dave goes back to the party with Sunny and I sit down in Nicky's room to sulk. She's knows him, so I confide in her.

"Brandy," she says shaking her head, "You don't even know that man. I've been his friend for nearly six years now and I've never been able to get under his skin. He's a very hard man. Extremely disciplined, creative and a little bit sick. I tried to warn you from the start, honey. He's a very kinky guy.

"You don't practice celibacy for a decade without getting a little perverted. He's developed certain other interests to keep himself satisfied. Personally, I never know what he's going to ask for next. I don't sleep with him but he likes to play games.

"All I want is little sex, Nicky," I whine. "I'm his wife. He's so good he drives me crazy."

"A little sex?" she laughs. "I don't think he knows what a little sex means. If you get any it's going to be a major production and it's going to be his way or the highway. That man has definitely got a Shiva complex. Shiva sets the rhythm for the whole world to dance, smashing egos and killing time.

"He likes to control the universe. I suggest you take a deep breath and wait for his instructions."

"What kind of games?" I ask.

"Pain is his favorite. Different levels of pain depending on what kosha he's playing with today. Could be physical, emotional, mental, disciplinary, he likes it all. I think it makes him feel like a tough guy. He's likes a fight especially if he thinks it's a fair one or a just one.

"I can't say I understand him, but intuition tells me he's trying to punish himself for some big karmic guilt. I've heard rumors and opinions, but I don't judge him. I'm just a friend trying to help him work things out without doing too much damage.

"I studied Tantra with him for years. He taught me how to have pranic sex without physical intercourse. But he also taught me one of my specialties, how to hurt him without leaving any marks."

"Oh," I'm shocked and confused. "He's definitely got marks on him now. He's got horrible scars on him."

"Yeah, I saw the gunshot scars in the bodybuilding photo. I'm very, very sorry to see him get hurt that bad."

"No, Nicky," I say. "He's got whip lashes on him, fresh. That's not in the paper. I just saw them yesterday, he's been hiding it from me."

She groans. "I hope he's not losing control with that. I'll talk to him. For now, I'd say be patient. Don't look at him or talk to him or touch him unless he asks."

Oh, shit, I think. I'm back to the beginning.

"Now, that one there," she continues, nodding towards the empty chair where Dave was sitting, "doesn't care one way or the other about pain. But he likes blood. The boys call him Dracula Junior because he gets turned on by it. S&M practically raised him so he's a strange one, too. He's not only celibate, he's a virgin," she sneers.

"I wouldn't count on that, Nicky," I laugh. "Kama Dave is the God of Love. I hear he's pretty damn good at it, too."

†

S&M

The moon is waning but it's big enough for us to howl at it for a few hours after the girls clear away the leftovers. Sage manages to quickly derail Beau and they leave early with the light of love burning. By the time all the guests are gone, Billy and I are about as drunk as it gets without falling down. Jain walks Billy back to the Fire House to crash in Kama Dave's room. I'm pretty sure Dave won't be sleeping there any time soon.

I have another drink alone and watch the moonlight spinning in big radiant circles down to Earth. I feel a tremendous malicious pleasure and satisfaction with myself as I sit there gloating over the whole universe sniffing the bottle of saffron. It's making me hungry for something more than the orgasms I'm getting from the moonlight.

I stand up and sway a little, find my balance, and then start walking slowly home, walking like Shiva, purposefully putting one foot down on the Earth after the other to make the planet spin and smash everything in my path. There's no one around to watch Shiva dancing like a slut stomping across the moonlit grass. That's too bad because I look so damn beautiful tonight.

I turn on all the lights in the bedroom. I turn on the whole universe. Brandy's sleeping but I don't give a damn because I'm better than any dream she could possibly be having. And I'm worse than any of her nightmares.

I want my handcuffs. Not the soft sissy hospital cuffs; I want the real ones, the ones that can hurt you if you try to use them for surgery. Dave's got the spare key. If I throw the key around my neck away, she'll be in real trouble. Fuck that, she's already in trouble.

I pull one of the kitchen chairs out into the bedroom and sit on it and have a pull on the saffron again. I can feel my blood pounding between my eyes, in my throat, in my heart, in my belly, in my cock. I'm feeling ravenously dangerously hungry.

After a couple minutes she wakes up and looks around and sees me sitting here leering at her with my top teeth biting down on my lip. I can taste a little blood on my lip.

"Oh, shit," she says sitting up in bed. "Sim. What time is it?"

"It's time," I snort. "It's fucking time I teach you some manners."

"Now?"

"I could wait until the end of the Universe if you want, honey, but the longer you make me fucking wait, the harder its going get for you."

I put my Om hand down on the front of my jeans to feel myself and laugh.

"Well, it probably couldn't get any harder, but it could get a lot more difficult. Do you want this or what?"

"Yes," she says. "Yes, please."

"All right then. That's better. What've you got on?"

She gets out of bed in her little pink silk kimono, the one I wore after Nat beat me. She's got nothing under it.

"Oh, yes. That works for me," I growl. "Nice. Get my handcuffs."

She reaches for the padded cuffs and I shake my head and point to the shelf. We've never used the real ones. I'm crazy to try them out.

She gets the metal police cuffs, hands them to me and stands there naked under the silk.

"Just wait," I say.

I count to ten for her full attention and then I pull my cock out of my jeans. It's so hard it hurts. She smiles and reaches out to pet me but I knock her hand away.

"Don't fucking touch me," I snarl. "I'm not feeling very nice. You wanted to sit on my lap when all my friends were here. Let's see how bad you want to do that now."

"I want to, Sim," she says. "Please."

"Then turn around," I order and handcuff her wrists together tight behind her back.

"Okay, now. There's only one way to do this. I'm not going to help you. If you do it like this, no hands, it's going to be hard. It's going to hurt. It's all or nothing, baby. Your choice."

She thinks it over. There's really no good strategy in her position, no easy way to sit on my cock gently or gradually. She has to take it all at once, and oh, gravity is going against her. I put my hands behind my head and lean back to enjoy the show.

"It's your choice, baby," I say again. "Do you want this or not?"

"It's going to hurt, Sim," she whines.

"Why do I get the feeling that you're going to like that very much?" I sneer.

She steps cautiously straddling my legs, her belly against my heart and puts her lips to my ear.

"Can I kiss you first?" she whispers.

"No, you can't kiss me. Just do it."

She takes a deep breath and slides herself down on me all at once and screams. It's the best pain I've ever felt and I come so hard it shocks me. Christmas lights up my brain and my head drops back in amazement.

When I open my eyes she's staring wide eyed, wondering what the fuck. She's helplessly stuck in chair pose and can't move without my help.

"Kiss me now, baby," I beg. "It's all right now. Kiss me please with sugar on it."

I put my arms around her and hug her tightly to me as she kisses my mouth, my ears, my neck. Then I put both hands on her ass and set the rhythm for a slow steady dance.

†

DJ

"Nico," I whisper. "I have something for you. Wake up."

She stirs.

"Nicky. Wake up. You'll like this."

"What?" she asks rolling over to look at me. "What now?"

"I have something for you. It will give you beautiful dreams."

"Don't tell me you're waking me up to help me sleep, DJ. You're crazy. You're scaring me.

"I'm Kama Dave, Nick. Please don't call me DJ. He was such a punk."

"I agree with you on that one. He betrayed his friends and turned into a junkie."

"Ouch, Nick. I fucked up. I might go to prison for a long while. But I'm very nice now. I'm controlled. I know how to be polite. S&M said pretend to care even if I don't, but I really do care about you. "

She doesn't answer. It's quiet in the house and everyone has gone to bed but me.

"Nicky, can I come in and show it to you or not?"

"Go away, Dave, or I'll yell for Dr. Jain."

"Don't do that. Let me show you and then I'll go away if you want. It's very, very nice." I hold up the little bottle of saffron so she can see I really have something and I'm not just trying to show her me. I'd like to show her me but only if she asks nicely.

"What is it?" she's awake now and curious.

"I have to show you. Can I come in?"

"Maybe for a minute but be quick."

That's the only permission I need. I sit on the side of her bed and twist the top off the bottle and show her how I do it. I close my right nostril and breath the saffron deeply through the left side. Then I close the left side and breath it through my right. She knows nadi shodhana and she smiles.

"Try it," I say.

She takes the little bottle and does a few rounds, breathing it deep and relaxing even deeper.

"This is how Nat taught me to do it," I continue when I'm done. "She's my new teacher. One drop on your crown chakra. One drop on your third eye. Let me do it for you. One on your heart, is that okay?

"Good. Now I should put some on the bottom of your feet. Is it okay if I touch your feet?"

She's getting very relaxed now and smiles. "Sure. That's nice, Kama Dave. Rub my feet with it. Annoint me."

I loosen the bottom of her blanket and uncover her beautiful feet. They're crusty with scars and bruises. Her little second toe is crooked and leaning away from the big toe. It looks painful.

Nat says the attars are too precious for massage and I should put them in the carrier oils but Nicky's toes are much more precious. I put the saffron attar on her feet full strength and massage it gently between her toes, on the arch of her soles, around her ankles.

Her eyes are closed and her mouth is wide with pleasure. She moans and purrs and I don't stop. I wait to see if the saffron can destroy her. If it doesn't work, I'll get the blue lotus to polish her off.

"Nick?" I whisper. "How does that feel?"

"Really nice, baby," she says. She's never called me baby. The saffron must be working. It's destroying her.

"Nick, Billy's sleeping in my room upstairs. He drank too much."

She purrs.

"I can hold you, Nick, if you like. I won't hurt you. I can sleep with you and keep you warm."

She doesn't say no, so I lie down next to her.

"Baby, you smell beautiful," she sighs. "You smell like heaven."

"I taste even better, Nicky. I taste like honey."

She laughs. "How would you know how you taste, silly boy?"

"I've been told," I assure her.

"Mmmm. Well don't try anything, Dave."

"I don't have to *try* anything, Nicky. I already know how," I laugh.

"What do you know?" she wonders. "You know nothing, little boy."

"I know Tantra now, Nicky. I know a lot more, too. I can come through my third eye but I like it a lot better when my heart comes."

"Since when?"

"I've had private lessons. I'm very, very nice. I could make you cry but it would be nicer to just sleep next to you tonight."

"Okay," she says. I lean my head against her shoulder and listen to her soft deep breath. I wait for the destruction. I think she might be melting into the pillow right now.

"Kama Dave?" she says at last.

"Yes, Nicky?"

"Can you really make me cry? I might like that."

"Oh, you would like that very much, Nick," I assure her. I turn my head so I can give her a taste of my mouth. I kiss her soft and controlled. I feel her heart racing and her prana pours into me like a river of pleasure.

"Honey?" I ask.

"Exactly like honey," she breathes hard. "You taste exactly like jasmine honey."

Part Three: NAUGHTY AND NICE

The only people for me are the mad ones,
the ones mad to live, mad to talk, mad to be saved
~ Jack Kerouac, "On the Road"

Part Three

NAUGHTY AND NICE

†

S&M

3am. The moon is at half mast and the tides are
even. I can smell it. I slip out of the pool house being
careful not to wake Brandy and sneak upstairs next
door.

"Billy. Let's go."

He reads me as clearly as if I'd texted. Now. Up.
Dressed. He knows the drill. Mack will kill me. Maybe
we should take Jain for protection. Probably not. We're
out the front of the house and into Billy's van before you
can say 'what the fuck?'

We're out of here.

Driving down the mountain in the dark, I watch
the shoulders of the earth against clear black space. I'm
sick with excitement. Every god, goddess, human,
animal, insect, plant and sentient being is quivering
with it. It's sick. I want it so bad my teeth hurt. Mother
of all energy, father of all discipline, the ocean is
sucking me hard.

Mmmm, it tastes like salt. It tastes like bitter tears. I'm crying with joy.

Billy has an extra wetsuit and board so we don't have to roust Sean at my house. Crap it hurts so bad even with a rash guard but once in the ocean I'm just sweet ice cream. I'm the most beautiful thing my mother ever dreamed.

We paddle out in the dark, pools of phosphorescent plankton lightening up under water with every stroke. The milky sea kisses us and the moon laughs at our audacious assault on her. Oh, mother ocean, sweet jasmine lake of milk dreaming me as I dream you. Oh, my mother. I suck sea foam and she comes all over me.

Night surf. Fuck. You can't see the swell coming in the dark, but you can see the white water break at the curl right before it explodes around you. It's as amusing as it gets. Sniff it. Listen for it. Higher consciousness works well on a night surf. It bombs us. We detonate it. We kiss the swell with our sticky wax feet.

We're so stoned with salt water and the rhythm of the sea that we could drown in delight. Then the sun rises on us and splashes us with blessings. Billy sees something dark on the shore, something black.

"Good view from here, Sammy," he says. "Little early in the day for it, but they never quit. That guy by the sewer pipe in the black beanie is the local Junko 7/11, the regional manager."

I sit on the board, legs cool in the ocean but fire rising up my spine.

"Nails," I suggest. "Hammer and nails."

We paddle in and strut up to the punk.

"Do you know me, honey?" I ask.

"Ahhhhh," he says. "Yaaaaa Ummmm."

"AhhhYaaaUmmm? Om on this, Sweetie," I laugh and put my Om knuckles into his mouth. Sean made me swear off guns and knives years ago, so my little right hand is all I've got. My bare foot works pretty nicely too. I give him a personal introduction to my foot in this third chakra.

"How's that taste for breakfast?" I spit.

"Ooofff," he groans, "Oooooofffuck."

He really seems to like the beach because he's kissing the sand and moaning like she's a hot date. Billy goes through his pockets. Money, money, money and smack. Smack and coke and maybe meth. I can't tell by looking at it but the little paper bindles are marked with H, C and M. Billy dumps the dope out on the sand and counts the money.

"This little fuck kindly donated $800 to the Point Guard for law enforcement," he laughs in amazement. "How fucking generous is he?"

He helps the lucky donor to his feet and brushes the sand off him.

"Steven Mack," the guy pants. "You're the fucking guy in the paper yesterday. We're going to roast your head for Christmas dinner. You're dead, S&M."

"Ooh, I'm looking pretty beautiful right now for a dead man. Who the fuck are you, sweetheart?"

"Prince Albert," he mocks. "Who do you think you are? That's an ounce you just dumped out."

"Mmm, 28 grams all packaged up for sale. I'd say that shows intent to commit a crime or two."

He starts to put a hand down his pants and I don't think he's reaching for his cock so I smack him with malicious pleasure. His head wheels back and he lands hard on one of the mudstone boulders splitting his skull open.

"Ooops, fuck," I swear. "I didn't mean to kill him."

Billy reaches under Prince Albert's belt and pulls out a gunmetal blue 22.

"I'm sure he would have done the same for you, Sam," he snarls. "Maybe we should get out of town."

I kneel down and check his breath then his pulse. Blood is spurting out of his head and he's choking on air, but he's alive. I peel the top of my wetsuit down and pull off the red rash guard, my hot, blood-and-guts red rashie. I wrap it around his head and gloat. I'm about 100 yards away from the spot where they shot me. Maybe I'm even. Nah, I decide. I'm not even close to even. Karma is such a slut.

"Should we call Sean?" Billy wonders. Sean is probably asleep in my house about 500 yards down the beach.

"Call him what?" I laugh. "I don't think I want to wake him up this early. You get his legs and I'll get the bloody end. I'm keeping him."

There's never been so much blood in Billy's van. It sucks and it rocks at the same time, just like the deep blue sea. I'm really confused about the karmic consequences of this so I roll them slowly like credits passed Billy.

"So I hit him. Not very nice but he would've killed us both if we gave him a chance.

"But I'm saving his life. I could've left him to bleed to death.

"Or maybe he'll bleed to death before I get him home. Then I've murdered him.

"Maybe we should have just surfed some more and ignored him."

Billy shakes his head.

"There's no point in thinking 'Maybe, baby'," he says. "You could die trying to figure out the karmic justice of the world. Everybody's karma is tangled up whether you like it or not. It was his karma to get his head smashed today. Someone else could have taken care of that. Car wreck, atom bomb, sniper. Fuck, Sam. You just happened to be the joker that showed up."

"Yeah. Go hard," I say. "I didn't mean to go that hard."

We pull into the driveway at the Fire House. It's exactly 9am on Monday, the most popular time of the week to drop dead. Jain's in the kitchen drinking coffee with Nat and Kama Dave is sitting with them, pulling the crusts off toast and dipping them in honey butter.

"Jain, I need some muscle," I beg. "I really hurt my back carrying this guy up from the beach. "Can you get him next door into IC?"

"Beach?" He raises an eyebrow. I've got the wetsuit half on. Nat looks at my feet and I notice I've tracked filth into the kitchen. My feet are gloriously anointed with dirty, caked sand.

Dave laughs, "You've got blood on you, Sim."

"We would have loved to take you with us, Jain, for our own protection, but I don't think you move as fast as me and Billy." I wink at Nat. "But actually, Jain, its fucking urgent. The guy might be dead by now."

"Shit," he says. It's the most appropriate word possible for the occasion.

Billy has the van side doors open and he's sitting next to Prince Albert's body.

"Breathing?" I ask. He nods.

"How did this happen?" Jain whistles taking the red rashie off Prince's head for an inspection.

"A rock right were God wanted it to be, I guess." Billy shows him the gun.

Jain picks the Prince of Darkness up and carries him over to Mack's house.

"You may be grounded, Sim. You may be kicked off the team, both of you."

"Hang on, Jain," I object. "We were training. I think we actually won the contest this morning before it even started. We surfed blindfold in overhead waves and then just cleaned the beach up on our way home. This Princess had an ounce of dope on him, 28 grams of white and brown stuff. And a gun. I'd do it again. I think we measured the karma out pretty nicely. "

"Right," Billy adds, just what you want to hear from your new best friend.

Jain gives me a glare I've seen before. The "I-can't-believe-you-believe-your-own-bullshit" glare. But who else believes me better than me? I'm pretty sure I'm right here. I know I want to be right.

Prince is still out cold, but he's alive.

"Maybe you should have dropped him at Emergency," Jain says. "This isn't why we're here."

"Nah," I say. "I want him."

Mack comes in to see what's cooking and I just say, "Surfing accident. The guy was accidentally dealing dope where we were surfing."

Mack laughs and I think he gets the cosmic joke, but then he puts both his hands on my shoulders and says, "You're sick, little brother. We need to talk."

Then the hardcore truth dawns on me. My heart sinks. I'm going to have to give this guy my toys. I hate to share, but he's definitely going to need the padded hospital restraining cuffs so they can stitch up his head. On the bright side, I've already taught my wife how to use the metal police cuffs. So I guess I'll live.

"By the way, Mack," I say. "Give the little fucker as much narcotics as you like."

†

DJ

It's Monday, Sim's religious holiday so he's blowing everything off and going back to bed. But Dr. Jain takes me and Nicky out to the gym after he finishes with surgery.

"Look. You're both kind of wrecked," he laughs. "So let's just do beginners' basic training and set a baseline. I need some fresh air. God that was a bloody train wreck Sim dragged home."

Nicky can't stand very nicely, so we're working upper body today.

I'm pretty sloppy on the bench press and I hate letting her see how crumbly weak I am but you can't get there from here unless you grovel. I don't get past 115 pounds. I suck. Nicky pushes 95.

She has big crusts of scars on her broken nose and her eyes are swollen black and blue. I kissed that pretty split lip. God, I'm ready to die of happiness. I kissed her. When she presses the barbell her chest gets pumped and her beautiful little triceps smile at me. I'm a dead man. She's murdered me in the first degree.

Jain laughs at me.

"Dave, get your mind back on this planet," he snorts.

Green glass. Emerald green eyes. Ooof.

"You know," she says to Jain, "I used to hate this little fuck. I mean he seriously annoyed me. He looks a little bit like S&M but he was such a punk. How did he suddenly turn into a human being?"

That might be a compliment coming from her. I try to show her all my teeth. She can have them all. She can wreck my car. She could burn my house down if I had one.

Jain says to do curls with the bar. There's nothing powerful about curls. They're just pretty. I can't use much weight with my hand hurt. Doesn't matter how much weight really, it's so specific that all the blood pumps into your biceps.

My arms are beautiful. I watch her watching me watching her. I do 12 reps with twenty pounds at the same time as I'm standing on two feet on a planet spinning through frozen space whilst I dive into her emerald eyes.

It's just a sweet piece of cake. Oh, give me a place to stand. I want to move the Earth. I flex my arm and ask her if she wants to touch it.

"Dave," Jain says. "I think we're done. I mean I think I'm done unless you guys want to do more triceps."

I'm really bored to tears with doing my arms. I want to do Nicky and she knows it. I push her back to the Fire House in the wheel chair and Jain lifts her into bed.

"Now, Nick," I say. "Do I still have to sit outside the door or what?"

"You should probably sit outside the house, Dave," she says. "You're really coming on too strong."

"Mmmm. Sorry. I don't know how else to come on," I sulk. "I could probably go back to my room and sniff the flowers."

"Jeez, honey," she says. "I'm sorry. You've been very kind. I'm not sure if I should run you off. It's just – "

"Just what?"

"Just what kind of flowers have you got in your room?" she asks.

"Jasmine, lotus, crocus. Pretty nice stuff," I lie. Maybe I'm exaggerating a little. I haven't been upstairs in two days and all the jasmine could be dead by now.

"You want to see my room?" I offer, but it's kind of a weak invitation for what I've got in mind.

"Why?" she says. "I'm sure it's beautiful up there but I can't do stairs. I'm safer down here. Bring your flowers down."

"I'll be right back," I smile then I go straight into the lab to see what kind of fresh flowers we really have today. Nat's got the usual bucket of jasmine, but she's also mixing in some nice dahlias and chrysanthemums.

"No lotus or crocus?" I whine.

"Not today, baby," she says. "But you know how to mix your own love potions. How was the gym?"

"I'm moving, Nat," I pronounce proudly.

"You just moved upstairs on Friday," she says surprised. "Why do you want to move out so soon? It's a beautiful private space, one of the nicest rooms in the house."

"She can't come up the stairs. I'm sure she wants me down here so I can take better care of her. I'm moving in with her. She told me to get my stuff."

"What?? What stuff?"

I grab half of her flowers. "This is all I've got and the stuff in my pocket. I need some more sandalwood but I'll worry about that later."

"I noticed she's wearing the blessing scarf I gave you, Kamadev. The best blessing is having one to give away. That was nice of you. Come on, I'll help you with the flowers."

She follows me into Nicky's room with a vase and a little lavender oil for the scars on Nicky's nose. While I fill the vase with water and arrange the flowers she sits on the bed and works on her nicked face. I can hear her whispering but can't hear what she says.

Then Nicky laughs, "Shit yes, he's bothering me. He's bothering me every second. He's an incessant little monster. But it's not the annoying kind of bother, it's the fussing kind. I'm actually enjoying it."

"This is all I've got, Nick," I tell her. "I'm really not going to be any trouble."

Nat whispers something else to her and Nick's eyes go big.

"Oh? He thinks he's moving into my room? That's amusing. Can I kick him out if he causes any trouble?"

Nat rolls her eyes. "He's beyond trouble, Nicky. I think you'll find he's actually pretty therapeutic."

†

PRINCE ALBERT

The room is dark and everything is far away. Far away pain, far beneath the river of hot dope in my head, splitting melon head wrapped and pounding with a dull pulse like a hammer against my temples. I can't move. My arms are strapped to the bed. When I move my feet, a muscle spasm shoots through my ribs so hard I have to stop breathing.

I try another easy breath and, yeah, broken ribs, dull pain, far away, as long as I don't move maybe I can ignore it. I open my eyes. Looks like a hospital, a little dark room and I've got a couple different IV drips and oxy.

"Good morning, Princess," he hisses and my heart skips hard. I'm in a horror show. He's sitting in the corner chair watching me like a bird of prey and I'm helpless.

"What do you think, honey?" he says to another person. "Is that your pusher?"

I try to see who he's talking to, but my head is strapped down, too.

"Prince Albert, yeah," I hear the other guy say. "The Kings of 36th Ave. He taught me how to shoot up.

"This is pretty fucking medieval even for me. This is wicked, Sim."

The younger guy picks my hand up and checks my 36 tattoo and looks down at me. I don't recognize him at first because now he's dressed up like a prom queen in a silk robe with flowers in his hair. He's even got a little smear of pink lipstick on the side of his mouth.

Christ, it's the little crybaby junkie from the beach house. He's supposed to be in jail, so I must be in the jail hospital locked up with these guys. I'm horrified.

"I cracked his skull open. I didn't mean to do that. Just wanted to scare him off the beach forever, but he tried to pull a gun on me."

"So what are you going to do with him?" the crybaby wonders.

"Not much right now," S&M says. "I thought Jain might fix him so I could beat him up again, but I'm out of luck. He's got a concussion and 38 stitches in his head and 4 cracked ribs. Plus, he really doesn't know how to fight. I reckon he's worthless to me.

"Apparently I'm not allowed to take any prisoners."

"You fucking robbed me," I groan. "I didn't do anything. I want my lawyer. I'm going to press charges. Where am I?"

"The Ice House dungeon," S&M sneers. "Don't worry. After we save your life, we'll put you back where the police can keep an eye on you. I've been on the phone with them for the last hour and they're ready to kill me right now. Maybe we'll all three end up in the same prison cell together. What a party, huh, Kama Dave?

"I knew I wasn't allowed to have guns or knives, but this ban against taking prisoners is a real shocker. You had an ounce of dope on you all packaged up for sale and a concealed weapon. And two of my friends identified you as the guy running the junk superstore out of my house. Where is the justice, I'm asking you?"

"I want my lawyer," I hiss. "I wasn't doing nothing but standing on the beach watching you guys surf. It looked like fun. You didn't even say 'hello'. You just hammered me and robbed me!"

"I wasn't very polite was I?" he sneers. "Where were my manners? I guess I was a little excited about getting a good surf after being locked up for weeks.

"So Sean wonders do ya got any warrants out or anything? We could still have a little fun with this. Otherwise, he wants to take you back down and arrest you properly when he sees you on the street again."

"For what? Standing on the beach? You took everything off me."

"I'll have to think about that. Are you a junkie, Prince Albert?"

"Nah. Junk is for suckers. It's just a business for me. And you really screwed my business up. I can't settle my account tonight."

"And this is just pleasure for me, Princess," he snorts. "My pleasure screwing up your business."

"Your friend there is the biggest junkie crybaby I've even seen in my life," I snarl back. "I've never seen anyone do that much heroin. Whenever it started to wear off he'd cry like a baby until we gave him more. Is he your little bitch?"

S&M gets slowly up to his feet like a big cat waking up and starts for the bed. I'm sorry I said it before the words hit him. He's my worst dream.

"What are you implying?"

"Fuck, I'm helpless here. I didn't mean anything by it. It's just... look at him. He looks like he's been playing dress-up with girls."

"That's because he has been," S&M laughs. "Women love to play with him. They play dress-up and undressing, too. I can assure you he didn't put that lipstick on with a tube. Wipe your face off, Dave. What are you on now? The third woman in four days?"

"Can I count Amber?" he asks innocently.

"Well she only did the centerfold shots, but that's money in the bank. You can count my wife if you like, even though you just slept with her. Who's to stop you from counting? I'll bet the red head hasn't kissed you yet."

"Fuck no. I don't want her. I'm training for the team, Sim. I moved in with Nicky."

With that they forget I'm even here. He punches the junkie in the arm and then bear hugs him and kisses him hard on the mouth. I'm shocked but I'm not saying another word about that department.

"Shit, cinnamon pearl lipstick, tasty," he says. "That's Nicky alright. You moved in with the goddess of the ocean, Sri Kamadev, you little fuck. I guess all those Tantra lessons paid off. What does Nat say about it?"

"She says I'm very therapeutic."

They're both laughing and shoving each other when the door opens and the Point Guard cop comes in. I know the bastard by sight. I know when to disappear but I can't. So I just close my eyes and pretend I'm dead.

"Okay, pal," he says to S&M. "Put a lid on it. The party was yesterday. This is serious stuff. Why didn't you call me?"

"It was kind of early. We went down at 3am and took him out at around 7."

"Bullshit, Sim. You thought you had a trophy. You wanted to keep him."

I open one eye. S&M puts his head down and snorts.

"I already heard your side of the story over the phone. Now I want to hear his. I know who you are, buddy," he says to me. "I know your business. What happened?"

"They robbed me, Officer," I say pathetically. After all dealers have rights, too. Pushers are people.

"I was watching him and Billy surfing this morning at sunrise and they were having a gas. I was a little jealous, having to sell all this — I mean having to work. I was just watching, not soliciting anyone; no one was around."

"And?"

"And they came out of the water and came straight up to me and hammered me and robbed me."

"They didn't say anything?"

"I think he said 'do you know me, honey?' and belted me in the mouth before I could answer."

"Is that right, Sim?" he asks.

"Right. I didn't say 'Good morning' or anything. I was just so happy to see him."

"Then he kicked me in the stomach when I was down. I think he broke a couple ribs."

"Four," S&M corrects me. "Right in the third chakra where you guys shot me."

"Billy emptied my pockets out and took my money, $800."

"Is he telling the truth? You guys just robbed him?"

"He had an ounce of smack, meth and coke in bindles, Sean, retail sales. We dumped them out on the beach. Then we helped him up and dusted him off. I thought it was pretty reasonable under the circumstances. Billy said he was the guy in my house."

"Reasonable? Legal? No way in hell. He's just standing there on the beach enjoying the view. You had no reasonable cause to suspect he's got dope on him. So then what? Prince, I want to hear your side. What happened?"

"They scared the crap out of me. There were two of them. I've heard S&M is a lunatic. Billy was a former client. I thought they were going to kill me. I reached for my gun in self-defense. He's a mean son-of-a-bitch, Officer. I didn't know where he was going with it."

"Did you threaten them, Prince? Any of those 'we should've shot you in the head' jokes we've been hearing?"

"No way! The only reason I had the gun was because of lunatics like him. I don't like to fight."

"Ain't that the truth?" S&M whistles. "He can't fight for shit, Sean. But he called me a dead man and some bullshit about roasting my head for dinner. That's a threat isn't it?"

"Really? Maybe you guys should have taken the gun off him instead of his money and then we'd all be having a nice Monday lunch right now."

"Where's the $800, Sim?"

"I gave it to Mack for the Point Guard."

"The gun?"

"Billy's got it. I'm not allowed to carry guns or knives."

"Damn straight you aren't," Sean hisses.

"What about the other stuff? About $1700 worth." I sniff.

Sean looks at me in amazement. "Would you really like to give me a written statement of exactly what other stuff is missing and press charges in court?"

"Concussion," S&M explains. "Better let him think about that."

"Listen. No judge is going to like any of this. It's my fricking day off so I'm not even going to report this. I'm up here as a friend. When he's stable I'll drive him back to town and keep an eye on his business. When *I* arrest him, it will stick.

"Prince, he saved your life. Count your blessings. Sim, you're not allowed to take any prisoners. I thought you were on my team, buddy. What did I tell you Saturday at the Point."

He hangs his head and says, "Let you do what you do best."

"Now both of you shake hands and apologize. I deserve one too. Mack woke me up."

"Sorry, for the trouble, Sean," he says crushing my hand. "Sorry I didn't knock your teeth out, Princess."

"I'm sorry I got out of bed this morning," I say. "Sorry, Officer. Can I get my money back and my gun?"

Sean nods. "Try that apology again, Sim," he says.

"Sorry you hit the rock, Prince Albert," he says. "I didn't mean to go that hard."

I feel a little better. It sounds like a sincere apology this time.

"Then if you boys are done spitting and snarling at each other, I'm leaving. I'll be in touch when Dr. Mack says you're better, Prince. You're not under arrest. The restraints are only to immobilize your concussion. Tell Dr. Mack if he harasses you." He puts his finger in S&M's chest and gives him a dirty glare.

"Don't be a punk, Steven," he snarls. "I'm warning you."

As soon as Officer Sean leaves the room S&M retracts his apology.

"Cock sucking little bitch!" he snarls.

"Mother fucking lunatic," I snap back.

"Too bad you can't fight, Prince Albert," he snorts. "We could've been friends."

†

JAIN

Mack and I sit with Steven for nearly two hours in the office and get nowhere fast. He's sullen and disturbed, crashed from the mania of this morning and driven into a deep ditch of depression. We're his business partners, but he doesn't want to talk about it.

"House arrest, Steven," Mack finally says in frustration, "unless you agree to therapy."

"Which house?" he smirks.

"Depends on how willing you are to cooperate. If you agree to get help, I'll put you upstairs in the Fire House. I hear the room is free. Then you can work with Nat. She's trained in this.

"Otherwise, I'll lock you up indefinitely in the old nurses' room. That's free, too. But I mean lock you up. Maybe chain you up until you shape up. No amenities. There goes your team, too. I'll suspend all of them. What's it going to be?"

"How about my wife?"

"You were celibate for 8 years, brother. I'm sure it won't kill you."

"You can't do that, Mack. I'm the fucking President of Sunrise"

"And Jain is CEO. Majority rules. Will you back me up on this, Jain?"

"Quit threatening him, Mack. He's upset. Let him think. I've got to go see a kid about a concussion. Chill out and have a drink, Steven. We've been watching you going off the rails for a while. Let's work on this, okay? We can help you."

I get up and leave them both to sulk over the bourbon. I tell Brandy I'll take over with the patient for now. Go home and don't wait up for Sim.

Prince's vitals are looking stable but he's moaning.

"You're going to be okay, buddy, I'm a doctor. I'm taking the restraints off. How do you feel?"

"What do you think?" he groans as I remove the cuffs and then free his head.

"Can you move?"

He turns his head but when he tries to move his arms he gasps in pain.

"Oooof. Back," he moans.

"Muscle spasms?"

He nods panting.

"Okay, I can help with that." I check his arms. No tracks. "You're not a user? That's a breath of fresh air here."

He shakes his head and moans, "I'm not a fan of narcotics. It's just my business, Doc."

"Alright then I won't give you very much." I pull a very small amount of morphine into a needle, just enough to dull the pain and stop his muscles from seizing.

"Let me know if you need more. I'd hate to get you strung out considering your profession. It's bad for business."

"This is already bad for business. I'm supposed to deliver $2500 tonight and I don't have it. I'm out of business getting robbed like that. I did nothing to hurt that lunatic. I paid $1000 a week to rent his house. No one forced his buddy to take all that dope. He loved it. I'm an honest businessman. Shady business, but I have integrity."

"Let's get you on your side so can I work on the muscle cramps."

When I try to turn him he screams so I decide to wait a few minutes to let the drugs work.

"Let's see if I can help you relax a little, buddy. First you have to set an intention, like making a wish. What do you want more than anything?"

"Freedom," he sighs. "I've seen that freak living in the beach house and he's got everything, time, money, chicks, friends, respect, front page photo. Hell, he doesn't even wear shoes. I heard he's a yogi queer.

"If I had money like him, I'd have freedom. I tried to talk to one of the surfer girls and she fucking hit me. I'm just trying to make a living."

"Okay, then. Think of freedom. Imagine you have all the freedom you desire in the bottom of your heart. Now just follow me. Put your attention on your right thumb, your index finger, middle finger, ring finger, just follow me and imagine freedom."

By the time I finish, he's breathing easier.

"What are you doing, Jain? Yoga nidra on that punk?"

I look up. Sim is in the doorway, confused and angry with tears in his eyes.

"Trying to fix him, Sim. So you can beat the shit out of him again. I'm a doctor. I try to help people. What are *you* doing, Sim?"

"I guess I'm looking for help, too. Mack says both Darrell and I were shot with a .357 not a .22. He said that's a pussy gun. They don't use them for hits. What would I know?"

"Oh, is that all?"

"I can't get even and I'm having trouble controlling myself. What do I have to do?"

"Did you hear me talking to him, Sim?"

"Yes. He hates me worse than I hate him. I don't even know him. I'm grateful I didn't kill him. Shit, even Nicky punched him, poor bastard. I'm feeling fucking sick, man."

†

NAT

Jain came in late with his arm around Sim. Both of them look like hell, but Sim looks like he'd been crying.

"Hey, Nat. Sim wants a little help with the control problem. He's going to stay with us tonight. Upstairs room still free?"

I nod. The lights are off in Nick's room but the door is open for her own protection. Kama Dave is sleeping with her, but there's nothing going on but a little kissing and foot massage, maybe a little sleight of hand, but they're quiet. She's not on his list.

"Talk to me, Sim," I say gently. "What happened today? I've heard all kinds of wild stuff from Kamadev about you breaking up a dope ring."

"I hurt a guy, Nat. I lost control. I almost killed him. I beat him up and robbed him. He's just a kid. I'm sick, Nat. What should I do?"

"For now? Have Jain give you a fistful of sleep aminos and we'll work on it in the morning. I know exactly what you should do."

I get up at seven and fix coffee, tea, croissants, fresh fruit and put flowers on the boardroom table. Then I wake everyone and invite them to a house meeting. Once they've settled down with their breakfast, I start.

"We're going to do something a little different today," I announce. "Group therapy." Everyone groans and Sim puts his head down on the table in despair.

"Before you start complaining, has anyone done this before? I didn't think so. This is your chance to help each other. Sim needs your help very much this morning. You owe it to him and you can all learn a lot by helping him."

Sim puts his head up and begs, "Not like this, Nat. Not in front of my friends."

He looks around the table helplessly from one face to another, horrified.

"Yes, like this, baby," I assure him. "This is what friends are. Shining mirrors reflecting your highest self back to you. Trust me."

"Oooooohhhhh," he groans face down again on the table. "Oh, fuck."

"Look, honey. This is so simple. Just look around and start with the person you've known the longest and tell me how they've helped you. This works."

He picks his head up and thinks. "Jain. Sixteen years. He always gives me good advice. He cares about me but he doesn't judge me like Mack."

"How painful was that? Go ahead; next longest."

"Kama Dave. Six years. He copies me so he inspires me to be a better person. This is killing me, Nat. He respects me and I don't want him to see this. Please. Please, don't make me do this."

"Stay with me. This will teach him more than if he thinks you walk on water. Next?"

"Nicky. Five years going on six. She's helped me a million times with control. I've missed her. She knows how to help me." He looks at Nick with a plea for mercy.

"And next? Must be me, because I'm the only one left," I laugh.

"A couple weeks. You saw me at my worst but you still respected me. And you didn't question me when I asked for, uh – Jesus, Nat! This is personal. I don't want to do this!"

"Of course it's personal. These are your friends. We can't help you if we don't get personal. You asked me to hit you and you asked me to take the paint off the walls. But you also asked me to teach you and work with you. I'm not judging you."

His head goes back down between his arms.

"Next, tell Sim how he's helped you. Same order, start with Jain."

"Well. I guess the best part of being your friend has been the way you've inspired me. You keep evolving. You take liberation seriously. You're your own man, never settling for less than epic. I like that. You inspired me to try to change my career here and now, not to put my dreams on the back burner. And you practically threw Nat at me."

"That's on my list, too, Jain," I laugh. "How about you, Kamadev?"

"You're my teacher. You taught me that feeling pain is educational, but causing pain is wrong. You taught me my koshas and the four noble truths and how to surf and drink and how to treat women. You took custody of me and you're trying to keep me out of prison."

He grins at me. "And you let Nat teach me kundalini."

Jain's eyes widen and I flush a little.

"Nicky?" I quickly push on, changing the subject.

"You taught me Tantric yoga. And without getting too specific, you taught me to how to get intimate without sex. Enough said."

He puts his head up and looks at her gratefully and she winks at him.

"As for me," I add, "you've been the best mirror I have regarding the work we do. You're the best boss I've ever dreamed of having."

Sim looks around and nods, "Thanks guys. Nice to hear all that stuff, but I don't see how it can help me with my control problem. I planned to get the snakes. I saw the issue with trashing the deck coming, but I didn't foresee hurting a kid like that." He shakes his head. "Can I go now?"

"Almost done, Sim. Just a few questions," I demand. "How does getting hit help you control yourself? What's the pain deal? And how does Nicky help you with that?"

Nick adds, "Yeah, I want to ask you about hurting yourself, too. I thought our deal was no harm, no marks, no emotional abuse. Brandy says you've got some bad belt welts on you."

Sim's face goes white and he stands up slowly with his hands on the boardroom table and hisses furiously, "That's fucking personal. I've had enough. Chain me up in the nurses' room if you want to. I'm fucking absolutely done with this. I'm out of here. This is not helping."

Nick says one word, "Down."

She taps the boardroom table once with the first fingernail on her right hand.

He sits down quickly and quietly and says, "Yes, Nick."

She pushes up from the boardroom table slowly and takes a few careful steps so she's standing behind his chair. Putting her left hand on the back of his heart and the other across his forehead, she leans down and whispers in his ear.

His eyes shut in relief and his face is suddenly peaceful. He puts his head back against her and relaxes as she kisses the top of his head and keeps her hands on him.

"A couple of you have known him longer than me, but I know my boy better than any of you, even better than his brother. So this may come as a shock to you."

Sim's smile is as soft as a sleeping baby and he keeps his eyes closed.

"He's a perfectly obedient boy. He's exquisitely obedient, aren't you, baby?"

He smiles wider and nods happily, eyes still closed.

"No one has ever told him what to do. But he loves it, don't you, baby?"

He nods again.

"Stay here and talk with us, baby."

"Yes, Nicky," he says. "Whatever you like, baby."

"And that, my friends, if you want to know how kinky he gets, is it. He's into it. You don't negotiate with him. You don't ask him. Just tell him. He loves it when you communicate and tell him what you want. But it's so important that you acknowledge and appreciate him. Throw the boy a bone when he pleases you.

"Nat, you could have stopped him from throwing the furniture off the deck with just one word. Billy could've stopped him from beating Prince the same way."

"What word?"

"'Stop.' You don't even have to say please. If you want to use two words you could try 'down, boy'. He's as well trained as a pedigreed show dog," she laughs.

"What did you just whisper to him, Nicky?" I wonder.

"I said 'Good boy'. That's better than sex to him. My sweet Shiva gets off on adoration."

†

NICK

It feels so good to have my hands on my boy again. I can literally feel him purring with pleasure. The rest of the house is staring at us but I don't care. I own him. He owns me.

"Kama Dave, beautiful, please make something nice for him," I order.

"Me too?" he asks jumping up.

"You too, baby. We'll wait for you," I lie.

As soon as he's out of earshot, I ask Nat, "Do you really want to go all the way with this in front of Dave? You know how suggestible he is."

She shakes her head. "I guess not, Nicky. I'm seriously concerned that you're going to hurt him beyond repair. We should move him back upstairs before this gets serious."

I pet his beautiful black hair and continue praising him.

"You're the strongest man alive, S&M. There's no man as strong as you on every level, body, energy, mind, heart and spirit. The whole kitchen sink."

Nat gasps when I say that.

"Are you controlling him, Nicky?"

I laugh.

"No, honey. I'm stroking him. It's very harmful to ask people to behave a certain way without giving them some positive strokes. If I don't reward him, he'll be frustrated and depressed. That's probably why he's run off the rails. He's trying to orchestrate the whole universe and not getting any thanks. It's not the control that gets him off, it's the adoration, right baby?"

"Right, baby," he purrs.

Kama Dave comes back with two tumblers of some mixture and tops them off with bourbon.

"My special cherry jam with blue lotus and lemon sour," he boasts putting them down on the table.

"Better get me one, too, Dave," Jain begs. "This is getting bizarre pretty fast."

When Dave goes back to the kitchen I tell S&M to open his eyes and talk to us. I hand him a drink and say, "Thank you, baby. You're so strong."

Nat says, "Damn. Kamadev copies everything Sim does. He wouldn't even talk to a woman until he found out Sim was married. Are you going to turn Dave into another pet, Nick? As a therapist, this is very disturbing to me."

"We could never have that kind of relationship, Nat. It's special. S&M is the only man I have this with. It can't be duplicated."

S&M takes a big swig of the bourbon sour and laughs. He looks composed, powerful, recharged. I've turned his lights back on.

"Blue lotus bourbon sour, where does he get these ideas? The boy is mad. But it's awesome. Taste it Nicky. Please, baby."

I taste it. It's the weirdest cocktail I've ever had. Alcohol is not my thing. But I say, "Thank you for sharing, baby. Do *you* like it?"

"I'd rather drink it straight but he likes it, so I'm drinking it for him. Thanks for tasting it, honey. You're so sweet." When Dave comes back he adds, "Good drink, Kama Dave. Thanks for making those for us. Nicky likes it but she doesn't want to fall on her face again."

Jain and Nat are watching us like we're insane, stroking each other in a three way.

"Kamadev, baby," Nat says, "why don't you go play with Brandy for a while? I think she has some new ideas for your hair."

Dave holds up his drink and grins.

"I'm just getting started," he growls. "Tell us about it, Nicky. What did you do to him? Did you trample him like Nat did?"

Jain winces and frowns.

"Why not let him stay, Nat?" S&M says. "I want him to know the score. You haven't always been so worried about disturbing him."

Kama Dave snorts back a laugh and nearly chokes on the Blue Lotus sour.

"Go for it, Nicky," S&M says. "Complete disclosure I think, honey. What the fuck do I care?"

Jain puts the whole drink down in one chug. "Go for it, Nick," he says.

"Well. Where to start? I guess I'll start at the start. When I moved here I just wanted to surf. But the boys were so mean, such hardcore locals, they kept trying to run me off. I got tired of it. I was strong and I trained hard but the Point Guard were so tight-knit and there were so many of them, it was hopeless. They didn't want to let girls surf the point.

"So I decided I needed an ally, the strongest of them to protect me. I started pitting them against each other. I was playing a game of chess for blood. I didn't need to fight them because they loved to fight each other. I just needed to steer."

"She caused a lot of trouble," S&M laughs and downs the drink. "Straight this time, Dave, if you don't mind." He pours a serious amount of bourbon in his glass. "But give me a few drops of the Blue Lotus."

Dave blushes and hands him the little bottle.

"You're so creative, Kama Dave," he praises him. "I can't wait to see what you think of next. Go ahead, Nicky."

"I flirted with them all and teased them. That was hard because they tended to ignore women. But I worked hard at it. I'd get them to fight each other to see who was stronger. And that was easy. They loved to fight, not out of anger but for sport.

"The winner would let me give him six lashes with a board leash to see just how strong he was. I wanted to see how far someone would go to please me, if they would be an ally I could trust."

"Oh, shit," Nat moans.

"Far out," Kama Dave nods with enthusiasm. Then he pours his next drink straight with a few drops of Blue Lotus, copying S&M.

"Nicky, did Sim win?" Dave wonders.

"Oh, yeah. He always won when he fought. He was top gun. And he found the whole thing very amusing to say the least. When some of the other guys fought, he even offered to take a whipping for the winner."

"Taking one for his brother," Jain connects the dots.

"He just didn't mind pain in the least. That's how he picked up the S&M nickname. He said pain was the best teacher on the planet."

"The Noble Truths of Buddha," Dave recites. "Pain is inevitable. Suffering is optional."

"Right. So he became my ally. He protected me and made sure no one hassled me and I got all the waves I wanted. Just like he did for you, Kama Dave, since you were 15.

"But he never wanted anything from me in return. He was celibate. He had all his bases covered. So what happened next was a karmic imbalance. I owed him so much that he owned me. I wanted to give it back to him and I wanted to be as strong as he was, so I started studying with him."

"You were the perfect student, Nicky," S&M says stroking me with praise. "I loved teaching you. I can take the story from here, Nat, from my side.

"I was done with second chakra sexual relationships at that point and I wanted to learn how to have a higher form of intimacy. Man, I used this woman," he laughs. "She had fight in her like I'd never seen and I figured I could teach her how to teach me what I wanted to learn. What I had in mind was a fifth chakra relationship that went way beyond sex."

"What the fuck?" Jain interrupts. "What the fuck is a fifth chakra relationship?"

"Vishuddha, the fifth chakra, is the seat of communication and self-expression, Jain. It has a higher vibration than the compassionate love of the heart chakra. The fifth chakra, in your throat, is a pre-requisite in Tantra for opening the third eye and fulfilling your dharma, your highest purpose."

"Oh, of course!" Jain says reaching for the bourbon bottle.

"What about the pain?" Kama Dave wonders.

"That was never my particular kink. It was always her kinkiness, testing people by beating on them. That's just basic first chakra stuff, fight or flight. I laughed at it. But that's where I went wrong with Prince yesterday. I never got off the ground, never even said hello. I just hammered him. It was a classic first chakra fucked up relationship. And now I owe him."

Nat whistles and finally asks in wonder, "You don't enjoy being whipped?"

"Nah. Why would I? I just missed impressing my fifth chakra girl. I missed being told how I walked on water and what a good boy I am.

"We've had a relationship for over five years based on respect and trust. We ask for things that don't violate our trust and we acknowledge our respect.

"We never hurt each other or ask for anything abusive or damaging, although we've definitely gotten creative with some special requests. The last thing she did before I got shot was save me from drowning myself.

"You're good, Nicky. You own me. I'd put Sri Kamadev in your hands with my unconditional trust if you want. Dave? She's on your list. Green light, baby."

I laugh nervously. "I don't know what I want. Don't push me, baby."

"No pressure, sugar. I'm here for you. Good to see you again, just in the fucking Nick of time before I dove off the deck," he laughs.

"Does that help, Sim?" Nat asks. She looks rattled. She thought she knew my boy after a couple weeks. Coldest day in hell she's ever seen.

"That really helps," he sighs. "I remember my dharma now, my highest purpose, turning all the fucking lights on."

Then he turns to me and says, "Nicky, you belted Prince Albert? He's just a kid. Maybe 19 years old max. I understand now why I did it, but why did *you* do that?"

"He asked me to kiss him. I hit him to see how willing he was to please me for a kiss. But he ran away before I could give him one."

"Well, maybe you should give him a kiss now for me. I hit him triple bad."

Kama Dave looks at me curiously and says, "Nicky, I don't want you to hit me. Why did you kiss me without belting me?"

"Baby Dave," I say, "You're special. I would never hit you unless you say 'Game On'."

Nat is glaring at me now in abject horror.

"How old are you, Nicky? You're way too fast for him."

"How old are *you*, Nat?" I sneer. She puts her head down and shuts up.

†

S&M

The sooner you take care of a karmic debt, the less interest, fees and penalties you'll have to pay. I push Nicky over to the Ice House to face Mack with me. I know exactly what to do now.

"Mack, I did the therapy like you asked. I can fix everything. Would you please ask Sean to come up again? And have him get the gun from Billy."

"You can fix everything after three hours of therapy and five shots of bourbon? I've got to see this."

"Give me 45 minutes, brother," I wink and wheel Nicky into IC.

Prince is sitting up in bed with Brandy watching over him. I give her a long deep kiss. I know she can taste the bourbon on me, but she doesn't object. Prince doesn't seem very happy to see me. He isn't thrilled to see Nicky either. In fact he's horrified.

"Don't let him near me, nurse. And don't let *her* hit me again. Please," he moans.

"Sim, you terrorist," Brandy says. "Since when did you start torturing minors? He's afraid of his own shadow."

"Good morning, Prince," I say humbly, ignoring her. "I brought you a peace offering."

I help Nicky stand. Prince raises his hands to protect his head but she just waits. When he finally gives up and takes a peek at her, she touches one finger to her lips and then puts it on his. His mouth opens in astonishment and she bends down and kisses him full on.

"I'm sorry I hit you, baby," she says. "I was just playing. You forgot to take this."

She kisses him again, longer and deeper.

"And that one's from S&M. He's really sorry, too. He'd kiss you himself but you already think he's gay. He's queer but not like that."

I make a face at Brandy and she reads me loud and clear. She gives Prince a kiss too, soft and easy without any heat. Prince's mouth is hanging open like a panting dog.

"I don't believe this," he says. "What kind of psycho game are you playing?"

"I'm dead serious, Prince Albert. You just kissed my wife and my girl friend. Which did you like better, the bourbon flavor or the cinnamon pearl?"

"Don't fuck with me," he swears. "I have friends."

I can see him considering how useless his connections are now that I've put him out of business.

"Like I said, honey, you kissed my wife, you kissed my girl. I'm here with my hand open." I put my palm up in the mudra of the Buddha. "'Ahimsa'. It means 'No Harm'. My hand is empty, no weapons. I owe you. I ruined your business. I want to ruin your business. I don't want you pushing dope on my beach again. But I caused damage and I want to fix it."

"You can't fix it," he hisses. "I owed $2500 last night and didn't show up. I lost my integrity. There's a $50,000 reward for taking you down and now there's probably a free drink reward for anyone who gets me. I was already in trouble for losing all of that heroin when they busted your house. I'm fucked."

"Mmmmm. $50K, nice. How much did they get for killing Darrell?"

"10K I think. It doesn't matter."

"Probably not. But I'm wondering, because you didn't show up last night, would it help to have a note from a doctor?"

"Fuck," he swears. "You fucking worthless bitch tease. A note from a doctor? How sick are you?"

"Not half as sick as yesterday," I laugh. "I'm going to buy all that dope Billy dumped out yesterday. Call your connection and tell them to pick up $2500 in full from Crystal at the Nest bar tonight with a note from Doctor Jain saying you were assaulted and you're in the hospital. You're free to go back into business. Is that what you want to do?"

He glares at me. "I haven't got a lot of choices. There's not a lot of business opportunities for a guy my age."

"Fine with me. I'm trying to give you a choice. Right now I'm covering your ass because I hurt you. Call your man and tell him to have some one pick up payment in full. I'd like to put a note in the envelope saying you quit. Think about it.

"I'll give you the gun back tonight, too, so if you want that $50,000 reward, I'm an easy target here. It's money in the bank if you're that desperate. If you want to talk about other options, I've got some."

He blows a big gusty sigh. I'm not sure if it's relief or disbelief. I wait.

"What do you want from me?" he says at last.

"Forgiveness. Maybe down the road, trust and respect, but for now forgiveness would be sufficient."

I hand him a tissue and add, "Wipe your face, Prince Albert. You've got lipstick on you."

†

NICK

"Mmmm, honey," I tease him. "You taste like 18. How old are you, Prince?"

He blushes and frowns. "I'm 28," he lies.

"Bull, sweetheart. S&M is 28. You're not a day over 18. Don't be embarrassed about it. You can't buy youth. It's more precious than gold."

"Look, Prince," S&M cuts in, "we've got some more business. Have you ever had a real job? I guess at your age you haven't got much experience, right?"

Prince Albert shakes his head and says, "This is my first job, sales. I wanted to be a chef but my father said it was a gay job."

"Is that where you got your homophobia, from you father?" I ask. "Where did you get those ideas about S&M being gay? He probably had 300 women before he was 21." My laugh cuts short when I see Brandy's face go white.

"Maybe 250," S&M winks at me and pretends to count on his fingers.

"That was what I heard on the street, that he hated women. Those photos in the paper posing with the cops and the handcuffs looked totally gay. And his junkie friend dresses like a girl. It added up."

"Are you a good cook, Prince?" S&M changes the subject. "Because I really want to see you change your profession. What would you do if you had the freedom to do anything?"

"I like to cook. I'd be a great chef."

"Listen. I'm giving you a couple choices. You can go back to pushing dope somewhere else and end up in prison. Or you can stay at my beach house with Sean until you get yourself together. Or you can work for us up here as our private chef, that is, if we like your food. We pay very well and I think you'd like working with us. So think about those options.

"I just need a favor from you."

"What do you want?" he looks very suspicious about all of it.

"I need a note for my brother saying that you forgive me so I can get out of hot water. Please."

"I don't know if I do. My head fucking hurts. My ribs are broken. You're saying you'll pay off my $2500 account, give me my gun back, and let me stay for free in the beach house or give me a job? I don't know. I need to think about it."

"And don't forget the kisses," I tease. "I can guarantee that you will be well supplied with attention and kisses every day. We've got some beautiful women up here who would enjoy helping you out in that department."

"Deal," Prince says. "Where do I sign?"

S&M takes me back to Mack's office. I haven't met him yet, but he knows who I am. I give him the note from Prince.

I forgive Steven Mack, aka S&M, for beating me up and robbing me yesterday. Signed, sincerely, Prince Albert
Witnessed by Brandy Petersen Mack
Witnessed by Nancy aka Nicky Dixon OXO

Mack is speechless then he starts laughing. "Is this genuine?"

"That's why we had it witnessed, Dr. Mack," I say. "You can ask him if he really means it."

"Amazing. I think your therapist deserves a raise."

"Actually, Mack," he says, "I don't think she's very happy with me at the moment. It's all really Nicky's doing."

"Whatever," Mack says. "I'm happy with this. Sean will be up to see you later. I think he'll like this very much, Steven. Nice save, brother. I guess I'm not going to have to lock you up after all."

"Speaking of that," S&M says groveling a little lower, "I'd still like to use the old nurses' room for some private business I have with my girl. Would that be possible?"

"Well, it's vacant, but don't damage anything, okay?" He winks at me.

I look at S&M and he's definitely just bit the head off a canary, he's grinning so hard.

"Come on, honey," he says, "We need to talk. Can you deal with the stairs if I help you?"

I nod and he helps me up to the nurses' room at the top of the stairs. I'm a little nervous about his intentions. Are we going to play a little? There's enough privacy up here to get rough if he's into that today. We sit on the bed and he holds my hands, gazing into my eyes with love.

"Nicky," he says. "I appreciate everything you do for me. You're the sexiest most beautiful woman in the whole world and that's not just a stroke. I'd like to show you how I feel, but the truth is I'm all over the map right now. You can ask my wife. I'm more erratic than erotic.

"But if you've got three hours to spare, I can send the God of Love over. Why do you think Nat is being so protective of him? She said he's redefined transcendental sex. She won't let you alone with him in the Fire House, but I can guarantee you'll have some privacy here."

I'm shocked. He's pimping Kama Dave.

"Nick?" he says when I don't answer.

"You mean pure and simple sex? With Dave? I don't know, honey."

"Omnivorous Kali, indiscriminate gourmet of all the world's flavors. You won't *ever* know if you don't have a taste. I don't think it will be pure or simple, but I highly recommend him. Why don't you give the boy a chance?"

I blush furiously. The fact is I'd really like a taste of that. It just seems too personal to do it this way. Then I remember how personal we got with S&M this morning, how good it turned out to be for him.

"Do you think he'd come if you asked him?" I wonder.

He roars, "I don't think he ever stops coming. But I guarantee you will, girlfriend."

†

DJ

Jain's helping me with my bicep curls but I don't care. Nicky's gone. Sim took her away this morning. I forgot how much she loves him and I've lost her. Nat is being very nice, putting some beautiful flowers upstairs in my old room so I can move back. She kisses me deep and not very controlled and says she's sorry she ever said good-bye. I thought she wasn't allowed upstairs.

Then Jain takes me out to the gym, but I don't care. He says just sit down for a minute and get your head screwed back on. We all had too much bourbon for breakfast. Just sit. Breathe. I see Sim walking across the lawn smiling like he won the lottery. He won so much more. I put my head down.

"Hey, Jain," he says. "I want to teach Dave some yoga. Are you done here?"

"Fine with me, Sim," he says. "His heart isn't into weights today."

"Baby Dave," Sim whispers in my ear. "Can you get me some saffron, blue lotus and sandalwood? I'll wait. Don't tell anyone."

I hate to give him my best love oils but I get them from my room. He's still my teacher. My heart is broken and I don't need them anymore. I bring them back outside and give them to him.

"No," he says. "Not for me. Nicky wants it. She was wondering if you could give her a massage. Do you have a couple hours?"

My heart stops. Sim puts his nose on my neck and sniffs.

"Yeah, you're solid gold, Kama Dave. What you got, she wants. Take this shit over to Mack's house. Up the stairs on the left. And lock the door behind you, honey. There are a lot of jealous women up here. Don't hurt yourself."

I stop breathing and he hits me on my back.

"Are you up to it or not, honey? Don't keep my girl waiting. I think she loves you."

"Me?"

"Sri Kamadeva, yes you. Take the paint off the walls, baby. I'll cover for you."

I don't believe it but then I don't care if I believe it or not. If Nicky wants the oils that's the least I can do. As I'm walking over to the Ice House, I start thinking about the most I can do if she asks me nicely. Oooof. I knock on the door at the top of the stairs and she opens it and lets me in. She locks the door and kisses me soft and controlled.

"I brought the oils, Nicky," I say. "S&M said you wanted a massage. Is that okay?"

"Everything you do is okay. Are you going to make me cry today, baby?"

I laugh. I think she's playing with me. But she puts her hands on my neck and slowly pushes the silk off my shoulders. She kisses my hickey and she makes it worse. She breathes me and tastes me. I can feel her heart beating against mine.

"Beautiful boy," she says, "what can I do for you?"

"Show me, Nick," I say. "Ask me nicely."

She takes her top off and says, "Please with sugar on it, Kama Dave. Kiss my heart, baby."

I forget about the massage, about the oils. I put my hands on her back and kiss her heart, her breasts, her mouth. She tastes like cinnamon sugar. She tastes like birthday cake and sea salt and moonlight. I put my right hand on her tailbone and send a whisper up her spine while I kiss her ear.

"You know this, don't you? I'm going to make you cry for mercy, Nicky. You can tell me to stop if I hurt you."

"You can have me," she says.

"I have to go slow, Nick," I explain. "I'll take your body but what I want is your heart and soul. It could take a long time. Have you got a couple days?"

"Yes, pretty please," she says.

"Then take it easy. Lie down and let me destroy you properly."

I get a glass and mix the sandalwood with lotus and saffron and start drizzling it drop by drop on her heart, her belly, smoothing it out like glass with my hands and then with my own belly on hers. Then there's no edge between us, no separation of her and me.

"You know Tantra." I put my hand behind her waist. "I like it best when my heart comes. Coming through the top of your head is nice, but through the heart is the best."

I move my hand up behind her back and roll her on top of me so I can rub more oil into her back. She hasn't got a scar around her heart. I think of my beautiful Kali on the futon in the jasmine moonlight and I feel her all around me. It's the same river that I felt in her flowing now in a current that doesn't care where or when I begin or end.

Nicky falls on me like rain. I can taste my own jasmine honey skin in her cinnamon mouth. I kiss her cherry jam cheeks.

"Show me, Kamadev," she begs with her hands clawing into my poor wrecked jeans, pulling the zip down. I take her hands off me and stand up so she can watch me undress. I can tell she loves me now. She watches me like she looks at Sim but even nicer. I pull her pants off and admire the outside of her. I've been waiting forever to see her and I could die happily if I stopped now. But I'm not stopping. The light's green.

I lie down next to her again and put her hand back on me and all the Christmas colored lights come on, red, orange, yellow, green, blue, violet and blinding white flashes.

"This is only the physical shit, baby," I assure her. "starting with the first kosha. Then I'm going to short circuit your prana. Don't scream when I start fucking your mind. I can slow it down anytime you ask."

She's done talking to me. It's all she's got just to keep breathing and biting me. She puts me inside her and tries to start me going, but I don't want animal sex. She knows kundalini and I just wait for her to beg nicely. Even then, I wait some more. There's no place to go, I'm in her. I can wait until the world ends before I move. When she starts to cry I release the prana, lighting her up from her root to the top of her tree.

The rivers of fire and ice begin to flow, calm on the surface with raging undertows and I pull her into the deep end with me. I take her down to the reef on the bottom of the ocean where waterfalls pour through shafts of light in liquid green glass.

I leave her beautiful body floating far above on the surface and dive into her mind, fucking her sanity. When she starts screaming, I fill her mouth with my tongue and smother the sound. I'm just starting.

One layer at a time, her body, energy, mind, heart and spirit, I take everything. Then I start doing all the layers at once, fucking the whole kitchen sink. I rearrange all the furniture in her house, repossess her heart and take a second mortgage on her soul. She's never going to look at Sim again. She's mine.

†

S&M

Sean brings the gun into Mack's office and sits down. He's tired so I want to keep it simple.

"First off, Sean," I begin, "I know I screwed up, but it's turned out for the best. A courier will come by the Nest tonight at 10 and ask for this. It's Prince's business investment."

I give him an envelope with $2500 cash and a couple of notes. One from Jain certifies that Prince Albert was assaulted and is under medical care. Another from Prince says that he is unable to continue in his position as regional sales manager for the Point. I also show him the note to Mack saying I've been forgiven.

"I'm really sorry, Sean. Do you want a word with him?"

It's late afternoon and the light is dim in IC. Prince Albert is resting with his eyes closed and Brandy is sitting with him, massaging his feet. Sean sits next to the bed and picks up another note on the bedside table, a shopping list in a feminine script.

Eggs, cream, sharp feta, greek yoghurt, parmesan, raddichio, eggplant.

"Moussaka," Brandy says. "We're working on some of his favorite recipes."

"Hmmph. Recipes, right," Sean mutters.

Prince opens his eyes and smiles. He's pretty stoned on Norco.

"How's it going, buddy?" Sean asks. "How's your head? Are you ready to go back to town yet?"

"Not now," he says.

Sean puts the gun on the bedside table.

"It's still loaded," he says. "Be careful with that. I got the money from Sim so the bartender can settle your account tonight. No strings attached. We won't hassle the courier."

"Thanks, officer," he says. "I apologize for the inconvenience. I quit."

"I saw the note. You quit dealing? You're not going back?"

"Nope," he says. "I'm working for S&M now. I'm staying here. I've got a better business opportunity."

Sean throws me an incredulous smile. "That's it? He works for you now?"

"Too easy, Sean," I smirk. "He's a pretty good businessman. His sales were $2500 a day, but I told him we raised a half million on Sunday. It would take him 7 months to do that at his rate, working 7 days a week.

"And he didn't really like that business much. Not enough freedom. I have nothing personal against him, just his product line. You won't have any more trouble from us. Are we good?"

"We're gold, Sim," Sean laughs. "I'll go back to doing what I do best and you keep doing what you do best, enlightening me."

We go back to the office and Sean says the words I love to hear, "Damn, he's good, Mack."

When he leaves, Mack motions for me to have a seat.

"You're not free yet, little brother," he laughs. "I've had a couple complaints from Sunny about the noise upstairs. Not bloody murder, but screams. What the fuck? Do I want to know what you've got going on in the nurses' room?"

"Ooops," I'm supposed to be covering that. I look at my watch, pick up the phone and dial 4. No one answers for 20 rings and then I hear Kama Dave say, "What."

"Three hours was up three hours ago. You're disrupting the house. Come down. It would be nice if you fed her."

"I'm not finished, Sim," he announces. "I've got her heart but I haven't got her soul quite yet."

"You don't need to do it all at once, Kamadev. She's not going to run away. How's her mind doing?"

"Uh, totally destroyed. She won't be hitting you again, Sim," he laughs. "I don't think she's going to be hitting anyone."

†

NICK

I like Sunny. She's got the same fire as I do. S&M asks her to give me a hand after he drags Kama Dave out of the nurses' room with that "I told you so" smirk of his.

"Did he live up to his warranty, Nicky?" he teases me mercilessly. "Do you want a refund?"

I hit him with a pillow and tell him to go fuck himself with my sweetest smile. My clothes were ripped when I got here, so I've just got the little yoga top and sweat pants that Nat gave me, and a silk kimono. Sunny draws me a bath in Dr. Mack's room and pulls out a few dresses for me to try.

The bath water is thick with the oils he put on my skin and the hot steam smells like Kama Dave. My mind is riveted on the thought of him. He put his little silver necklace on me, but he kept the handcuff key around his own neck. He said he's got the key to me now.

Everything S&M taught me about pranic sex, Kama Dave knows. But Dave took it a lot further than kundalini. He went all the way with it. I've done a lot of stuff but I've never had sex in all five koshas at once. The boy has definitely redefined transcendental sex. S&M did not exaggerate in his promotional advertising.

"I don't know him, but Brandy does," Sunny says. "Be careful with him, Nicky. He was addicted to heroin less than a week ago and he was arrested on two felonies. He's dangerous and he's facing a prison term. Both those boys are far too fast for safety. And both are out of their minds. Brandy says Sim is getting violent."

I start laughing and get out of the tub. Hmm. Brandy says S&M is violent?

"Sunny, S&M is a perfect pet. He's not normally violent. We're helping him with that. And Dave is a puppy. I've known those guys for almost six years. I trust them. Brandy doesn't know them very well yet. They're really very good boys."

"Nicky," she reminds me, "didn't you see what Sim did to that boy downstairs in IC? I assisted Dr. Jain with the surgery. Thirty-eight stitches in his head. It was horrible. And I helped stitch Dave's hand before you got here. He attacked Nat, smashed a window and tried to beat Dr. Jain with a drip stand pole."

I think about it for a minute but my heart isn't listening. I pick the green dress and while she helps me with my hair I decide to quit using the wheel chair. I'm going to start walking again. I'm on the team. I'll crawl up the stairs if I have to, to get to Dave's room.

†

DJ

Sim and I are meditating on the futon at the top of the world, breathing the natural juice of the forest and blowing smoke at the evening star. I've stuck another handful of jasmine buds behind my ear because they intoxicate me when they're so close to my nose.

"Kamadeva, you freak," he teases me. "You're giving me a bad reputation by running around with all the flowers, silk, jewelry and perfumes. Prince thought you were my boyfriend."

"I am," I laugh. "I'm everybody's boyfriend. But the God of Love knows what's sexy and doesn't give a damn what anyone else thinks. Try it."

I put some of the jasmine behind his ear and tell him to shut up and do nadi shodhana. I've never told my teacher what to do before, but after eight rounds, he says, "Shit. You're right, Kamadev. You're on to something."

"Yeah, it's important to put the flowers on the left side because you're breathing directly into the right brain, you know, the mad side. It unlocks the door to your soul. That's where it starts getting seriously sexy."

"Maybe I should start taking Tantra lessons from you, Dave," he sighs. "My sex life is bizarre. I think all those years of celibacy have confused me."

"Nah, Sim," I tease him, "You're just getting old. I'm sure you were just as hot as me when you were my age."

His mouth falls open and he looks wounded.

"Fuck, I'm teasing, Sim. You're a sexual legend. Bizarre and confused are just fine when it comes to sex. Don't ever try to straighten it out. Sex likes a good twist."

"Thanks, buddy," he says, "I'd kiss you, but I've already done that once today and I don't want to make a habit of it. Anyway, I don't think I taste as nice as Nicky."

"No you don't. And you don't have the electrical wiring she's got either."

I start thinking about Nicky's pranic circuit diagrams and her cardio-respiratory system. I've always loved her little muscles and sea green eyes, but now I realize I was in love with the frosting and didn't even know there was cake involved. I start to get a little hungry again. I still have a lot of business to take care of with her.

"Calm down," he says reading me, "She'll call when she's ready. She knows you're here. I hope this isn't too much to ask from the God of Love, baby, but do you think you could be a little more discreet about it? You'll break Nat's heart."

"Maybe I should move back to the Ice House," I suggest thinking I'd like to just lock myself up in the nurses' room with her for a couple weeks.

"Your court date is in two more weeks. If you and Mack fuck up one more time with the morphine, it's all over for you. You've only been clean for a week. Won't prison hurt that much harder now that you've got a beautiful woman? Ouch. Concentrate on behaving. I'm not letting you screw this up."

Ooops, I forgot about prison. I've been too busy thinking about sex to think about prison. Except when we went in to look at Prince I remembered what we were doing with two bricks of heroin in the closet and a couple bags of coke. Needles and dreams and smoke on a permanent vacation I almost forgot I took. Oh, shit.

I start to tell him to just lock me up with her, but that's not what he wants to hear.

"Control," I say. "I've got complete control, Sim. Discretion. You can call me Discreet Dave."

I'll behave like a perfectly obedient boy, just like him. I know what he wants to see now. I shake his hand. I mean it. Even Nicky can't knock me off this pedestal.

When the phone rings, I want to run to it, but I'm watching my control now, like I'm standing back watching a movie of myself. I don't move. S&M smiles, gets up slowly and goes into the bedroom to answer.

"Nicky's on her way over with Sunny," he says coming back with a little smirk.

"Nice," I say, very nice and controlled. Game on.

Nicky takes forever getting here. She's trying to walk but even with Sunny helping her she's pretty slow. I'm thinking about what Nat said, that Nicky is too fast for me, and I start laughing out loud.

I stop laughing pretty quickly when I see her. Sunny has given her a long green dress the color of her eyes. Little gold stars are woven into the fabric, floating as soft as the breeze on her fragrant skin. She's looking at me differently, shy for the first time, and my toes start to melt. Sim gets up from the futon to make room for her next to me.

Just don't fucking touch her, Kama Dave, I tell myself, or you won't be able to stop. Control. I stand up, too, and help her sit down.

"That dress looks beautiful on you, Nicky," I say. "I mean you make the dress look beautiful."

She laughs and blushes. She's got my little silver handcuff necklace around her neck.

"Thank you, baby," she says. "My clothes are wrecked. Sunny helped me out."

I offer my spot on the futon to Sunny and ask if she'd like to sit down. I'm so polite I almost have to laugh at myself, but I don't. I just watch myself behaving perfectly. Sim is snickering a little, though.

"I'm sorry if I disturbed you, Sunny," I apologize. "I got carried away with the noise."

She looks at me shocked and embarrassed and then in amazement. She hasn't talked to me since I punched out the cabinet door when I was loaded and she helped Dr. Jain stitch me up. She doesn't even know me. But she takes my Om hand and accepts my offer to sit down. She holds it and takes a close look at the scar and my little tattoo and then looks me in the eyes for the first time.

"It's very beautiful here," she says. "I haven't been over here since the morning the police brought you up. You look like a different person now, Dave," she adds. "You look a lot better without all the snot and blood on you."

"Thanks, Sunny. I feel pretty nice now, too, without the dope. I feel a lot better."

I taste a lot better and smell better too, but it's probably not polite to say.

†

BRANDY

Prince Albert reaches for his gun when Nat comes in. He's still got that primitive reactive response to anything unexpected that's commonly seen with traumatic head injuries. I learned that in nursing school. Any sudden movement and he goes for the loaded gun.

Nat raises both hands in Ahimsa and says, "Oh my God, honey!" and starts walking backwards towards the door.

He glares at her suspiciously and says, "Who are you?" the gun still leveled at her chest.

"I'm Nat," she says calmly. "I'm a therapist. I came to help you."

He holds the gun steady and thinks about it.

"I work for Sim, he's my boss," she adds.

"Oh, all right then," he says putting the gun back on the table. "I work for him, too. I'm his personal chef."

Nat's eyes widen and she looks at me and taps her head.

"Yes, he's got a concussion," I say, "but he's not delirious. Sim hired him. I think he's going to be moving into your house. Prince Albert, Nat can help with your broken ribs. She went through the same thing. I'm mean, Sim didn't kick her in the ribs, but she broke a few."

"Same problem that Nicky had," she laughs. "Gravity attacked me."

He's still staring at her cautiously so I whisper to her that Sim said he needs extra physical attention because he's traumatized. Kiss him, I instruct her. It doesn't have to be a heavy kiss, just let him know he can trust you.

"Really?" she wonders, "Boss's orders? That's not a problem for me."

She bends down and gives him a very sweet kiss that changes the electrical charge of the room. He likes it and he smiles up at her like the teacher's pet. She seems to like it very much herself and she shows him a lot of her teeth. He's nearly half her age but I don't think she's counting.

"He's a lot easier than Dave, Nat," I assure her, knowing my words can be construed suggestively as well as professionally. I don't care if she takes a sexual interest in the patient as long as she takes him. I'm tired.

She tears her eyes off him long enough to ask me if I know what happened to everyone. Both her patients have been missing all day. I tell her what I saw leaving out the innuendo of what I know.

"Dave's doing yoga with Sim and Sunny's taking care of Nicky," I say with all veracity.

She breathes a sigh of relief and turns her attention back to Prince Albert, planning all of the things she knows to make him feel better.

I tell her I'll be at the pool house. Dial 5 if you need me.

It's been a long day. I leave her sitting next to his bed, holding his hand and I pick up the leather restraining cuffs on my way out.

†

S&M

Brandy comes through the kitchen door brandishing the padded hospital cuffs. She doesn't say a word but holds them out to me laughing. I'm sitting on the floor of the deck and pretend to reach up to grab them, but I take her wrist instead and pull her down on top of me pinning her to my heart in a submission lock.

"Oh my God, Sim," she protests, "Your friends are here."

"It's okay, baby, when I say it's okay," I instruct her.

Nicky cheers and looks at the cuffs curiously, then stares at me.

"And?" I challenge her. "I'm just playing with them."

I toss the cuffs over to the futon and she picks them up.

"Beginners' version," I say. "I've got the police regulation ones I took off Kama Dave in my bedroom. For more experienced complicated stuff," I wink at her.

She smiles and takes a sly look at Dave and I can hear the gears hammering in her head.

"Go ahead," I offer. "Take them home and have some fun with them. I got married because of those. If you need anything more complicated, just ask the nurses. Surgical tubing, rubber gloves, scalpels, masking tape, oxygen, Sunny can get it, right baby?"

Sunny laughs nervously, not sure if I'm teasing or not.

"No hypodermic syringes for Dave though," I add.

"Prince Albert just pulled a gun on Nat," Brandy says. "He's a little jumpy. Is it loaded? Shouldn't we lock that up?"

"Nah, its okay. I destroyed his equilibrium. He needs the gun to help ground him again. He's still scared. And yeah, it's loaded, but it's loaded with blanks. Sean took care of that. I didn't think he'd try to use it. I bet he's never fired a gun in his life."

"Good to know," she says and then she turns to Nicky who's still examining the leather cuffs. "Here, honey." She takes a split ring out of her pocket and shows Nicky how to rig the cuffs together.

"Sunny," I laugh at the horror on the nurse's face, "you really should hang out with us more often. You might be able to teach my brother some new tricks."

Her face drains of color and now she's thinking how much she wants to kill me, so I tell her there's a $50,000 reward for doing that. She can get real bullets from Mack if she's serious. I can see her considering her options and then she blushes.

"Shit, I'm sorry, Sim," she apologizes. "I need to lighten up, don't I?"

Nicky is trying to put one of the cuffs on Dave but he shakes his head and whispers something in her ear. She stops fooling around in a heartbeat and hands him the cuffs. He winks at me and mouths the word "discreet."

"So, Nicky," I say, "I want to move Prince Albert into your room. He's going to cook for us and that's closest to the kitchen. So I've got a couple ideas for you. You can sleep with him," I tease, "or you could move into the old nurses' room next to Sunny and Mack – "

Before I go any further, she interrupts me. "How about Dave's room?"

"That's not very discreet," I observe. "I don't want to disrupt the house."

"My room's got a bath, Nicky," Dave offers. "The nurses' room doesn't. I like a hot oil bath. Why don't you take my room and I'll sleep on the couch."

"S&M," Nicky begs, "Dave needs 24/7 supervision for the next two weeks. Brandy and you must be tired of it. You can trust me to watch him. I'll sleep on the sofa like Brandy was doing. You've known me for six years, sugar. I invented discretion."

Kama Dave smiles at his Om tattoo while he pets her hair. "Good girl," he purrs.

†

NAT

Sim taps on the doorframe and asks Prince for permission to enter before coming in, a wise move I will keep in mind for the future.

"Hey, Prince," he says, "I've got a private room for you next door, next to our dining room and kitchen. You can move in anytime you want. The only deal is no narcotics in our house, so no Norco or morphine over there.

"You know how much junk Dave was doing before he was arrested. He can't be around it. We've got a hearing soon to see if he goes back to jail.

"It's your choice when you want to get out of here. Nat's experimenting with some interesting alternative painkillers and she can teach you about nutrition and medicinal herbs. I'm sure you're a good chef, but she can help elevate you to celebrity Ayurvedic bodybuilding chef. She's a very good teacher.

"How's your head doing?"

"It hurts somewhere in the distance. I can see why people like narcotics, but its kind of dull, like the volume's turned down on everything."

"Does that suit you, Nat?" he asks me, knowing he's the boss and doesn't negotiate. "I'm going to have Nicky take Brandy's place on the sofa so she can watch Dave this week and let us get some sleep. She can help you with Prince, too.

"Sure, boss," I say. "How's your back doing today?"

"Much better, thanks," he smirks. "I might even be done with this kimono. I can go back to doing what I do best, walking around half naked."

He takes it off and shows me the snakes. They've faded into broad red welts without any discoloration or blistering. There won't be any scars.

"Let me work on that some more after dinner," I offer. "I'll bet I can make you forget about them tonight."

"Cool. I can't tell you how fixated I am on having sex in an actual bed. That kind of thing never used to turn me on, but now it's all I can think about. I haven't slept in a bed for days. I'm a psychotic wreck, Nat," he laughs.

†

S&M

Prince is in such filthy pain that I have to ask Jake to bring the ambulance gurney up to move him. My assistant witch doctor, Nat, has been working with her own pain and has convinced him to try her alternative painkillers, the psycho-neurological-immune system's internal endogenous drugs.

Simply put, the body is a whorehouse of chemistry that makes a traditional pharmacy look like a cheap date. Your body can synthesize almost any drug known to man—painkillers, sedatives, steroids, aphrodisiacs—just by thinking about it and providing the right ingredients for synthesis. The pharmaceutical versions are actually copies of the stuff you can make but you can't buy.

Your psycho-neurological receptors are a perfect fit for the natural versions. They were designed for this. But there's no endogenous drug dealer. You've got to make your own.

"Anandamide," she enthuses. "I'm really on to something with this, Sim. It's the chemical that fits perfectly into the morphine receptors of the brain, an endogenous cannabinoid neurotransmitter. Anandamide, the natural brain chemical Arachidonoylethanolamide, was only identified in 2006, and was named after its effect on the body, Ananda, Sanskrit for bliss."

"I'm going with you on this, Nat," I say. "Put me in the guinea pig pool for homemade morphine. I've got enough pain to sink a ship."

"The seriously kinky thing about this biochemical is that pain actually contributes to its production," she explains. "Pain can create a painkiller that's as nice as morphine. Pain is a messenger, a neuro-transmitter. If your mind becomes very efficient at anandamide production, you might even start to like pain."

"It won't be very popular, Nat, if you have to cause pain to produce it."

"No, but that's just a benefit for people already in pain. Other things that produce it are very pleasurable. The stimuli for anadamide production include orgasms, hugs, kisses, yoga, meditation, exercise, beautiful music, the things that give you 'the chills'."

I think immediately of little Alex getting off to Beethoven's Ninth in The Clockwork Orange.

"The chemical precursors are found in eggs, ice cream and chocolate: choline and inositol or lecithin. We can have some fun with this, boss."

"Ananda, blissful non-attachment, is the key that unlocks Vishhudhi the fifth chakra, my favorite. I reckon heroin and morphine short circuit enlightenment. True bliss opens the third eye."

"Anandamide has given me a lot of insight into the way conventional pain killers work," she explains. "The trouble with anandamide is that it's very short lived in the body, usually just a flash, so you need to help it out a little. Acetaminophen, the common painkiller, works because it is a re-uptake inhibitor of anandamide. What that means is it keeps the bliss molecules around longer. Tylenol and paracetamol don't kill pain, they just help increase anandamide levels.

"Pain, exercise, meditation, music and love create it. Lecithin and calcium feed it. Acetaminophen preserves it."

"Try it out on Kamadev," I suggest. "He's got anandamide production going on. He's an orgasm factory. Give him a bunch of the ingredients and see how high he gets," I laugh.

Nicky will like playing with Kamadev's fifth chakra.

†

S&M

It's late by the time I get home, but Brandy is still sitting out on the deck quietly counting the stars. When I walk out, she gets to her feet and then kneels down on the wooden deck. She's got the police handcuffs locked around her wrists and she doesn't have a key.

"How can I please you, Sir?" she says very seriously with her head bowed.

I'm shocked. I think I've probably been a little too rough on her emotionally and maybe not nearly nice enough physically. She really doesn't know me very well. I was fucked up when she met me and I'm still sorting myself out. It's time to make myself perfectly clear.

"Uh, first off, get off your fucking knees, Brandy." I help her to her feet and unlock the cuffs with the key around my neck. "If you're going to fool around with these, I'll have to get the spare key back from Kama Dave. It'll break his heart."

I give her one of my best kisses, the kind that comes from the bottom of my feet.

"On second thought, why don't you take this?" I take the key off and put it around her neck. "I wish it had a diamond on it. Jain told me you passed your exams with a perfect score. You deserve a reward.

"Tell me what you want. Ask me nice and you can have anything," I purr.

"Anything I want?" her imagination takes off and I can feel it flying around the room, then around the house, down the mountain and out into space, skipping from star to star.

"What I want," she smiles, "is you, Sim. Body, heart and soul or any little bit of you I can have. I want to look into your eyes and see myself."

"Well, I'm completely available at the moment, Brandy, every last bit of me," I offer. "Nat just finished working on my back and its much better. I don't mind if you hold me now. I wouldn't mind if it involved a bed. Would you like that?"

She puts her arms around me with her hands gently feeling my back, my shoulders and down behind my waist.

"Does that hurt, Sim?" she whispers.

"It always hurts," I confess. "It hurts everywhere on the outside and deep inside. But your hands on me don't hurt. They heal me, baby. You're pumping me full of painkillers when you look at me. Kiss me and fix me, Bran."

Nat gave me one gram of acetaminophen and two grams of pure crystal choline and inositol. Brandy gives me ninety-seven-plus kisses and eighteen or so orgasms. My mind pumps out rivers of anandamide. Pure bliss nonattachment molecules flood the opiate receptors in my brain. When the emptiness of space isn't big enough to contain me any longer, my seventh chakra reaches open like a lotus flower at sunrise.

It makes a fentanyl rush blush. It makes morphine seem heavy and dull. Nat's Rx makes the Kings of 36th Ave pushers look like ice cream peddlers.

†

DJ

The Fire House never seems to run out of hot water. I just keep running it on a steady trickle so the bathwater doesn't cool down. I've got all the windows and doors shut, steaming the whole upstairs suite with sandalwood, jasmine, blue lotus, saffron, and palo santo.

I'm just soaking in it, meditating on pranic orgasms and overdosing on pranayama. Nat gave me six caps of vitamins and told me to have some fun. Whatever gets you off, Kamadev, she said. Just chill out. Start with this, she laughs giving me one of her end of the world kisses. She's forgotten all about control. It's a good start but it won't end here. For the first time, I break a house rule. I lock the fucking door when she leaves. Arrest me.

Nat and Nicky have been fussing over the little Prince all evening and ignoring me but I don't mind much. I can have a lot of fun on my own. Anyway, he's just a baby. He called me a crybaby but he's not even old enough to drink. He wouldn't last three minutes with either of them. Oops, he can't even move or have a hug. Sim really fucked him up.

Whatever gets you off, Kamadev, she said. The hot water is giving me chills and the snorts of steam are stoning me. I'm humming in the tub and I can feel the mantras vibrating my spine and releasing pleasurable waves of prana out to my fingers and toes.

Once I've got the physical body happy and the energetic body is coming, I drop down into my mental layer, manomaya kosha. The mind is the easiest part to amuse. I just think of Nicky screaming with joy into my mouth, resonating my throat chakra. My koshas are stacking up like a perfectly baked lasagna as all the layers melt into a delicious integrated whole.

Nat says the vitamins will intensify any pleasure I enjoy. She's testing them out as painkillers to replace narcotics. So far, so good. It's not making me cry like heroin did and its much smoother. I don't even mind that Nicky's not sitting on my lap in the bathtub because my mind has already enlisted Kali, Nicky and Sage all in the hot water with me, kissing my neck, petting and stroking my happy body.

Like I said, the mental layer is pretty damn easy to manipulate, especially if you dangle some interesting sex in front of it. Your mind is even willing to believe all this shit is real, but the next layer down knows its all Maya. Nothing is real. Have fun with the sensations, play with them, feel them and then watch Kali crush them into submission under the heel of her foot. Time is a whore. Everything disappears into the black transcendence of Kali like dust in the wind.

I hear tapping on the door and then hard knocking, so I shut the water off.

"Are you okay, Kamadev?" I hear Nat. "You're not supposed to lock the door."

"And you're not supposed to come upstairs, Kali baby," I scold. "I need my privacy."

"Okay," she apologizes. "Just wondering how you feel."

"You know how I feel, Nat. I feel like the best fucking thing you ever put your hands on," I laugh. "But the vitamins are nice, too. I like it very much."

"Are you coming down for dinner, honey?" she tries. "I'm making one of Prince Albert's recipes."

"Nope. I'm dope. I'll come up here. Too busy meditating to eat, Nat. Save me some leftovers."

After she leaves, I get out of the tub and turn the hot water full on, steaming fragrant vapor and then I open up all the windows so I can perfume the universe with it. It's dark out and the stars are filthy beautiful. Orion's big sword, or maybe his cock, hangs down from his belt and points toward the smear of the Milky Way's sperm shooting across heaven.

I listen for the roar of Om in the background cosmic noise but all I hear is Sim laughing and Brandy screaming in pleasure down at the pool house. You know its love when it makes you happy to see someone else happy. I fucking love him. I come over the noise.

I unlock the door but leave it closed and lie down on the bed to count stars and let my mind go. I'm done watching imaginary bathtub fantasies and the clouds of thought.

Now I'm just sitting in a theater chair at the back row of my head behind the pituitary gland and shining my eyes on the projection screen right behind my forehead. I see fire reflected back from my third eye, candle flames and nuclear fission.

The starlight is coming from millions of miles away, exploding in space and shooting through the lens of my eyes into the stream of my consciousness. I'm sitting in the back of my head very amused by the cosmic fireworks projecting on the screen of Maya.

The longer I look at the Milky Way, the more it starts to look like diamonds than come. I see something moving on the edge of the galaxy and then I can see that all the constellations are spinning in space. Finally I hear the hum of Om in between the screams.

There's a tap on the door and it opens a little.

"Baby Dave, are you okay?" I hear Nicky and my mouth automatically spreads into a knowing smile. I know there is cake behind the sound of her voice and my mouth waters.

"I'm stoned out of my mind, Nicky," I laugh.

"Do you need anything, baby? Just checking."

"Are you crazy? I'm naked. Do you need a written invitation?"

"You said to be discreet."

"I'll show you discreet, Nicky. It's called the door lock. Sim is making so much noise that no one will notice us," I guarantee. I've got some ancient cosmic starlight to share with her and I'll double her money back if she's not satisfied.

†

NICK

How in hell did I ever overlook him? I shake my head. I ignored him for six years, but he was just a baby then, he was never like this. I made him sit outside my door for three days before S&M opened my eyes. Now I spend the evening sitting at the bottom of the stairway to his room.

He doesn't come down for dinner and I lose my appetite. Nat goes up to check on him but he won't open the door. She makes beautiful vegetarian moussaka and leaves a plate by his door, but after everyone's gone to bed I go up to check and it's still untouched.

I can smell the fragrances coming from his room though, and I have an idea what's going on in there. I try the door and it's open. He's laughing about being stoned on starlight and steam and sandalwood and invites me in. This afternoon he insisted on discretion but apparently it's all just evaporated out the window into the starlight.

I don't argue about it. I'm infatuated, intoxicated. I'm blind now. It's chilly in the room but when I touch his feet they're burning with warmth. I kiss his beautiful toes and then his belly, his heart, his neck and his third eye. He giggles like a little boy in delight.

"Now where was I when I was so cruelly interrupted by Sim?" he laughs. "I've been waiting for you, baby. Should I start all over again or just go straight for your soul?"

"You should do whatever you please, Kama Dave," I whisper. "Surprise me."

"Hmmm," he hums, "I think I'll invent something completely new for you tonight. Have you got six hours?"

"It's after midnight, baby," I tell him. "Nat will be up by six."

"Don't worry about her, sugar," he purrs. "I've got dirt on her. She won't talk."

What he's got for me surpasses anything I could ever hope to find in sleep or dreams. By the time the sun rises behind the pool house, I'm ravenous. I hear footsteps on the stairs and someone tries the door but he ignores it and reaches into a drawer next to the bed for the restraining cuffs.

"Oh, no, baby Dave!" I protest. I need a break.

"Not for sex, Nicky," he grins, "I want your hands free for that. I'm just going to take you for my prisoner now. No one said *I* can't take prisoners.

"It would be very indiscreet if we had breakfast at the boardroom table because I can't keep my eyes or my hands or my mouth off you. But I'll serve you breakfast in bed if it's okay. Sim said not to restrain anyone unless they consent. So I'm asking please."

I look at the little cuffs and realize they have no lock or key. They're just leather straps. Then I look in baby Dave's eyes and see he has the true lock and the key, pure love and adoration.

"Please," I say. "Go ahead."

He wraps me in his silk kimono then puts one of the cuffs around my left wrist and the other end around the bed headboard and smiles, "Don't go anywhere. Orange juice with no bourbon, croissants and jam. Eggs? Tea or coffee?"

"All of the above with black coffee, thank you."

He dresses in nothing but his ratty jeans and the white prayer scarf. Fifteen minutes later he comes back with a tray full of breakfast and rolls his eyes.

"I'm in deep shit apparently," he sighs getting back out of his jeans. "Worth every inch of it though don't you think? She's fucking pissed at me. She called Sim but he told her to stay out of it. He wants to deal with me personally. That is gonna hurt."

Since he's got one of my hands restrained, he spreads the cherry jam on my croissant and tears off little bites to feed me. I handle the coffee and he gives me forkfuls of scrambled eggs in between his own mouthfuls. We're both ravenous and laughing and I tell him a story about how an elephant can be trained to believe it's restrained with a simple stick and a piece of string. It's not the physical restraint that's powerful enough to hold an elephant, it's the power that the elephant bestows upon its master.

"You could tie me up with a piece of thread," I tease him, "and I could not escape from your breakfast in bed."

"Good girl," he says, feeding me the last mouthful of eggs.

"Discreet Dave," Sim says opening the door and taking in the scene. "That didn't last 24 hours, honey. What have you got to say for yourself?"

"I'm training her for the team, Sim," he explains. "She's got to eat."

"Alright," he nods looking at me, at the handcuffs, the breakfast tray and our state of undress. "You okay with this, Nicky? Did you agree?"

"Yes, sir," I answer. "I'm very good with this."

"Cool," he says. "Then I have no problem with a little consensual naked breakfast. I'll see you at the gym at 10. I'll pour some cold water on Nat. She's got her eyes on four men at the moment and she's only got four hands."

"Oh, that really hurt!" I laugh sarcastically after S&M leaves with a approving smile. "How much pain can you handle, baby?

†

S&M

I'm on deck at the gym at 9:59 sharp and the team is all squared up waiting for me. That is Nicky, Kama Dave, Jake, Billy and me, the team captain. Jain is working down at the hospital. Even considering three of us have been up all night, we've got a lot of fuel to throw on the fire.

Dave has released his prisoner long enough so she can train and since she is the most experienced bodybuilder besides Jain I put her in charge today. I'm amused by the blossoming codependency between my two old friends. He's got her so tightly wrapped around his little finger that he orbits around her. She shines so brightly from the heat of his love that he consumes her.

If Kama Dave's upstairs room were a prison cell and Nicky were the warden, he'd volunteer to be locked up permanently. Same goes for her. It's not clear which one has captured the other, which one is the jailer and which one the prisoner. From where I stand, it looks like a life sentence without parole.

"What's it going to be, Nicky?" I ask.

"Legs and back," she says. "The surfing muscles. Squats, dead lifts, rows and pull downs. If I can't destroy you with those, we'll throw in a few of the pretty muscles, delts and traps."

Nick can't work legs yet with her broken toes so she plays ringmaster for us with precision, pairing me with Dave on squats while Jake and Billy trade off dead lifts. Then we switch. With no injuries in the lower body department, the team gets some serious lifting done. My squats are still pitiful, but I'm doing them with a fierce pleasure.

She throws us some yoga warrior poses to stretch and balance before she joins us for upper back. And there she kills us. She goes hard on the rows and pull downs but I'm still in excruciating pain working my back. Dave drops down on the weights too because of the injury to his hand. Jake and Billy are healthy dogs and they give her hell, but it's clear as glass that Nicky's running the show.

Her emaciated body is brimming with new nourishment emanating from the core of her soul and she can barely contain her flashing teeth. The veins in her arms pump up in delight, her chest swells and her eyes twinkle. She's on fire.

Finally she shows a little mercy and let's us work on shoulders, light and pretty. It's a good day for us and we end up flat out on our backs on the lawn. It's been two days since I've talked to Billy and I bring him up to speed on my new personal chef, the former regional manager of my beachfront heroin Quick Stop.

"Ouch," he says. "You paid for all that junk we dumped on the beach?"

"I haven't quit paying yet," I say. "He won't actually be able to move much let alone cook for me for a few weeks. Nat's picking up the slack for him."

"Nice moussaka last night," Nicky says. "I believe there are leftovers."

Suddenly everybody is revved up and revived and on their feet at the prospect of a good feed. There are five of us, and probably only a little bit of leftovers so I'm thinking there could be blood in the kitchen if it comes down to knives and forks.

Nat's in the lab when we barge into the house, but she comes into the kitchen when she hears the voracious clamor. Billy doesn't hesitate to give her some pathetic grief about starving but he quickly changes his story and starts in on some fairly aggressive molestation, fingering a beautiful crystal pendant she's wearing around her throat.

He puts his arm around her neck and purrs, "Now that would look very beautiful on me, sister. I'll bet you would like what I could do in trade for that."

Her eyes widen and she looks to me for protection, but I'm just a poor amused witness. Kama Dave goes to her rescue putting his nose right up against hers and says, "I'll take care of that for you, Nat." He takes the necklace off her and puts it around his own neck and snarls at Billy.

"After lunch, Nat," Dave promises. "We're just starving animals. Did you save me some moussaka? I'm first in line aren't I?"

I watch my poor assistant turn red then white as she realizes she's now got six men on her poor hands, me, Kama Dave, Prince Albert, Billy, Jake and her absentee fiancée Dr. Jain. I wonder if that's enough for her.

"Let me help you, Nat," Nicky volunteers as she shoves us physically out of the kitchen into the boardroom. Dave grabs the bourbon but she takes it away from him.

"Down, baby Dave," she commands. "You're in training."

Nat and Nicky start bringing in plates. There's not really enough moussaka for us to kill over but they bring enough tahini and fig jam and whole wheat bread and egg salad and icy black tea that no one gets stabbed by a fork or dies of hunger.

Billy keeps leering at Nat's emerald earrings enviously, but his appetite subsides with every bite. I'm getting soft and careless and start thinking about going off where I can catch the sleep I missed last night.

"Nat," I beg, "I need abhyanga and yoga nidra. Please? Take me there and I'll never let these boys in your kitchen again unless you say so."

†

S&M

"What am I going to do with you, Nat?" I tease her as I strip and lie on her massage table. "You were supposed to give him up. I smell jealousy as thick as fumes."

She doesn't even bother to cover me and she doesn't follow her usual plan of starting on my fingers. Instead, she goes straight for my heart and my throat and I wonder if she's thinking about squeezing the life out of me.

"I love him, Sim," she sighs.

"More than Jain?" I wonder. "More than me?" I'm thinking it's a damn good plan that I never slept with her.

"Differently," she says. "I love Jain like a husband. But Kamadev is different. I love him like he's my baby boy."

"And me?" I whine.

"I can't even go there, boss. I worship you."

"Oh. I like that," I smile. "I do really well with worship."

She pours sweet oil into her palms and works on my tired shoulders.

"You know Hafiz?" I quote,

Even after all this time
the Sun never says to the Earth
'you owe me'
Look what happens with a love like that.
It lights the whole sky.

"That's true love, honey. Give that to Kamadev. You taught him well. If you really love him as much as I love him, you would be squealing with joy. Nicky is his heart's desire. He's loved her since he was fifteen. He loved her when he was still clueless about love.

"I've had hundreds of women I didn't care about. Dave has only had two but he has me hands down when it comes to passion. He'll always love you. You were his first."

She kisses me on my forehead and then sweetly on my lips. I open my eyes, all three of them, to ignite the fire that's laid in her heart.

"You'll never get that necklace back from him," I laugh. "Omnivorous Kali with an appetite that can eat the whole world! I wouldn't have thrown Jain under your feet if I didn't think he could handle you. You just can't eat all the cake in the house, baby."

"I'm worried she's too old for him and much too fast," she groans.

"Obviously not as fast as you are, Nat. She won't hurt him. After you got your hands on him he can blow the doors off any woman. You're a legend, honey. Jealousy is so far beneath you."

I can feel her hands relaxing a little as she works down towards my feet so I keep teaching.

"You know the four pillars of wisdom? Patanjali summed it up nicely in the Yoga Sutras. Maitri. Karuna. Mudita. Opeksha."

"Yes, boss," she sighs. "Love, compassion, joy and equanimity."

"Right. But the joy, Mudita, is a very special kind of joy. It's the love of other people's happiness and achievements. It's not a selfish joy. It's the unbounded joy of seeing your friends and even your enemies happy. Very powerful stuff, Nat. It's the recipe for freedom.

"Never mind finishing me," I say. "Let me give you some joy."

I get up and put my jeans back on and take her dress off gently. I help her onto the massage table, cover her ass with a sheet and spread sandalwood on her beautiful back.

The scar around her heart is deep and dark and nothing will likely ever make it disappear. But the scars deep inside her heart are light and I feel them start to melt under my hands.

†

PRINCE ALBERT

"What's this mess?" I hear voices in my room, and when I open my eyes, there's the punk surf star Billy with the cinnamon girl and the crybaby. I reach for my gun but not fast enough. She grabs my hand and holds it tight.

"It's okay, Prince," she says.

Billy saunters over to the bed threateningly and sneers, "Didn't we already give you gun lessons on Monday? Lesson One: never pull a gun unless you intend to use it. And Lesson Two: be prepared to get killed if you do. Which part of that don't you comprehend?"

"Be nice to him, Billy," she says. "You might even want to apologize."

"For what? I never touched him. I might have robbed him but Sammy did the damages. I reckon he had it coming. What the fuck is he doing with the gun?"

He picks it up, unloads it and examines the bullets closely.

"Shit, man, blanks," he laughs at me and puts everything into the bedside drawer. "Get over it. Don't get me started."

The beautiful woman sits on the edge of my bed and puts a hand on my head. "How is it, Prince honey?" she says sweetly. "Can I get you anything? Tea, meds?"

My head is throbbing and my ribs ache but I got some good sleep and feel a little better. "Yeah," I say. "Sure."

"Dave, baby," she says to the junkie, "would you mind? Tea with a lot of cream in it and the pain vitamins." When he leaves the room she kisses me nicely. "I apologize for Billy," she says. "He can be an aggressive asshole, especially when he's all pumped up."

She gives Billy a serious stink-eye glare, daring him to cross her.

"Sorry Prince," he pouts. "If Sam says he's called a truce, that's good enough for me."

"Who's Sam?" I ask, confused.

"Sim, S&M. We go way back before Nicky started raising hell. It was just me, Sammy and Darrell before Nicky showed up and started organizing all the punch outs and thrashings. You can blame her for encouraging us."

The junkie kid Dave comes back with milky tea and more pills for me. Then he puts his arms around Nicky and pets her. She looks about ten years older than him and I'm shocked that she lets him touch her like that. Billy's eyes widen and his mouth gapes.

"Nicky?" he questions her. "Nicky, no way!"

Dave laughs and sneers at Billy. He doesn't say a word but he bends down and bites her on the neck. She purrs up at him.

"Shit, Nick," Billy swears. "Have you lost your mind?"

"It's totally gone, Billy," Dave laughs. "Totally destroyed. She's my prisoner. Look, we've been up all night and after that workout and all the food, I think I need a nap. If you want to keep Prince company that's fine. Sim will be out soon or you can hang out in the boardroom with Jake.

"But Nicky's going to be tied up for a few hours. Or maybe just handcuffed. Are you coming, baby?"

He walks out the door and she follows him with a wicked satisfied smile. Billy stares after them speechless and stands there sulking. I laugh. "I thought the fucker was gay. How does a little junkie score like that?"

Billy crashes into the chair by the bed. "Man, I didn't see that coming," he shakes his head. "I never." He thinks hard and then asks me, "How old are you, man?"

"Eighteen," I answer.

"I'm ten years older than you and she's even older than me by a few."

"But she's really nice," I tell him. "I mean, she hit me a few weeks ago, but now she's so sweet. I don't care how old she is. The other one, too, Nat. She's very sexy."

"He took Nat's necklace, too, that pimp." Billy looks stunned like someone just smacked him in the face. Then he stares at me and asks, "What kind of name is Prince Albert anyway? Are you some kind of royalty?"

"It's a street name. I don't use my parents' name anymore. I divorced them. My father was a real brutal bastard. S&M, Sam, Sim, whatever he calls himself, they're all made up names. Nicky signed her name Nancy. Dave was DJ when I rented the house from him. People here seem to call themselves whatever the fuck nom de plume they feel like. Why are you just Billy? Is that your real name? William?"

"I'm a pro," he says. "At least I was before I got suspended from the surf tour for heroin. Pros tend to like our real names for publicity purposes. I've been called worse things. 'Bully Billy' has been very popular but more often 'Fang' because I eat like a ravenous wolf most of the time."

I laugh. "I'm a real fine chef, Billy. S&M wants me to cook for the team when I get better. What kind of food do you like best?" I'm starting to think food might be my best and only defense against Billy.

"Everything!" he laughs. "Anything that sits still long enough to let me get a fork into it. Sam's more of a picky eater, vegetarian healthy stuff. He likes some lamb and fish really well, but he's happy with rice and beans, eggs – "

"Give me a tahini and fig jam sandwich any day," S&M interrupts coming into the room with Nat. "Do you know how many millions of sesame seeds have to be crushed to make a jar of tahini?"

"I can make some monstrous tahini oatmeal cookies for you, S&M," I volunteer. "I can add figs or dates and walnuts, whatever you like. It's pretty nice stuff. I'll give the recipe to Nat."

Nat starts fussing over me. I tell her Nicky gave me more meds and tea. I'm feeling better. I'm feeling a little safer, too, even without my gun loaded.

"Fucking Nick," Billy whines to S&M. "What's going on with her, Sammy? DJ said he's going to tie her up so he can get some sleep. He had his hands all over her. I've never seen her let anyone touch her."

S&M looks at Nat and puts his arm around her. She nods, a little sad nod, and shrugs. "Joy," she says. "Good for him. I'm happy."

†

JAIN

It's nearly midnight when I get back from the hospital but all the lights are blazing in the Fire House and it looks like a party.

"Yay, Jain," Sim cheers when I walk into the den of iniquity. "My good old brother, Dr. Jain."

There's a mob sitting around the boardroom table and I stand there absorbing the culture shock after spending the day at the hospital in surgery.

"Sit down, lover," he commands. He's not my lover and I don't sit. For a guy that doesn't like narcotics, he looks completely stoned. But there's no bourbon on the table, just cookies and milk.

Nat gets up and gives me an intimate kiss. She tastes like sweet vanilla and cream. She's got nothing on but a pearl necklace, bra and panties. I'm embarrassed.

"I'm out," she announces to the room and they answer her with boo's.

"Traitor! Loser! Coward!" Sim howls.

He's got nothing on that I can see but a green feather boa, but thankfully he's seated at the far end of the table so I don't know about the rest.

Billy's dressed in nothing but board shorts. Kama Dave's wearing jeans with Nat's favorite crystal around his neck. I don't want to know how it got there. There are things that you see but don't want to see, and things that you know but don't want to know.

Nicky is wearing Dave's little silver handcuff necklace and the white blessing scarf hides her naked breasts. Brandy has nothing except a sarong draped around her like a bath towel.

"I'm out too," Brandy laughs. "Sim's a cheater. His house rules and scoring provisions are twisted. We had him beat a long time ago."

"With all apologies to Einstein," Sim hisses, "God loves to play dice. Strip dice is very nice."

Sim throws a pair of dice across the boardroom table and sneers. "Pair of deuces. Immunity. I can't lose."

"Pair of what the fuck? I had double sixes," Dave growls.

"God loves to play dice alright," Nicky snarls. "And hates to lose and doesn't mind cheating."

She throws a one and a two. "Oh yeah! By your rules, that's a straight! Baby Dave you lose your jeans with double sixes."

Dave growls. "The jeans or the crystal? Tough call."

There's a pile of jewelry in the middle of the table, some gold, a few emeralds, a ruby earring, Sim's silver handcuffs. There's a pile of clothing on floor. I'm really tired but something's weird about this.

"Sim," `I wonder. "Why on Earth would you let your silver necklace go and keep the feather boa? That's pretty trashy."

"Um, my wife gave it to me," he laughs. "She found it in a junktique shop and thought it looked like seaweed. It's for the stripper in me. But I will never lose. I will have all of this. The dice are loaded."

"The dice are fair, boss," Nat says. "You and your rules are loaded." She picks up one of the kimonos and covers herself. "We know where you're coming from, boss."

Sim snorts and looks around the table.

"I DO NOT LOSE," he growls and throws the dice again. "Snake eyes. Double Shiva immunity."

"Cheater," Brandy whispers and pulls the boa off his neck leaving him as bare as a baby. "You beautiful cheater."

Nat throws him a tea towel to cover his best bits.

"Crap," I swear, too tired for serious cussing. "It can wait until tomorrow but I need some blood from Dave for the court documentation. How's that going to look?"

Dave says, "Have at it, Jain. I've got some beautiful blood. I overdosed on anandamide but no narcotics. I didn't touch Prince's tahini oatmeal bhang cookies. I heard they're good but I didn't have any. The judge is going to love me."

"How about your blood alcohol level?" I wonder.

"Clean," Nicky says. "I took him off bourbon today for training. I'm taking care of him," she laughs and winks. She gets up and puts her hands on his shoulders. "I'm on him 24/7."

"I'll bet you are," Sim laughs.

"Can I have the green dress back, S&M?" Nicky begs. "I don't think it will fit you."

He makes a face and then concedes, "Okay, but you'll owe me. A lot."

She picks it out of the heap of clothing and steps into it. She puts the white blessing scarf around Sim's naked shoulders, kisses his hair and whispers some strokes in his ear.

"I'm keeping the jeans and the crystal, Sim. I need them," Dave says getting up to follow me into the lab for the blood work. "I'll owe you, too."

"Game over," Sim declares. "If all the women are out, it's just too twisted."

I pick up Nat's emerald earrings from the pile. "I owe you, Sim," I smirk.

Billy leers at me and objects that he's still in and part of the loot should be his, but I'm much bigger than him. Sim grabs his silver necklace and tosses Brandy's ruby earring to Billy.

"Thanks for bringing the bhang, Billy," he laughs and then turns to me seriously and adds, "We're not smoking it, Jain. Nat says the medicinal effects are much healthier if we eat it."

I roll my eyes and point to Dave. "Lab. Now." Nicky follows us in.

I get the vials and hypodermic needle out of the lab cabinets and turn around to see Dave grinning like a happy idiot. At first I think he's fooling around with Nick, but then I realize he's excited about the needle.

"Geez, buddy. You like this?"

He nods with enthusiasm.

"I can draw it if you like, Doc," he says. "I know how. I've got some beautiful blood for you tonight."

"What have you got, a couple weeks practice shooting up? Trust me, buddy, I've been doing this for a lot longer. I don't want you playing with needles."

I look at Nicky for a little help as I draw the blood. I don't really know Dave. He worries me. I've only seen him on narcotics and for the last week he's been extremely delusional. I don't buy that mad innocence. When I suggested to Nat that he could use a little group therapy of his own, she was clearly nervous enough to worry me.

"Nicky, you've known him a long time. Is he behaving at all normally?"

"No," she laughs. "He's nuts. But I like him very much like this."

"I'm nuts?" Dave wonders but then his mind changes the page in a flash and his face goes dark. "You *like* me, Nicky? You fucking *like* me? Is that all?"

"No, baby Dave," she rushes to calm him down. "I like it that you're nuts. I *love* you, baby. I LOVE you!"

"Well, alright then," he pouts. "I'm not interested in fooling around. I've got forty-seven marriage proposals and I haven't got time for that 'like' stuff."

"Forty-eight," she teases him.

"Well, I'm tired," I interject before they get too personal, although I'm slightly relieved that he's chasing after her now instead of Nat.

"I happy enough if he's got clean blood work. But the team missed workouts for two days. Did you guys get anything done while I was gone today? I mean besides eating dope cookies and gambling?"

"You would have been proud of us, Doc," she says, "S&M let me stand in for you and we all trained hard. Legs and back. Then we ate healthy, had a nap, swam and sunbathed. The games only came later. Trust me, Doc, these guys need to let off some steam or they'll implode."

"Fine," I say. "We'll see what happens tomorrow at 10. Chest and arms."

Dave's playing with the arm I drew blood from, flexing his bicep and trying to pump himself. Nicky's watching and she puts her hand on his arm at the same time as he puts his eyes on her chest.

"Chest and arms, Nicky," he grins. "I'm imploding."

†

NAT

The dew is still wet on the grass when I walk over to the pool house for yoga at 7:30. Sim opens the front door and puts his hands together in Anjali, the prayer mudra.

"Namaste, Nat," he bows. "Thank you for coming."

He's teaching the first yoga class for the team at 8 and has asked me to be his teaching assistant. He's already set up the mats on the deck, four of them facing east towards the warm sun rising over the forest and two set perpendicular along the far edge of the deck for the teachers. We sit together with Brandy and drink tea, discussing the class plan.

"On Thursdays, I focus on the 3rd chakra," he explains. "Since it's the seat of power and control, the spiritual practice concentrates on our intentions and desires. The physical practice focuses on spinal twists and lateral bends like Fish, Dolphin and Triangle.

"This one's a bitch for me, Nat," he complains, "so I really appreciate your help demonstrating the asanas. I know you have some of the same third chakra issues as I do, but between us I think we can show them what's therapeutic, even if it's limited.

"Injuries are just as good teachers as pain," he laughs. "Maybe even better."

He picks up a little pocket watch from the edge of his mat and puts it back down next to his Tingsha meditation bells.

"One of the new students needs a personal invitation," he laughs and goes into the bedroom to use the phone.

He returns with his star students, Kamadev and Nicky and he sits down to check the watch again while they settle in the front row.

"Namaste, Sri Dev," he bows. "Namaste, Nick. We've got one more on the way. Just hang loose and start pranayama while we wait."

Dave sets his kimono aside, takes a little bottle out of the pocket of his sweatpants and starts doing nadi shodana with his oil. Nicky sits in lotus position, closes her eyes and breathes soft ujayii breaths. Brandy sits in easy pose cross-legged behind them.

While we wait, I watch myself watching them. It's hard for me to see Kamadev sitting next to her. I took the last of the scabs off her nose last night with lavender oil and for the first time I see how beautiful she is without the scars. I also see his innocence and absorption as he inhales the sweet perfume of his oil. I can nearly taste the subtle smell of his sandalwood mingling with the jasmine flowers dripping from the rafters of the deck.

At exactly 8am, Sim picks up the Tingshas and swings them together once. The sweet sound of the bells resonates through the morning. When it disappears in thin air he begins.

"Namaste. Today we'll focus on Manipura, the energy chakra. The third chakra is located in the solar plexus and associated with the digestive system, our personal fire and the seat of our power in the world. Just as we transform our food into our personal body by digestion, we transform our experience into our desires through our intentions."

"Hey, Sam, am I late?" Billy asks as he struts out onto the deck.

"Namaste, Billy," he says with a nod. "Thanks for coming."

Billy takes the empty mat in the back row next to Brandy and gives her a little leer. He's wearing her ruby earring and his board shorts and he fidgets on the mat while Sim continues.

"Our desires create our world. When the third chakra is open, your intentions and desires become reality without effort. When it's blocked, you become frustrated and ineffectual. Real power arises from knowledge. If you don't know exactly what you want, if you aren't crystal clear about it, you will never be able to manifest what you desire.

"We'll start our practice today by becoming aware of what it is we desire and setting an intention. An intention is like a seed. You plant it and keep watering it and nourishing it. But once you set your intention, trust it will grow and detach from the outcome. Don't keep digging it up every day to see if it's sprouted.

"I'll start. My intention is for integrated strength in all the koshas: body, energy, mind, heart and spirit."

He shuts his eyes for a few seconds and then turns to me. "Nat?"

I have a new intention now. I don't have to think twice. My old intention was for wisdom, but now I'm refining it to be crystal clear.

"Joy," I say. "A very particular kind of joy, Mudita."

He laughs and purrs, "Good girl! That's pretty powerful stuff, Nat." He turns to the class and explains, "Mudita is a key ingredient of wisdom, finding joy in the success and good fortune of others. How about you, Sri Kamadev?"

"I'll go with the same as you, Sim. Strength in all the koshas."

Sim smiles and says, "Kamadev, you set an intention the first day you were here. Remember? How's that been working for you? Do you really want to just copy me?"

Dave thinks for a moment and then looks directly into my eyes. I feel a rushing wall of prana hit me like a tidal wave so powerful that it would knock me over if I wasn't already seated on my mat. Kama. He's remembering it now, the first time I met him when he was so sick in IC.

"Oh, yeah. I forgot. Love. I want love in me and all around me. I guess I want to stick to that one. I like being the God of Love. It's working very nicely, thank you."

"Good," Sim continues. "How about you, Nicky?"

"Freedom," she says without missing a beat. "Liberation. The jewel of discrimination is freedom from attachment to desire."

"Oh, nice" he laughs and teases her. "Studied Tantra much, Nicky?"

She bows her head in gratitude for his recognition, but Kamadev objects.

"You can't have freedom, Nicky!" he hisses. "You said you're my prisoner."

"Of course I can, baby," she says raising a remanding eyebrow. "I'm free to be your prisoner."

Dev looks helplessly at Sim.

"It's okay, Kamadev," he explains. "She can still be your sex slave and have freedom, as long as it's a discrete choice and not an attachment. That's much more enlightened than bondage."

Brandy nearly chokes on her laughter. Billy's hand shoots up for permission to speak but he doesn't wait for it to be granted. "What the fuck? Sex slave?" he demands.

"Um," Sim thinks. "I meant consensual submissive intercourse. Sexual games, Billy, that's all. Can we get back to yoga? Brandy?"

"Love," she says. "Pure love. Not just consensual sex games, Sim. I want love, baby."

"Good choice, Bran. I'm listening. How about you, Billy?"

"Me what?" Billy stammers, having lost the class plan.

"What's your deepest intention and desire?" Sim repeats.

"Money," Billy answers. "Maybe fame but if it was a choice between money and fame, I'm definitely down with the money."

"Spoken like a pro, Billy," Sim laughs. "That's the third chakra alright: power, control, money, and desire. We'll work on all of it. Now take a deep breath in and envision your intention filling your heart. Pause. And exhale, releasing any obstacles in your path. Nice.

"We'll start the physical practice with Sun Salutations. Nat, would you give Billy some extra attention with this. He's my best and most important student today, a perfect beginner."

†

JAIN

I'm grateful for the extra sleep and some quiet time in the house while those lunatics do yoga. I drink almost a full pot of coffee and then give Mack a call to say I think we're due for another board meeting. Just me, Mack and Sim.

"How's it going over there, Jain?" he asks. "You've got a pretty full house now. We let Billy stay in our spare room last night. Nice not to have any overdoses or bloodshed in the last 72 hours. God, I'm knocking on wood."

"Probably why we need a meeting, Mack," I growl. "Were we planning to run a wellness center, an asylum or a strip club?"

"You sound...annoyed?"

"Tired, angry, frustrated, disturbed, jealous. Yeah, I'd say annoyed, too."

"Jealous? Of who?"

"How would *you* feel if you came home and found Sunny playing strip poker with three boys nearly naked half her age. Or even older men, what's the difference? I'm jealous of Nat, Steven, Billy and even the little teenager Albert. And I'm going to bury that fucker Dave in the forest.

"If any of those guys go missing, just look for fresh dirt in the yard. Have we got a shovel up here, buddy?"

"Hang on, I'm coming over, Jain," he says and hangs up before I can say 'leave me the fuck alone.'

I make a fresh pot of coffee and sit down. I know exactly what I'm going to do about this. I'm going to bury them all.

Mack comes in, looks around and frowns.

"The place looks nice. I haven't been over for a while. If there was a wild orgy here last night, you could fool me. But you look like a train wreck, Jain. Hard day at the hospital yesterday?"

"Yeah, I had a couple rough surgeries but it was a walk in the park compared to this place."

"Okay, man. Tell me what's going on. It can't just be a little gambling and nudity to get you so worked up. Or is that all there is? Your fiancée was playing some risqué house game?"

I blow all the air out my lungs like a bad taste and shake my head.

"No, Mack That's not all there is. You don't see what's going on. Steven sweeps a lot under the rug. The little junkie attacked Nat in the lab last week. He tried to hit me with the rack pole and smashed the glass on purpose. We cleaned it up. We hid it. I have tried and tried to be cool about it but he should have stayed in jail. He's guilty. Even Steven didn't want to help him, but Nat talked him into it.

"Last Friday when Dave came to the house meeting all clean and dressed up, he was wearing Nat's scarf. Something wasn't right. 'Doing yoga,' fuck he says. I don't buy that innocent act.

"When we got back from the beach Saturday, he was fucking the girl from the apothecary in the boardroom. Well not quite in the act but close enough for horseshoes. Bet you didn't hear about that.

"And there's something twisted going on between Steven and Nat. She beat him with a belt pretty bad. You didn't see that shit either. He covered it up with the kimono.

"Now Dave's got the new girl in his room all night, but I don't think that makes any of the other women any safer. It just proves he has no boundaries. He ought to be locked up, Mack. Jail suits him. He's a sleazy punk.

"Last night when I came home he was wearing Nat's favorite crystal necklace. That's what finally set me off. She had it on when I kissed her goodbye in the morning."

"Wow," Mack whistles. "There's a shovel in the shed next to the pool house. And I've got the bullets for Albert's gun. But Jain, Nat loves you. Dave can't compete with you on any level. He's still a kid. A pretty fucked up kid. She's probably just being nice to him."

"But women love bad boys. He's going to hurt her."

"Well just back off for a second, Jain, and take a look at it from the outside. How did you get started up with Nat? You brought her up here to help Steven, right? Were you romantically involved then?"

"Of course not. She was a patient. But Steven insisted she give me some private lessons after she started working for him. And she was... very nice."

"Right. Steven set you up with her. I could see it. Like he set up Sean and Crystal, me and Sunny, Beau and Sage, Dave and Nicky.

"And guess what? I started the whole fucking game because I wanted to see him happy. I set him up with Brandy because he was so depressed when we brought him up here. Now he's playing that game on everybody he knows because he wants to see everyone else happy."

"Fuck," I say. "I've been played."

"You've been played in a very nice way, Jain. He loves you. There's a very traditional yoga quality called Mudita. It's the joy that comes from seeing the happiness and good fortune of others. He's not going to like seeing his friends buried in the forest."

It's ten minutes to 10, so I tell him I've got a team to train. I'm on a new cycle and the least I can do to celebrate is to start by burying all the bastards in the gym.

†

NICK

The yoga was so good that my broken toes are smiling. I've missed my teacher for so long and I loved seeing him back in his element. Freedom! Strength! Love! Joy! And even money! God, I love him. I love to hear him unravel knots by pouring light on their little twists.

Nat was an excellent assistant and I'm really starting to like her. I had trouble with Dolphin because of my broken foot, but she was very kind and said, "Nicky, ease your front leg back out to the point where there is no pain and then let it go, like a rag doll. Rest there. And when I wobbled in Triangle, she showed me how to back off again. The point isn't to form a perfect shape but to create a lateral twist. She had me put one hand on my hip and an elbow on my knee for stability and then focus on turning my head up to the jasmine above us.

She didn't even touch Dave. His poses are textbook perfect. He hasn't got a twisted bone in his body or any physical aches or pains. All his injuries are mental, emotional and energetic, the standard injuries of addiction. I tried not to look, but he's so sweet on the eyes. There's no apparent damage when you look at him. Just divine perfection. The closer we get, the more I'm convinced he's made out of sugar.

At the end of the class, when we did Sivasana, the corpse pose, Billy tried to leave, saying if we were done he couldn't see the point in lying there doing nothing. Typical beginner. But S&M persuaded him that it was the most important part.

"Don't just do something, Billy Boy," he laughed. "Lie there!"

Brandy served us some beautifully fermented tea with leftover bhang cookies and berries before we headed over to the gym. Dave pulled handfuls of jasmine from the vines and handed them out.

"Put it behind your left ear," S&M advised us. "It opens your soul according to Sri Kamadev. I recommend it."

When we head over to the gym with flowers in our hair and time to spare, Jain is already going hard at it. He looks like an animal, a big predatory alpha animal. I slow down a little in my tracks, instinctively watching his moves. He gets up from the bench and sees us and spits.

I feel fear and put my hand out to hold Dave's.

"Hey, Jain," S&M hails him. "Looking like a beast, brother!"

Jain snorts at him, flexing his chest with a grim smirk.

"Doc," I say, "what kind of cookies are you eating? You look like an Olympian contender."

"Hey," he sneers at me, "are we going to play or are we going to get serious today?"

"Serious!" Dave says, "Chest and arms, right?"

If looks could kill, Dave would be in a coma, but S&M ignores it and says, "Jain, can you use Nick for your assistant? She's pretty good."

The doctor looks at me like I'm a piece of pie and he's on a diet: disdain and lust wrapped up in a package to go. I know that look. I've been in gyms a long, long time. He's on a cycle. He's on a heavy cycle.

"Alright then, Ms. Nicky, who wrecks cars and bites the heads off men," he sniffs, "Where do we start?"

He motions to the bench press where he's already got 225 loaded.

"We'll start with the bar, Doc," I say. "45 pounds for everyone to warm up."

He laughs with scorn and pity.

"Doc, we are injured some of us. It's not funny," I scold. The only way to appease an alpha beast is to admit to your inferiority, roll over and play dead or injured. But the truth is, we are hurt, all of us except Billy. Dr. Jain scares me a little but I know where he's coming from. Knowledge is power. Knowledge is greater than strength.

We all warm up with the naked 45-pound bar then it goes to 65, 95, 115, and 135. I miss on 135 and need a spot so I'm out. So does Dave. We sit on the sofa with Nat to watch while S&M and Billy go on to press 155. S&M fluffs it on 175 and swears. Billy keeps going and barely manages 195.

"That's all you've got?" Jain snorts. "Well, spot me then while we're at it."

He puts 295 on the bar and slams it. Then he goes 315 with ease. Yeah, that man is on a serious cycle. He was only doing 275 a week ago. I take S&M by the arm and whisper in his ear. "Careful. There are things going on you don't know about. Trust me, baby."

†

S&M

Mack calls a Bored Meeting at noon. Ugh. Incredible waste of the noon hour when Agni is burning so hot but thankfully Sunny brings in a pile of egg salad sandwiches. I nearly drown in them. She put saffron and nutmeg and paprika and crushed coriander in the eggs with white pepper and aioli. Never mind. I can die happy now.

"Steven?"

Oh, God, that's always a bad beginning being called by my Christian name.

"Call me Sam," I joke. "Most of my friends call me Sim. They used to call me Nim, short for S&M. But never mind, just call me," I tease them. But they are horribly serious, fiercely inviolable. I can't poke a chink in their armor.

"Steven, are you high?" Mack wonders.

"Aren't you, brother?" I challenge him. "Are all your cards on the table?"

"Or all the dice," Jain sneers at me.

"All the dice, okay, okay! I ate a cookie with bhang butter in it but I'm really high on my friends, my beautiful wife, yoga, the intoxicating forest around my house and a nice pump. And how's the morphine going for you, oh my brother?"

Mack flushes.

"Sorry, Mack," I say. "Didn't mean to hit the soft spot but the vibrations are really low in this room. I mean the drug vibe is dense. What can I do for you?"

Jain leers at me and says, "I don't like your friends, pal. I don't like Billy and I'm thinking of killing Dave."

"Ouch. Is this corporate business? Or is this like a crucifixion? Because I can go both ways."

Jain glares and neither one answers so I think I've permanently shut them up but that's not always a good thing. It's much better to talk than to let your friends stew in poisonous juices.

Sunny comes back into the room to see how we're doing.

"Sister, you've killed me with those beautiful sandwiches," I thank her. "I was hungry but now I'm free. Have you met my personal chef yet? You and Prince Albert could rock the house. Nat's teaching him Ayurveda and nutrition. You are what you eat, right?"

She smiles at me for the first time and I remember the day she punched me in the face. Now she loves Mack and I feel the rush of Mudita. It's the best drug on the planet.

"Mack, please. Trust me. If I fuck up it's only because I'm trying to do what's inhumanly possible. You're my teacher. Trust me to be a teacher."

Mack looks at me like his sweet little brother and I know I'm forgiven. Now is the time to take his heart in my hands.

"Tomorrow's Friday," I yawn. "Have Sunny invite Croft, Sage and anyone else who's on the front burner up here tomorrow for lunch. I'm going to announce the rules and scoring provisions for the contest. I've got them nailed down. I cannot lose.

"Wake up, Mack. It's a half million dollars and that's just a start. We're giving it away to the community. We're giving it to the beautiful beach.

†

DJ

It doesn't seem fair that I have to negotiate with my prisoner, but she says all is fair in love and war. I want to take her upstairs and invent something to put her teeth on edge, but she's busy fanging on oranges.

"Wait, baby Dave," she laughs. "I'm worth the wait." I'll wait until all the stars fall out of the sky.

Dr. Jain comes in from the kitchen and stares at us. Nicky stops pulling her orange apart and I can hear her breath stop.

"Good job running the show, Nicky," he says. "I was trying to bury all of you."

"Yeah," she laughs. "You did. You were getting serious there, Doc. Amazing bench, honey. But you can't expect all of us to do the same – yet! That's my favorite word: 'yet'. Be patient with us."

He looks at her for a long time, like he's looking for a key.

"Nat did a nice job on your face," he smiles. "No scars. You're very pretty. You look much nicer like this."

"Thanks, Doc. She's a jewel. You're a very lucky man."

"Yeah, I'm lucky. Hey, I wonder if I can have a word with Karma Dave. Alone."

"I think he's busy," she says but I'm not and I tell him fine, let's go. He's my bodyguard. He's Sim's oldest friend. I want to know what his favorite word is.

"Come on, Dave, buddy" he says very chummy. "Let's go for a walk."

We walk out past the gym and he laughs.

"What was it on the bench press? You couldn't quite get 135?"

"Nah. I never lifted seriously. Sim and Nicky did weights but I was a slacker I guess. I like yoga better. This is new to me. But I want to. I see how she looks at you, Doc. You're a machine. I want to have all that muscle."

I look at his arms. They look like hams with all the fat trimmed off, if hams had veins. I touch his arm to see if it's real.

"Don't fucking touch me," he snarls. "Don't even think about touching me."

"Sorry," I say. I'm really sorry. I like him. I don't want to piss him off. We walk past the pool house and he motions toward a little trail leading down through the forest.

"I'm not supposed to go off the grounds, Doc," I explain. "Because of my trial."

"You're fine," he says. "I've got you."

It's beautiful in the forest, cool and dark. It smells like juniper and eucalyptus and some scents I don't know but I want to know. There are huge shrubs with brilliant flowers on them, crimson and white and red. Rhododendrons he says. I've got to take Nicky down here. It blows the jasmine deck out of the water. It looks soft and sweet on the forest floor with a thick blanket of pine needles.

"Okay, Dave," he says stopping on the trail. "Tell me what the fuck is up with you."

"Me?" I'm not sure what he means. "Everything is up. I'm in love. I've got the prison thing, but I'm not worried. I'm not attached to the outcome. Sim taught me that. Detachment."

He glares at me. His face is darker than the shadows surrounding us.

"You stupid fuck," he swears. "I'm not talking about your fucking philosophy. I'm talking about your dick, you little whore."

Ooh. That's definitely not up right now. I tell him so and he hits me so hard I fall down. I don't want to get up. All I can think about is Nat. I don't love her that way. He can have her. But that's what he doesn't know. How would he know?

"Did you touch her?" he snarls. "Did you sleep with her?"

I feel the red stuff running down my mouth and wipe it off with my hand. Blood. Hot. I lick it.

"You like blood? I'll show you some more where that came from."

He kicks me then picks me up with one hand and knocks me back down with the other. I taste it. I don't really like blood as much anymore. A little goes a long way. This much blood really sucks.

"I'm sorry," I whine. "I didn't sleep with her. I, uh – "

"Let's re-phrase that then, honey," he threatens. "Did you fuck her?"

And I can't answer that one with any chivalry. There's no good story to be told. She was so complicated I couldn't even give him the outline of the plot. She tore my heart out. And then when I don't answer him he starts to tear the rest of me apart. The last thing I see is the blood red rhododendrons hanging underneath the sky.

†

S&M

"Sim, it's fucked," Nat whines. "I don't know who else to talk to. He's not himself. Can I talk to you about it, in confidence?" We're sitting on the sofa on the lawn next to the gym, with the sun on our shoulders and back. It's peaceful and it's private.

"Sure Nat. Trust me. Talk to me."

"There's no sex lately. I found some little blue pills in the pocket of his lab coat. So if it's not with me, then who? Nicky? Is there someone else? God, I love him, Sim. I don't want to lose him. Now I'm jealous of Jain and Nicky and jealous of Kamadev and Nicky. I'm hurt."

"Uh, I wouldn't be worried about Nicky. She's got her hands full. Plus she doesn't screw around unless she's dead set. You would be the first to know. Someone else? Maybe at the hospital? I don't think so or he'd be gone a lot more. Maybe he's not taking the blue pills. Maybe he's hanging on to them for a special occasion. Are they still in the pocket?"

"I can check," she says but before she gets to her feet, Sean comes around the corner of the house. He doesn't wave. He's in full uniform and looks seriously official.

"Hey," he says. "I didn't get the blood today. You know the deal. As long as he's testing clean, I'm good for him to be here. I had the hearing moved up a week but I have no blood. You've got custody, but I paid the bail. It's a lot of money, Steven."

Oh, shit. I don't like the tone of my name. I don't even like having a name.

"No blood? That's not like Jain. I happen to know he drew Dave's blood last night, right Nat?"

She nods. I'll bet my life Dave is clean. I wouldn't bet on Mack, but Dave has got some beautiful clean blood.

"I'm taking him in, Steven," he says. "We'll run the tests down at the station. Where is he?"

Nat jumps up and takes Sean's arm.

"I'm sure it's a mistake, officer. Let's check the fridge in the lab. I'm sure we've got what you need."

We walk over to the Fire House and sure as shit there's a vial of blood in the fridge. In fact there are two vials, both with yesterday's date. Nat gives them to Sean and he frowns.

"There's no documentation. They've got the serial numbers but no tracking. I can't use this. Where's Jain? This isn't like him."

"He isn't like himself," Nat whines.

"Look, Sean," I explain, "Take the blood, run the tests and I'll get the documentation down to the lab later today. Trust me, buddy. I'll take care of it."

He puts his finger on my heart. God, he just did that on Monday when he threatened me for beating up on the Prince.

"I'm warning you, Steven," he growls. "We'll be in touch."

"Absolutely, brother," I promise. "I'm on top of this."

I walk him out to his car and keep up a nice front even as I notice Jain's car is gone.

†

NICK

I'm waiting. I'm waiting not so patiently. I know he wanted to play so I'm getting a little pissed off about waiting so long. Then I hear feet on the stairs. S&M peeks his head in the door and looks around.

"Where is my little shadow, Nicky?" he asks.

"I'm waiting for him," I say with a sweetness that borders on homicide. "If you find him, tell him I'm going to tear his little heart out and feed it to his rearranged third eye."

"Hang on, Nicky. You're supposed to be watching him 24/7."

"I was. But Dr. Jain took him about two hours ago. I would think Jain's bored to tears entertaining him after – "

"Shit, baby," I cut her off. "Jain's gone. And Dave can't leave, so this is screwed."

I get up and walk to the window, put both hands on the sill leaning out as if I can smell him from here.

"Sean was just here about the blood tests. Everything is going south fast," he says. "Are you coming, honey, or are you just breathing hard?"

I laugh. I'm coming. I think we can find baby Dave just by following our noses. He smells like a bouquet of flowers.

He's not in the Ice House. We check all the rooms. Mack is reading in his office with his feet up on the desk.

"Seen Dave or Jain?" I ask.

"Jain had an emergency at the hospital. He said don't bother him. What's up?"

"I'm looking for Dave. Last seen with Jain. Any clues, brother?"

He shakes his head and turns a page.

"This is such a trashy book," he scoffs. "William S. Burroughs. Did you know that a junkie gets a huge increased sex drive when he quits? So quitting heroin is better than Viagra. I really don't like this book but I'm learning a lot. I might just clean myself up."

"Oh, fuck. You do that, Mack, you sick fuck, brother."

He pulls the door softly shut but I can feel that he wants to slam it. He looks at me and I can taste the pain in his eyes. I would do anything to soften it for him.

We walk over to the pool house where Brandy is tending to some young herbs on the deck. Holy basil, thyme, rosemary and bacopa.

"Yeah, I saw them," she says. "Jain and Dave went by here a couple hours ago towards the forest trail. Can I walk with you?"

We go down the trail and the forest kisses us with its heady scents. The smell of the forest is so overwhelming that I couldn't smell Dave unless I tripped over him. And then we nearly do.

He's crushed, bleeding, and out cold in the middle of the trail, sucking on his knuckles like a baby.

†

DJ

This is weird, the damn IC again, drips, needles, nurses and pain. I'm so fucking amused I want to laugh. Sunny is stitching my head up, but Sean is staring at me.

I've got handcuffs on me.

"Okay, let's go, Dave," he says when she's finished.

"What?" I say. "What the fuck have I done?"

"The blood was nasty," he snarls. "I'm not sure which sample was yours but one came up loaded with morphine and the other sample tested positive for steroids. We're done here. I'm taking you back to jail. We'll sort it out downtown."

Jail? It's not fair. I look around the room searching for some place safe to hide. I want to be dead. I wish I were buried in the forest under the pine needles and the rhododendrons. I pull at my hands and the metal bites my wrists. I've got the more complicated serious version on, not the sexy leather cuffs. I don't know a word strong enough to spit at him. I hold my breath and bite my lip.

He takes the handcuff key off my neck and puts it on the table. Where is the beautiful crystal? It's gone.

Then he pulls me up to my feet and takes me out into the night. Where is Sim? Where is Nicky? Where is Nat? Where is Jain? Who has me? Who has me?

"Fucking don't cry," Sean says. "Don't cry. You're old enough to know better. What's the matter with you, boy? Quit your sniveling."

But I cry. This is exactly why God made tears. This is what they're for. I cry so hard I drink the salt and snot. I cry the whole ocean all the way to jail.

†

S&M

Nat is crying her eyes out. Brandy is weeping like a baby with a broken toy. But Nicky is howling so hard I'm worried she might choke on her tears.

"Nico," I try to soothe her, "We'll get him back. Trust me honey. Have you ever cried over a boy before? I've never seen this side of you."

"Shit, S&M," she says. "I never had such a beautiful boy to cry over. Not even you." And then the tears fall like rain and Nat and Brandy pump up the volume like a fire hose.

"Come on," I try to soothe them, "It's not like he's dead. He's just – in fucking jail."

And then the snot and tears pour out like renaissance fountains.

I can't deal with it anymore. I get up and go into Prince's room and slam the door behind me.

"How's your life going, honey?" I smirk. "No woman, no cry."

He smiles.

"I'm feeling better. Maybe I can get up soon and start cooking. I'm a little bored but I'm thinking about crème fraiche on pumpkin soup. Maybe some toasted pistachios on top with lavender salt. But please don't call me honey. It scares me."

"Sorry, honey," I say and then I want to slap myself. "Sorry. How's your head?"

He nods. "It's still there on the top of my neck. Right where I want it. Please don't ever touch it again."

"Sorry. Triple sorry. I'm having some guests up tomorrow, kind of important press stuff. I don't think you can serve them but I'd appreciate it if you'd collaborate with Sunny on the menu. Nothing fancy but real sexy. Are you up to it?"

"Oh, yeah," he laughs. "I'm up. Send Sunny over in the morning. What's all the noise going on out there?"

"Don't worry about it," I say. "Just some tear jerk movie the girls are on to. Get some sleep."

I wink at him and probably scare him but hell is in me and all around me. I'm moving fast so it doesn't scorch my heels. I feel a lot stronger when I go back into the boardroom. The ladies are still sitting around the table but the snot and tears have been wiped away.

"Trust me, they'll let him go after they find out he's clean," I reassure them. That's what Sean promised me.

"So, Nat," I wonder. "The little blue submarines you were talking about. Have you got any of them?"

She gets up and goes into the bedroom and when she comes back she throws a couple of blue pills on the table. I'm thinking of crushing them into a powder and putting them up my nose but I restrain myself.

"Mmmm," I snort air instead. "Never needed it. I'm hard enough."

"Never needed it? What are you thinking about, baby?" Nicky rolls one of the blue pills between her fingers.

"I don't know much about aphrodisiacs, honey," she laughs. "I *am* the Viagra. I would worry about a man I couldn't raise from the dead. So I don't know what Viagra looks like. But I know this little blue pill very well. It's Dianabol, methandrostenolone, a very powerful steroid. It makes men big and strong, but it also makes them mean and wicked as a side effect. And it makes them totally useless in bed. Not getting much lately, Nat? A very nasty little drug, this one."

†

S&M

It's after midnight when we hear the car pull in. Sean hits the siren once to announce himself and I open the front door. He helps Dave out from the back seat but drops him and he crashes onto the driveway.

"Crap, Steven," he complains. "Give me a hand. He's useless on his feet."

"Down, girls," I say, shooing them out of the doorway. "Go to bed. I've got this. Brandy, it's just you and Sean. Let's get him out of this house right now.

"And Nat, I suggest you keep your hands off Prince. Nicky, you're in charge. Keep an eye on them. All three of you are under house arrest until I say so."

I've seen too much blood and tears today. I want to put my hand through the window, but I'm thinking I'm going to need it if I want to beat the living shit out of the good doctor.

"Steven," Sean warns, "I'm sorry. Cool down. It was just normal procedure. His blood tested clean after all. I don't know whose samples you gave me, but it wasn't his. Narcotics and steroids? Shit!" He whistles.

"The doctors," I snarl. "Fucking doctors both of them. You might as well lock me up right now for intent to commit murder."

"Don't make me do that, Sim. You guys have given me enough trouble today. Jain is in jail. I don't want to see you get within a mile of the police station tonight."

†

SEAN

Brandy pulls the covers back and we tuck Dave into the big bed in the pool house. He's not unconscious but he's totally blank. Sim motions me to the chair and I'm grateful to get off my feet. It's the third time I've had to drive up here today, none of it for pleasure.

Brandy checks his eyes, his pulse, and his blood pressure.

"I'm sorry," I start, "he was all cleaned up when I took him in but it got rough."

"Tea, Sean?" she asks, "You look almost as bad as he does."

"Please," I say, "I'm beat. He's checked out but I'm still wide awake. I would appreciate a break. He wouldn't listen to me.

"I couldn't explain anything to him the whole way down because he was bawling so hard. I tried to tell him the plan was to get him right back up here tonight if we got a clean test, but he just went off about how she was waiting for him and not being able to say goodbye to her. Who is she? Nicky?"

"Yeah," Sim says. "It's not puppy love this time. It's terminal."

Brandy brings me the tea and starts washing his face, cleaning up the fresh blood on top of the stitches.

"He thought he was going to prison permanently. The guys got a little rough on him because of all the noise and crying and locked him up in time out while I got the test done. He bashed his head some more in there. Then he shut up and he hasn't said a word to anyone. Even after we took him out and told him everything was good.

"I took the cuffs off him, but he still wouldn't talk to me. At least he's not howling now."

"He's catatonic," Brandy says. "It's different than physical shock. I can tell because his blood pressure is fine. This is emotional post-traumatic shock. We should have Mack take a look."

"Mack's probably nodding out by now," Sim swears. "Call Sunny. I don't want anyone else touching him right now. See if you've got some non-narcotic sedatives."

Dave is staring at the ceiling with his eyes wide open like he's watching a nice movie.

"Lorazepam will bring him out of it without hurting him. A slow intravenous dose. 2 mg every six hours, maybe less. If I'm right, he'll be okay," she advises and calls Sunny. As soon as she hangs up, the phone rings. Sim picks it up and swears some more.

"No, fuck no. Absolutely no. Stay there and watch those two. I need you there, Nicky. Dave's out to lunch anyway. We're going to put him out. There's nothing you can do to help. We've got him. Oh, yeah, and Jain's in jail, so just lock all the fucking doors and go to bed. No body leaves. We'll talk tomorrow."

He turns to me and whistles, "So Jain is locked up?"

"Yeah, that was a wild scene. Just as I'm dragging Dave back to my car to bring him back here, three other officers pull up with Jain very drunk and disorderly. Jain looked at Dave like he saw a ghost, like he thought he was dead. He sobered up on the spot.

"But Dave just walked past like he didn't recognize him. Like there was no else on the planet but him, in the state of grace so to speak. I didn't stop to exchange pleasantries. I called back to the station and found out Jain started a big fight at the Nest. They'll release him in the morning. Unless Dave wants to press assault charges."

"Dave doesn't look like he's pressing anything," Sim sniffs. "but I might. I have to decide which is sweeter, murder or prosecution."

"Tough guy," I suggest, "consider the third alternative. Forgiveness. He could lose his medical license if you push it and he's been working with me as Dave's legal advocate for rehabilitation. Sleep on that, Sim. Sleep on that one very seriously."

"Hmmm," Sim grunts. "Good point. Can we talk in the morning? There's a free room next to Mack. It might be nice for my big brother to wake up with a cop in the house again. I'll keep Dave in my room with us for now."

"Yes. Please. I'm finished off tonight. You guys are killing me. I might be your next catatonic patient if this keeps up."

Sunny comes in the front door, takes a look and grumbles about her beautiful stitches being messed up. She's got syringes and ampules and an IC chart. "Lorazepam," she tells me. "Not an opiate. It's an anti-psychotic. But he looks pretty heavily sedated already. What did you give him?"

"A big dose of reality," Sim snarls. "His bodyguard tries to kill him and then he gets hauled off by the police. I wonder what scared him more, Jain or jail?"

†

BRANDY

Sunny leads Sean out and says to phone if we need any thing else. Get him to sleep she says. Sim is pacing up and down the room furiously.

I put a little yoga eye pillow over Dave's open eyes and a hand on his forehead. I feel his wrist and his pulse is soft and steady but he's twitching. When I put a little bottle of spirit oil under his nose, he pushes my hand away hard.

If it were physical shock, I'd put him on a saline drip but his blood pressure is good. For emotional trauma, he needs to talk about it and process it. Yoga nidra will help but a good sleep is the best start. I wait for the sedative to kick in.

"Will you talk to me, baby?" I whisper. He barely shakes his head, just a twitch. I pick his hand up to hold it but he grabs me so tight it hurts. "Ouch, honey!" I say. "Don't hurt me."

I pull his fingers off my hand one by one and put my hand over his, flat on his heart so he can't crush my fingers.

"You're okay, we've got you. Sim's here. You're safe. Can you hear me?"

He shakes his head 'no'. I giggle and look at Sim.

"Come to bed, Sim. Nurse's orders. I think you need this as much as he does," I point to the sedatives. "This will help you. Just a little bit ok?"

Sim shakes his head 'no' too, but he lets me take his arm and give him some.

†

DJ

"Nim," I whisper. "Nim."

He opens one eye and laughs. "Nim? You haven't called me that since you were a teen-ager. What's up, DJ? You're talking now?"

"No. Just whispering," I beg. "Can you hide me?"

"Of course I can. I'm hiding you right now. How do you feel?"

"Scared I think."

"Scared of what?"

"The forest. The police." I think and then I tell him the truth. "Women. She beat me up."

"How about the woman with her arm around you, buddy? Scared of her?"

I feel warmth hugging my back and her hand is in my hair. She's snoring softly and I feel safe with her holding me.

"You're sleeping with my wife again. You can't make a habit of this," he teases. "But you came home pretty trashed last night."

"Are you going to kill me?"

"For sleeping with Brandy? Not unless she asks me to. Which woman beat you up?" he asks opening the other eye and getting up on his elbow. "Has Nicky hit you?"

"It was Nat. She beat me up with a belt in the forest."

378

"Nah, that was a bad dream," he says. "Do you want me to fire Nat? Does she still scare you?"

I don't know. I don't know. I can't talk about it anymore. I pull the cover over my head and feel Brandy's arm tighten around me. "Are we awake?" she yawns.

"You ain't seen crazy yet, honey," he laughs. "I think it's time to give Kamadev some more lorazepam."

She lets go of me and gets a needle and I yell 'no drugs!' but he says, "This is okay today, Dave," and she shoots me into a kind of hazy and not so scared place but not the stoned place.

"Listen," he says. "Jain hit you. Jain went crazy and lost his temper. He's in jail. Do you want me to keep him in jail?"

I don't know. I don't know. I need Jain to protect me. I don't like jail.

"Is he finished hitting me?" I whisper.

"Oh, definitely," he promises. "He won't ever touch you again or let anybody else touch you, especially Nat. You are very safe here. A lot of people fucked up. Nicky was supposed to watch you. Mack was stoned. Nat crossed the line. Sean couldn't wait a day. But you didn't do anything wrong, baby. You don't need to hide."

He pulls the cover off my face. "You don't need to hide, but you need to rest. Brandy will take care of you and give you a couple shots, but they're good shots. I have to take care of some business but I'll just be next door. Rest and I'll take you surfing with Nicky on Monday."

"Surfing? Off the grounds?" I don't believe him.

"Well, we haven't got any waves up here. I'll arrange for a police escort and a bodyguard. Sean owes you. Jain owes you, too. And Bran, honey? No one gets in here but Sunny for now. Period. Failure to obey is grounds for divorce. I'll be in Mack's office. Give him some tea and I'll send over breakfast in bed."

†

S&M

"I hope you got some sleep, Sunshine," I don't give her my lady killer smile because she won't buy it. Instead I give her my pathetic poor boy smile, which is very out of practice. "I need your help, please."

"Sure, Sim," Sunny beams. She's sitting in the office with Mack and Sean drinking coffee. "What can I do for you?"

"Can you give me a head count on the teams entered, not counting the ones just contributing but how many have actual teams competing? I need that before lunch."

She nods. "I think its twelve, eight competing and four just sponsoring, but I'll check to be sure."

"And before that, Brandy and Dave need breakfast. No one's allowed in my house except you. It's a psychiatric ward at the moment. See if he needs more lorazepam. And then I'd really appreciate if you'd work with Prince on a lunch menu for the guests. You can work at Nat's and she'll do the cooking. She's got a karmic debt to settle."

"Right away," she says and takes her coffee to the kitchen.

"Lorazepam?" Mack questions me. "What the fuck now?"

"For catatonia, brother. Brandy is very good with her diagnoses," I brag. "Perfect test scores."

His face goes a little red. "Is he schizophrenic?" he wonders as the neurologist in him kicks in. "Jain said he's delusional and he's been crying and screaming a lot. He thought it was because he's an out of control punk, but those are schizoid symptoms. I don't think we're trained to treat a catatonic schizophrenic."

"You tell me, Doc. He could go permanently that way if he's not treated right. Bran says catatonia isn't a disease; it's a symptom of an underlying mental disorder. She thinks its post-traumatic shock from drug withdrawal and, yeah, getting the shit beat out of him by someone he trusts."

"Geez," Mack moans. "Jain's in jail for beating up a mentally ill psychotic kid?"

Sean interjects with all due political correction, "I never thought he was psycho, Mack, just special needs."

"First things first, boys," I say. "I came to talk about blood." I lean back and wait for some explanations.

They look at each other and gulp the coffee in unison.

"I'm not touching those blood samples, Sim," Sean says. "They weren't entered into evidence legally. Morphine is a Schedule II controlled substance in medical practice; prescriptions are very strictly limited and monitored by the DEA except for emergency situations. I doubt addiction and recreation are emergencies.

"Steroids are Schedule III drugs and the laws are very specific and extremely clear; a valid medical prescription is not enough; you must have a valid medical purpose. Performance enhancement does not meet this requirement.

"It's a felony to abuse prescriptions. You are skating on ice so thin a joke could crack it. It's a fine line legally but it makes Dave look like a boy scout. I don't want to touch it if I don't have to. I don't want to shut you guys down, but I'm warning you."

"And why were you taking your own blood samples?" I wonder at their apparent stupidity.

"Monitoring each other's scripts," Mack says in a voice so low I can barely hear him.

I get up from the table and get more coffee and a bunch of the bran muffins from the kitchen. I go back into the office and put the shit on the table.

"After I finish with the rules for the surf contest, we're going to sit down together and write some new house rules and provisions for the board members and staff. I promise you," I hiss. "I suspected what was going on, but I didn't know I'm in business with a couple of alleged felons."

I'm getting my appetite back. I stuff half a muffin in my mouth and chew it. Finally Sean breaks the silence. "What about Jain? Is Dave going to press charges? Are you?"

"Dave isn't doing anything. He's fucking catatonic. Just see that Jain finishes the documentation for the hearing and makes it sparkle. Or fucking else. I will press charges if he doesn't. I'm not even worried about prison now. Dave will end up in a mental hospital if we can't keep him here."

Sean picks up the phone and calls the station, looking me in the eyes. "Okay to release Dr. Jain. The bartender at the Nest already dropped the charges and the assault victim is not pressing charges right now. Right."

I hold my finger up. "Tell him to come home. He's got work to do."

†

NICK

We've got Prince sitting up at the boardroom table with Sunny and Nat and me working on the party plan. He seems very proud to have a team of three female assistants to execute his menu. Crudités with tzatziki, shrimp and vegetarian satay skewers with coconut tahini sauce, avocado stuffed with crab-mango salad, a carrot cake and merlot sangria.

Sim comes though the back door and smiles, "Good little minions, working for a change." He looks at the menu and shows some teeth. "Prince, you are right up my alley, my man. I'm keeping you."

"Sunny is going shopping, boss," Nat says, "since I assume the rest of us are still under house arrest."

"Damn straight. But it's just until the party is over. Do a nice job and I'll set all of you prisoners free. Nick, you don't need to help unless you want to. Why don't we have a word upstairs while Nat starts on the sauces and the cake?"

"Boss?" Nat begs. "Can't you talk to me, too?"

"Separate issues, honey. You don't need to know what you don't know. I'll talk to you separately."

I follow him up to Dave's room. He lies down on the bed and I take a chair.

"It's not so good, Nico," he says. "You can't see him right now. He's on anti-psychotic meds and we're treating him at my house. Bran knows what she's doing. Trust me, honey."

"Can I talk to him? At least on the phone?" I plead.

"He can't talk, Nicky. If you called he couldn't even hold the phone. Give us a day or two and you'll be the first person to see him, I promise you. It would only hurt you to try right now. He's good physically, just some stitches on his face. The nice thing about a fight like that is a small guy goes down so easily. Little guys are hard to kill on soft ground."

He laughs. I don't think it's very funny.

"Dave doesn't fight. He didn't fight back. Then the jail thing flipped him out. He's mentally disturbed. He's, um, yeah fucked. I don't want to get medical on you and scare you. It's just everything that's been going on for the last six weeks since the day I last saw you guys on the beach. I want to take him back there, take him surfing. If he's better in a couple days, we'll go on Monday, just us. You'll see him before then though, I promise you.

"And no more fucking crying. Don't get all emotional on us. You're hardcore, Nicky."

"What's he doing?" I ask. "What's the treatment?"

"He's lying in my bed in corpse pose with an eye pillow so he doesn't have to see the ceiling. He's doing the fifth limb of yoga, pratyahara, total withdrawal of the senses to restore calm. And he's getting shot up with sedatives every six hours. We can't even do yoga nidra with him at this point. Trust me, honey, there's nothing to see. There's nothing to say. It's better this way.

"Stay busy, get strong and I'll let you talk to him soon. Fair enough?"

"What about Jain? Is he still in jail?"

"Oh, yeah that. He'll be back today but he'll be staying at Mack's. The Dianabol will be out of his system. He's going to be fucking sorry and I'm going to make him even sorrier. I like a good fight. I'll be sure he gets one. See you at the party."

He swings his feet over the side of the bed and starts to get up to go.

"S&M, thanks. But tell me something, honey. I used to ignore Dave because he was kind of weird. I thought he had ADHD or something. Is he crazy? I need to know."

"He's always been a special kid, Nick, but he was doing really well in the beach environment before I got shot. I don't think he ever had a clinical diagnosis because he was a street kid, but he got pretty disturbed when he didn't have any guidance. So I taught him. I'd tell him what to do and I looked after him as much as I could. Darrell and Sean looked after him, too, but mostly me.

"People thought he was my little brother because of the resemblance and he acted like one. He was my shadow. He annoyed the shit out of me because he would copy everything I did. But when I realized it gave him guidance to have someone to copy, I tried to be a better person. I quit screwing around. I quit fighting except for fun, to entertain you.

"I love him, Nicky. He's a beautiful soul. I thought you would, too, if you ever got close enough to know him."

He gets to his feet and I can see tears on his cheeks, so I stand up and hold him.

"He's made out of sugar, isn't he, baby?" I whisper. I don't cry because he told me not to.

"Sugar or honey. Or cherry jam. I'm not sure which, but he's sweet," he smiles.

†

S&M

When I get home, Brandy is lying in bed with Dave, holding one arm tight against his chest. The breakfast tray is slightly touched but not much. Dave's breathing hard and fast like he's coming, but he's not moving a muscle.

"How's it, baby? Need help? A break maybe?" I offer.

"Yeah, I need a break," she sighs, "He went into the repetitive motion phase, first just tapping himself on the shoulder and then punching it over and over. Pretty normal at this stage of processing things, but it's hard to watch."

"Finish your breakfast, or go for a walk, Bran. They're making a beautiful lunch for the party. I'll hang here until then. Is he talking to you at all?"

She shakes her head. "He'll repeat some things. He likes 'no' very much. Otherwise he's ignoring me. We don't want to give him any more sedative than necessary because he'd just stay like this forever. I've been reading a lot more about it. Medication is just the first line of treatment. He won't get better unless he processes the underlying cause."

"That's a lot of shit to process," I sigh. "I'm glad he trusts you because one of his big issues now is women. I just had a talk with Nick. He's had problems since I've known him. It goes way back when."

"I figured that," she smiles. "He's definitely on his own planet from what I've seen. At first I thought it was the heroin but then I realized he's a little bit like churros, twisted with a sugar coating."

I laugh. It's a pretty astute summary. She sits in the chair and bites on a muffin. "Hmm, tea is cold, I'll heat some more water. How are you doing with all this?"

"I'm staying busy like a madman. I'm going to rewrite the planetary rules and make sure the stars keep shining. I'm getting my Shiva on, Bran. You'll love the way I get worked up," I wink. She's laughs and goes into the kitchen.

I lay down on the bed and punch Kamadev's shoulder a couple times. "Do you like that, honey?" I tease him. "Maybe I'll teach you how to fight now. I mean, now that you know how to fuck."

I can see his lips twitch, but there's no answer.

"Shit, I got nobody to talk to. I lost my shadow. Where the fuck is it? I thought I had it sewed to the bottom of my feet! I'm fucked without my shadow."

I give him another little love tap punch on his shoulder. "I'm fucked!" I whine, sniveling and pretending to cry. "Who's got me? Who's got me?"

"Nim," he whispers.

"I can't hear you," I tease.

"Nim. I'm here."

"Oh, fucking thank God," I moan, "I thought I was going to be in so much trouble if I lost my shadow. I was really scared all my friends would kill me."

"No," he says. "No. It's safe."

"Thank you, baby. I'm so relieved it's safe now. I had no one to talk to. Who's got me?"

Brandy is back in the chair by the bed, watching with a thin smile.

"Nim. I'm here."

"Close enough for rock-n-roll, little brother. Keep talking. Where have you been hiding?"

"In the forest. Underground. In the dark. No one would know."

I smile at Brandy. We're getting some longer phrases. But I keep the eye pillow on his face so he can feel safe in the darkness.

"Nicky knows where you are, buddy," I say. "She knows you're safe underground. She will wait. She told me you could take your time and rest."

He frowns. "No. No. Nim, no."

"Yes. Yes, yes," I laugh. "You, Kamadev. She loves you very much. She'll wait forever. She would never hurt you. She said you are made out of honey."

He smiles, a big toothy lovely smile. "I taste like honey. She loves me, Nim. I lost her. I can sew her to my feet, can't I?"

Bingo. We've got sentences and even a question. We're back in business. I pick up a corner of the eye pillow just to let a crack of light in.

"No. No. No. No. No." He grabs my hand.

"Never mind then. I thought you wanted me to teach you how to fight. Some other time."

He smiles again and pulls the eye pillow off and looks around. "I'm in the fucking pool house!" he wonders amazed. "I'm sleeping with your wife again!"

"I won't tell anyone if you don't, Dave. Save your intergalactic transcendental sex for Ms. Nicky, but it's okay to sleep with my wife if you're just resting."

"Sleeping is okay. Save the sex. Fine. Can I look at her or talk to her?"

"Yes! Look at her and talk to her as much as you can, okay? She's your nurse."

"Hi, Kamadev," she says. "Nice to see you again. Do you want some tea?"

"Nice. Thank you."

And it's nice to have him back on Earth. Not all in one piece, but close enough for rock-n-roll.

"So let me run this past you, Kamadev. You're very good with math. I have a meeting soon and I need help with the rules for our team. okay?"

"Okay, Nim."

"We've got 32 surfers, 8 teams of 4. I want to use the format from the original Duke Kahanamoku big wave contest at Sunset. It's a simple format but they weren't doing team surfing and they only had 24 guys. So it's been keeping me awake at night trying to figure it out.

"They had 24 guys in four 6-man heats. Only the top 2 in each heat got to be in the final, an 8-man final. It's almost a brawl compared to modern surf comps. Throw in the team element, with only one team member in each qualifying heat, and it's going to be more twisted than Shiva strip dice."

Dave laughs and his eyes light up.

"Four 8-man heats! It's a fucking brawl, Nim," he laughs.

"That's my boy. I like it really well. I cannot lose. If all of my team goes through to the final, we'll shut them down with 50% of the surfers dominating the break. We will kill them."

"Bloody murder, Nim," he snarls and takes a cup of tea from Bran. "Murder in the first degree."

†

BRANDY

The lunch is on the lawn so I can hear the laughter from the pool house. It sounds like a good crowd, but I don't feel bad about missing it. There's more entertainment value in the bed.

After Sim leaves to greet the guests, I give Dave his shot of lorazepam and ask him to roll over so I can hold him. I put the little pillow back over his eyes and snuggle up behind him like spoons in a drawer with my hand holding the pillow in place.

"Fine, Brandy," he says. "But no sex."

"No sex," I promise.

"Just like Nim and Nicky. Intimate without sex."

"Oh?" My ears pick up. "Where did you come up with that? What about Nim and Nicky?"

"I know everything. We had group therapy for Nim. He was so disturbed. We gave him special drinks and told him thank you. Nat said what about pain and whippings? Then he got very, very more disturbed. Nicky tapped her finger and he obeyed. He's perfectly obedient. He's a pedigree boy. If he gets a bone he won't be sad. She said 'Good boy' and he was very, very happy, so happy. We all helped him. Then fighting and whippings so Nicky and Dave could surf and intimacy way beyond sex so Nim could turn on the universal lights. Then he took her away and I lost her."

Speech is spitting out of him like a faucet without an aerator filter. I don't know Sim very well and the kid is spilling the beans. I couldn't do better with the truth serum, sodium pentothal.

"What about whippings? Does he like that?"

"No. It's not him. Nicky likes to hit them then kiss them. She doesn't hit me but she kisses me because I taste sweet. Nim said get the love oils and I cried but he's my teacher. Give Nicky a massage in the nurses' room. Lock the door. Jealous women are everywhere. She asked me to make her cry. She asked nicely with sugar on it. I thought she was the frosting, but her heart is made out of cake. Nim gave me a warranty now. I have control."

Ooofuck, I think. I knew but I didn't know how twisted it was. Maybe he's dreaming this. Just to be clear I ask, "You and Nicky are having sex?"

"Dave and Nicky are married like Nim and Brandy. I took everything. I handcuffed her and fed her. She's my sex slave. She's a good girl, pedigreed. Obedient. She won't hit anyone now."

I laugh, "You were playing with those leather cuffs? I got married because of them. I'll tell you a funny story, Dave. I loved Sim so much I took him for my prisoner and I did such a bad job of sex, he says he had to marry me to teach me to do it right. I'm still learning."

"I don't have to teach her anything, Bran. She knows. Did you go three minutes?"

"Ten I think."

"That's very, very bad. Three hours is better. Three days."

"Are you sure you're married, baby?"

"She has to ask me," he laughs. "She has to ask nicely maybe ninety-nine times. I'll wait. She might have to get down on her knees and beg before I say yes."

And then I know I'm stepping way over the line of my profession and taking advantage of his situation, but I may never have this opportunity again.

"Kama Dave, can you tell me, which one is better in bed, Nat or Nick?"

"In bed or the futon or bathtub?" he asks seriously. "I never went to bed with Nat. And Sage is the best on a chair because I never yet – "

"Shit, come on, baby. You know what I mean. Sex any way. Even standing up."

I know they're both much more experienced than me, Tantrika sex goddesses who know kundalini and can tear men's heads off. Which one would win?

"Don't be silly, Brandy. They both have the same wiring circuits and chakras and koshas."

"Oh," I say, a little disappointed.

"But, silly Brandy," he goes on. "Nicky's heart is made out of birthday cake. I could never get enough of that."

†

S&M

"That's wild, Sim," Chris says. "I'm not sure if that can work. It sounds like of a free for all. Are we going to be able to judge it using the normal criteria?"

"Of course not," I say. "It's going to be so twisted they'll be talking about it until next year. But it's damn fair. There's no team advantage until the finals and then bloody hell will break loose. I can already see it. It's based on a classic format though, Chris. If it's good enough for the Hawaiians, no one can complain."

"Fair enough. The team that rules the most qualifying heats will kill everyone else in the finals. It's kind of like loading the dice, hey?"

"Sure, but any of the teams can get loaded. It's fair."

"Then why do you have all these scoring provisions for the finals? *If one team rider scores a wave directly after another member of the same team, it's a 'straight' and counts for double points. The third consecutive team ride counts triple and if there are four consecutive team waves, the contest is forfeited to that team.*"

"That's good, huh? That's sick," I snort.

"I guess. But it could end up like 400 to 10. If one poor guy got a perfect score on his own he'd lose badly."

"Yeah right, you got it. It's a team challenge, not a fucking man on man final. Anyone could do that. And anyway it's a charity fundraiser not a professional contest. Who really cares who wins? The community wins. Just as long as I'm not the poor fucker with the perfect score who loses because my team sucks. I will put them all under house arrest and thrash them daily."

The thought makes me lose my appetite for a moment but only until I take the next bite of mango-crab avocado. I didn't know I liked crab. The sangria is inspiring me to never touch bourbon again.

"It sounds perfectly reasonable, S&M," Sage purrs. "Of course I don't surf, but my team will do whatever I tell them." She's eating carrot cake out of Beau's hand and washing it down with sangria. She pulls all the fruit slices out of the drink and eats them, peel and all, just to get me to watch her I think. I'm watching.

"Alright, deal, "Chris says. "Point Guard rules. Take a ride on the wild side."

Crystal is captain for the Nest team. She says it's a go. Sean is staying out of it because of conflicting interests. The police have a separate team and they've sent a couple of pretty fit guys up to represent them, Neil and Wally.

"We're good with bloody hell," Wally laughs. "We deal with it every day. We're fine with the rules. The money is all going to law enforcement and rehabilitation so it's just going to make our lives a little easier."

Big Mel is the captain from the Fire Department team. "Whatever," he says. "You can use Texas Hold'Em poker rules or spin the bottle. We're going to kill you whatever you do."

"Hit me with your best shot, honey," I laugh.

Team six is from the Marine Mammal Rescue Center. "Sure, bro," captain Mike says. "We'll rescue all you drowning animals after Mel runs over you."

Like I said, it's going to be a brawl. The other two teams aren't here but we've got a majority. Game on. We finish off the sangria and shake hands on it. We set a contest window six weeks from now on the first solid swell. I need six weeks because my team is so messed up.

When everyone has left but Chris, I tell the prisoners they're free to attack the leftovers. I ask Nicky to sit with us, but Chris says he's got something personal he didn't want to bring up in front of the other guests.

"There's nothing's too personal to talk about in front of my girl, Chris. Come on, Nick, sit down a while."

Chris opens up his big reporter's satchel and pulls out a six-inch pile of letters. I look at the addresses and hand a

bunch of them to Nicky. They're all addressed c/o Chris Croft at the newspaper. Some are opened but the majority of them are still sealed.

"It seems it's all for you and Kama Dave. This is just a sample. I've got bags more. I opened a couple to see if it was important and I almost died laughing. Maybe you won't find it so funny, though. Do you want my assistant to sort them for you?"

"Oh!" Nicky screams. "Beautiful! Oh, S&M."

"It sometimes happens when you make front-page news, Sim, but not usually this extreme. They just came pouring in after we ran the story. This could make a front-page story of it's own."

And sure as shit, letter after letter is either a picture of some woman wanting to marry Kama Dave or a picture of somebody's nine year old kid who looks a lot like me. Nice looking kids, mostly boys but some pretty girls as well. I go get the bourbon.

†

NICK

"Yah," he says chugging down a water tumbler half full, probably 4 shots. "Probably best if you keep these, Chris, and blackmail me down the road."

He glares at me but I can't stop laughing. He could start a small army with those boys. He could populate a medium sized island.

"Nicky, get your dirty little nose out of the gutter. You didn't see that. We've got things to do." He stands up, finds his balance and whacks Chris hard on the back. "Fuck you, brother. I'm still not letting you win. I'll pay the blackmail before I do."

I shake hands with Chris and I'm still laughing when he's gone.

"I only did it to amuse you, Nicky. Four years before I ever met you, I thought you'd get a really good laugh out of it one day when you needed one. And now I think we should do this thing. Let's see if the God of Love would like some carrot cake."

My heart jumps and my stomach gets a little pang. But I've got to know. He makes a big plate of food for Brandy and I make a plate of cake for baby Dave. I cross my fingers as we walk over to the pool house.

"Wow," he says when he opens the door. "Well come on in, Ms. Nicky. The patient is looking much better."

Dave is sitting up in bed talking to Bran, sniffing on his Blue Lotus bottle but he just shuts up in mid sentence when he sees me.

"Cake?" I offer.

"Oh, fuck. No. No," he stiffens then his whole body shudders with an orgasm. "Nim and Nick. No."

"Oh, he's been talking about you two," Brandy says. "He's been talking non-stop, Sim. I've listened to the entire transcript of the group therapy session with Nat, the complete S&M course on the transmission of pain through the koshas, and the pranic structure of the chakra system, which I already knew, but he explains it beautifully. And then I've got the mathematical probability of your team winning using the provisional scoring system.

"Nice to see you, Nicky. I've got a lot of dirt on you too, sister, highly complimentary but almost too fantastic to take without a grain of salt."

"We'll have to trade notes, Brandy," I say teasing S&M, but I will never betray his secrets. Then I turn to Dave who's as white as a ghost. "Don't you want the cake, baby? We made it just for you. It's very sweet, honey."

"Not now," he hisses. "My friends are here, Nicky."

S&M whispers to me, "He's not very coherent but this is a thousand times better than this morning. This is awesome."

I sit on the edge of the bed and try to look in his eyes but he won't look up. He's staring at the carrot cake. Finally he says, "This is not my favorite cake, Nicky."

I put my hand on his forehead and place his hand on my heart. "Look at me, baby. Please. I've been waiting for you."

He pulls his hand away and sticks it into the cake, breaking off a big piece and stuffing it in his mouth. He chews on it with a frown and looks up at me defiantly. Then he takes another piece and another, still frowning at me.

"It's nice, isn't it?" I say. "Carrot cake. Prince Albert gave us the recipe."

When he finishes the whole thing, a huge portion, he says, "I don't like it."

"I'm sorry, baby. What is your favorite cake?"

"Wedding cake," he smiles, a really mean wicked little smile. For the first time I feel the big difference in our age. He's acting like a little boy throwing a tantrum. But I remember he's ill. So I try.

"Okay, honey," I promise, "I'll find some wedding cake for you tomorrow. Are you happy now?"

"No," he sneers. "No. No. Ninety-eight times no."

I look helplessly at S&M and he shrugs. But Brandy laughs.

"Are you getting married, Kama Dave?" she teases.

"Yes," he says. "I have forty-eight marriage proposals."

"Oh," I don't know what to say.

"Ask me."

"Who are you going to marry?" I ask.

"No," he demands angrily. "Ask me nicely."

Bran is looking at me with her eyebrows raised. "Ask him, Nicky," she suggests.

"What? What?" I'm getting disturbed and want to cry. Brandy puts her hands together and rolls her eyes like she's praying as a clue.

"Oh! Kama Dave, will you marry me?"

"No," he says and he breaks into a sweet smile, laughing with delight.

"Too bad," I say. "Who are you going to marry then?" He frowns.

"No. No. Ask me again."

"Will you marry me, baby?" I try.

He laughs with a snarl, "NO!"

Brandy can see my pain and frustration and she says, "Nicky, he wants to hear you say that over and over again. If he says yes, you won't ask him again. Understand?"

"No! Is he playing with me?"

"Yes!" Dave laughs. "I'm playing with you. Consensual submission. Sexual games. Ask me nicely, Nicky."

"Will you marry me, baby?"

"NO!" he roars with laughter.

"Oh, you sick fuck," S&M laughs. "You little pervert!" Then he looks at me and says, "Nicky, on your knees."

"What? Oh, hell." I kneel down next to the bed and put my head down and say softly, "Honey, cherry jam, sugar, will you marry me?"

"No," he purrs this time. He's getting aroused. I can tell. He strokes the top of my head softly. He's playing me hard now but he's so happy, I don't mind. I'm even amused now that I know the rules of the game.

"Please marry me?" He just shakes his head now and smiles at me. He's looking deep into my eyes and he takes my hand and puts it on his heart.

"Nicky?" he whispers. "I'm waiting."

S&M breaks it up. "How long does this game go on, Sri Dev?"

"As long as it takes, Nim," he smiles innocently. "As long as she'll play."

"It's your bedtime now. Can you finish this up tomorrow?"

"I can finish it any day, Nim. What time can you play, Nicky? I get up early."

I look at S&M and shake my head sadly. He winks and nods his head 'yes'.

"Call me when you're ready to play, baby Dave," I say and then I kiss him softly on his sweet twisted perverted lips. "Call me as early as you want, sugar."

He purrs, "No."

"Sri Kamadev," S&M tells him kindly, "Nicky can stay until you fall asleep but the game has to end now. You have to get your rest. You can dream about her, okay?"

"I'll dream about her, okay."

Brandy gives him a shot of his anti-psychotics and puts the eye pillow on his face. His lips are wide with a smile and I imagine he's counting all the marriage proposals he's had tonight. He'll dream about me all right.

I sit in the chair and watch him until we hear soft snores. S&M points to the door. He walks me back to the Fire House under the evening stars.

"A barrel of laughs, isn't he?" he sighs. "Tell me. What's going to happen when you ask him 99 times and he finally says 'yes'?"

"When or if he says 'yes'? I wouldn't ask him even once if I didn't want to. He's the most beautiful twisted little thing I've ever seen. I could have a lot of fun with him. We could adopt a couple of nine-year old street punks who look like our teacher. Do you think he's going to go to prison?"

"No," he says, and he puts his arm around me. "He's going to get better and he's going to be a very happy man."

He walks me to the door and gives me a soft kiss. He picks a little piece of jasmine from the pot on the porch and tucks it behind my ear.

"Sweet dreams, Nicky," he whispers. "The whole universe revolves around you."

†

S&M

Before the sun even thinks of showing its face, I'm out on the yoga deck daring it to fuck with me. This morning my practice is simple: sitting in padmasana, lotus position, setting an intention and releasing it to the universe. My intention is crystal clear. I need my bed back, I need my wife back, and I need my house back.

As much as I love that boy, I need to kick him out. I watch the stars fade until there's none left but one and then I close my eyes. I envision my bed with nothing in it but Brandy and nothing on her but a suntan. I set that intention and then I breathe it all out and let it go.

By the time the sun comes up, I'm crashed on the futon catching a few more snores before I unleash the power of Shiva and reorganize Sunrise Wellbeing Inc. I'm burning.

Brandy is curled around Dave and I nudge her shoulder gently. She opens her eyes and I put my finger to my lips. I point to Dave and then signal with my thumb and fingers against my inner arm: shoot him. I need a head start and he should be sedated for what I've got planned.

The lawn is wet and the birds are singing little Kapha tunes as I stroll over to the Fire House with my best porn star gait. I'm watching myself picking up the imploded shrapnel of my life.

Nat is already up in the kitchen. I give her a kiss on the forehead and ask her to make me a tray of croissants with jam and eggs to go for four. I promise I'll talk to her later. Then I go up the stairs and rap on Dave's door. After a minute, Nicky opens dressed in her corporate issue saffron silk kimono.

"Games already?" she yawns.

"Yep. New rules today. Are you ready to play? Meet me in the kitchen in ten and I'll explain on the way over."

Brandy is up and dressed when I get back with the tray and Dave is nodding in and out, half asleep, but when he sees us, he sits up in bed and grins.

"Nim and Nick! Good morning!"

Nicky sets the tray down on the bedside table and Dave's eyes light up when he sees his favorite breakfast foods with a side order of hospital restraining cuffs. His mouth drops open in awe and he pants like a hungry dog.

I just smile at Bran and she gets the tea. Nicky sits down on the bed and whispers in Dave's ear. He blushes and shakes his head furiously, laughing. Game on. Nicky puts one of the cuffs on his wrist, attaches the other to the bed headboard and proceeds to smear jam on the croissant and feed him. After each bite, she whispers another sweet proposition in his ear and he laughs and spits tea and shakes his head.

I give Brandy the chair and sit on the other side of the bed chewing on a croissant. "Today, my little brother, I'm going to take you for a walk and then later on, I'm going to teach you and Prince Albert how to fight. How does that sound?"

Brandy gasps. "Sim! No!"

I give her a sharp glare. "*They* are not going to fight. They're going to learn." And then I mutter some horrible curses under my breath about lack of respect and trust.

"Yeah!" Dave says. "Cool!"

I shovel eggs in my mouth and shoot daggers at Brandy until she blushes and laughs. "You, my dear wife, have the day off today. Unless you want to learn how to fight, too, in which case you can meet us at the gym around – uh, let's see. I think 4pm is a damn good time to fight. Peak Vata time.

"Dave?" I ask, "Can you shower by yourself? Are you good to stand up or do you need a nurse?"

"Nicky?" he asks.

"Not a choice," I command. "By yourself or have a nurse help. Otherwise you'll be in there for three hours."

"I can do it, Nim," he says. Nicky unleashes him and helps him to his feet and he heads for the shower.

"We're just going to take him for walk, Bran. Nicky can play with him while I take care of business. Whether she wants to play infinite propositions and proposals or teach him Sanskrit, I don't care. Just so he feels safe again.

"How'd this wedding cake game start anyway?"

She blushes and looks at Nick wondering if she wants to say it and then she spits it out. "He said sex is better with her because her heart is made out of cake."

"The creative little pervert amazes me," S&M laughs. "Don't let that innocent act fool you. He doesn't miss a beat. This isn't a psychotic game, Brandy. It's a 5th chakra sadomasochistic game. The really kinky stuff isn't done with whips and chains and clamps; that's so fucking Victorian. It's done with hearts and minds."

"I don't understand, Sim."

"Nah, you wouldn't. The subtler it is the less obvious. He wants the cake. If he just smacked her around until he got it or tried to take it away from her, it would be pretty low level. But if he plays it from a higher frequency he'll have her heart served to him on a silver plate. He knows what he's doing."

"I'm still drawing a blank, guys. I don't play these kind of games."

"Of coure you do, Brandy," Nicky offers. "All humans do. Have you studied yoga at all? A little? All you need to know to understand human nature are the basic tenets. It's very simple.

"Suffering is caused by ignorance, by not understanding where pain and pleasure come from. Pain and pleasure are two sides of the same coin, aversion and desire.

"Both can cause you to suffer. You get what you don't want; you don't get what you do want. Even if you get what you want, it's painful because nothing lasts.

"Pain and pleasure, fear and desire, and the subtler expressions: telling and asking. At a little more extreme is commanding and begging.

"That's what baby Dave is up to. Commanding that I beg. And oh, I will play. I like to play. It's more evolutionary than most relationships. Dave had a good teacher. One of your husband's big kinks, by the way, is that he loves to be begged. Try it. You can get almost anything you desire."

"Nick!" I scold, but I'm proud of her. I've got my feet up on my bed drinking tea and Nicky's training my wife for me. It's a piece of cake I muse.

Dave comes back in the room sparkling clean and distraught.

"I haven't got any jewelry," he moans. "Sean took my handcuff key!"

"Poor suffering boy," Brandy says. "Take mine."

†

DJ

Nim and Nick take me past the pool house, out into the sunshine. My legs scream with pleasure. We're due for legs and back. Our chest and arms are done. I remember imploding in the gym and then she pulled the oranges apart and sunk her teeth into the wedges and said, wait, I'm worth the wait. Shit. Here is the trail and I stop. I won't go.

She takes my hand and says come on, honey, but I won't. Nim stops and puts his arm on my shoulder.

"No, I can't go off the grounds, Nim. No."

He smiles. "Breathe, Kamadev," he purrs. "Through your mouth this time. Can you taste the forest?"

"It tastes like a grave," I say. "I don't like it. Let's go home."

"Nicky, go ahead, we'll meet you down at the grove," he says and she leaves us, disappearing down the trail. Oh, Nicky don't go, it's so dark down there underground.

"How's your list, Dev? Do you remember? I know you do, you little fucker, you don't miss a thing. Breathe. I'll give you another list. It's okay to go off the grounds with me or Nick or Brandy. It's very bad to go down there with Jain or Nat or by yourself.

"But there's nothing bad down there, it's beautiful. The only thing to fear is here."

He taps my third eye.

"There's a beautiful woman down there who wants to play consensual games with you. Do you trust me to take you down?"

When he puts it that way, and I know there's cake in the forest, I want to go.

"I'll go, Nim."

And then the forest becomes enchanted again. The rhododendrons don't drip blood; they drip with cherry jam. The smell of earth and pine and honeysuckle and jasmine start to wrap their fingers through my hair.

She says, Good boy, when she sees me coming down the trail. What can I do for you, beautiful boy? She's sitting on the forest floor on soft pine needles, barefoot with her beautiful broken toes wiggling in the sunlight. She shines like an angel. I turn to see what Nim says but he's walking back up the trail.

"I've got work to do, honey," he calls. "Take the paint off."

†

MACK

I've been waiting for him to show up and drop the other shoe, so I'm not surprised when he knocks on the office door. "Good morning, brother," I say and then I add, "I'm clean." But I'm not ready for where he goes next.

"Cool. Hey, Mack, did you ever have a kid when you were younger, I mean really young before you knew any better?"

"No," I say. "I knew better. Our parents were still alive when I was young.

"Are you sure? I mean if you had a kid when you were 15, he'd be Dave's age now. I know 15 is awful young and I didn't have any kids until I was 18 but he looks so fucking like me, I swear brother, he could be your son. My nephew. Just saying."

"What the fuck are you talking about?" I swear back.

"So no chance you had unprotected sex when you were 14 or so? I guess not. Well he can't be mine because I know I didn't father any kids when I was 7. I'm pretty sure of that."

"Well, I'm damn sure I don't have any 21-year old kids," I huff. "When I was 14 the only thing I knew how to do with girls was pull their hair."

He sits on the leather couch and puts his bare feet up on the table and broods. The soles of his feet are dusted with forest floor, soft peat and crushed pine.

"You've got kids?" I manage to choke out.

"Just between you and me? There may be a hundred or so bastards. I might need a legal team. But so far, it's just fan mail, no threats," he laughs and the laughter dies into deep panting like he's lost his breath.

"Uh, sorry. Just tripping a little, lots of stress. Can you get Sunny in here?"

"I'm really not sure I want to," I say.

"And I am really sure you do. She's the executive assistant for the board and I want to execute."

He draws himself up like a big cat and pulls his feet under him cross-legged, getting dirt on the couch but I say nothing. I pick up the phone and ask Sunny to come down.

"Sunshine, thank you for making that party a hit yesterday," he smiles. "Everyone was blown away. When Prince is better, I won't impose on you like that."

She beams at him, "No problem, Sim. What else can I do?"

"Simple stuff today. I want a legal document drawn up to amend the board rules stating that all prescriptive drugs dispensed by any physicians at Sunrise must be monitored and authorized by you. See that Sean gets a copy as a member of the screening committee. That's it."

She blushes. I nod. Fair enough. I need boundaries.

"Also just wondering if we've got all the legal documentation for Dave."

I push a file across the desk and he opens it. I know it sparkles. Jain worked on it for ten hours and Sean wrote a brilliant personal recommendation. We even have a statement from Prince Albert on the condition of his 5th amendment rights that Dave was not involved in the sale of illicit drugs for financial profit. He just rented the house.

He smirks at it. "What does Sean say?"

"He says it's going to be no contest. He's already talked to the judge and he's willing to grant probation under the terms we proposed for rehabilitation. Probably six months up here with supervised leave."

"Fair enough."

"How is he, by the way?"

"Right now? I don't think he's feeling any pain."

He stares at me. There's an elephant waiting in the room.

"Jain is sorry," I add.

"Not yet, he isn't. Would you tell him to meet us at the gym at 4 for training? And ask him not to wear anything nice, okay?"

†

NICK

His royal haughtiness is frozen in his tracks on the forest trail standing in the sunny spotlight that sneaks through the treetops. I feel his fear, excitement, confusion, and delight refusing to mix into anything palatable, curdling and separating like cheese and whey. He could go in any direction.

I reach my hand out and he takes the last few steps until he's looking down at me. The commanding tantrums and pretentious cockiness have softened into something like wonder.

I take his hand and pull it down so I can kiss the pretty little Omkara tattoo on his knuckles, then I put his hand on the crown of my head. I draw on the river of sexual desire and pure love that starts in my toes and send it spiraling upwards through the top of my head into his hand so that it floods into him.

"Oh fucking yes!" he moans.

"I can't hear you, baby," I tease. "What did you say?"

"Yes! Yes! Yes!"

"Then ask me nicely."

"Nicky, will you marry me?" he whispers.

"No," I tease. "Aren't you going to beg?"

"Yes," he says. "I'm begging you, Nicky. I'm begging you with my body, my heart and my soul."

"Alright then, yes. What kind of cake would you like Prince Albert to make for our wedding?"

"Carrot cake please, Nicky. I love carrot cake. I always did."

"Good boy," I say pulling him down into the dirt and pine needles, because the prisoner is really the one who is the object of desire. Great prisons have been built just to contain the prisoner and the only purpose of the jailer is to guard her.

†

S&M

So it's Kama Dave and Nicky, Prince Albert, Nat, Brandy and me sitting on the lawn waiting nicely at 4pm for Jain to show up for fight lessons. We see him dragging his feet, looking a bit sheepish and I've already got him beat.

"First thing, class, it's always a bad idea to fight out of anger. It's much more fun to fight with your friends. And second, there's a big difference between fighting and beating some one up."

I give Prince a little apologetic nod and then I get up to give Jain a hug before I bury him.

"Most of you have been studying human engineering with me, the rest of you, listen and learn. Everything you do is either evolutionary or not. Same goes for fighting."

"Fighting?" Jain wonders. "I thought we were going to train."

"Well, kind of. A different training exercise today, buddy. I'm going to teach them how to fight."

Jain groans but I can't be deterred. I continue with the class.

"Evolutionary fighting means you are using more than your body. You're using your prana, mind, heart and soul. I'm going to teach you how to elevate fighting to the highest level, like anything you do, including sex," I wink at Dev, "by using your higher consciousness based on the chakra model.

"The fight starts before it begins. Starting at the root chakra, fight or flight, is the awareness that every choice has consequences. It's just a brawl if you don't take it to a higher level.

"At the second chakra there should be an effortless, unerring right choice. Then, based on your present moment awareness, at the third level is your intention. Are you with me so far?

"At the heart, the fourth level, is the energy of give and take. A good fight has got to be an exchange. Fifth chakra energy is detachment from the outcome, being flexible and accepting uncertainty – even though I know once I'm fighting at this level I cannot lose. And that's the sixth chakra, confidence, because I know when my foundation is balanced I've got an impeccable purpose.

"After that, anything goes, everything is pure potential. Your true self is beyond the ego's need for approval, power and control. Game on, brother."

Jain's mouth is hanging wide open, speechless. Then he shakes his head and says, "I don't want to fight you, Sim. I don't want to hurt you."

"Oh, you can't hurt me, brother. I never lose because I pick my fights. I'm picking this one, not out of anger but purely for educational purposes."

"Fight!" Dave cheers.

"I can't fight by myself, Jain," I whine. "It has to be an exchange. You owe me."

I give him a few love taps on his shoulder to pique his interest. "Pretty please," I tease. He pulls a little punch to my chest and I kick him in the ribs nicely. His face goes dark and I know now he's fighting from the lowest level. He hasn't thought it out and he hasn't got a good reason or purpose to fight me.

He hits me really hard this time and knocks me flat. Nice! I pop back up like a weighted pin and smack him in the face so fast it stuns him. He's a really big guy but he never has to fight in the hospital. He hasn't got fight. No one would want to give him a go after they took a look at all that muscle.

Me, I grew up scrapping with anybody who wanted to go to the beach, short ones, tall ones, big ones, bad ones, armed ones, dangerous ones, fast ones, and ones who never showed their faces again.

My favorite fights though were with Darrell and Sean. Sean's older now but he's got some serious moves and Sean taught me everything he knows. Darrell was dead serious, too, even though it was for fun, but now he's just plain dead. I land a couple more to the body and kick him in the ribs again, trying not to break anything.

He's so pissed off at that he breaks my nose and flattens me. I'm lying there looking up at the sky and laughing with the taste of blood in my mouth and he says, "Give up, Sim. I don't want to hurt you."

"You're joking," I laugh. "I'm way ahead on points. I do not lose."

I jump up and show him how Darrell does it, ring style, jabs and upper cuts and hooks and he smacks me again like a giant trying to squash an annoying fly. He splits my lip and it hurts my teeth. I wink at Dave. He's grinning enormously at the gratuitous blood flow.

I hold a hand up for a pause and turn to the class and count off on my fingers.

"One. Consequences. Two. Unerring choice. Three. Intention. Four. Give and Take." I point to my broken nose and laugh when I say 'Take'.

"Five. Flexibility. Six. Confidence." I laugh and turn back to Jain.

He's shaking his head. But I'm nodding my beautiful bleeding head, snarling.

"Come on, honey. Come fucking on to me," I tease.

He takes a wild swing and I duck under it and plough into his solar plexus and hear, 'Ooofff. Ooofffuck!' And the crowd goes wild.

"One for Dave," I tease. "Can I get you anything else, sir?"

He's bent over with his hands on his thighs. There's not a drop of blood on him, but I can see he's done.

"No thanks," he smiles. "I don't have any room for dessert."

I take a bow to the class and Jain laughs, "Sim, you may have won but no one could tell by looking at you. You look like a train wreck, brother."

I'm bloody, but I feel phenomenal, like I've just straightened out the cosmic slate and balanced the karmic checkbook. I wish Billy would've been here to see it, but I know he'll hear about it for a long, long time. I know Darrell is kicking over it in his grave.

Jain sucks some big breaths of air and then walks over to the side where the class is sitting cross-legged. He puts his hand out to Dave, pulls him to his feet and hugs him.

"I am so sorry, man," he says. "I was so fucked. I thought I killed you, baby brother. How can I ever make it up to you."

Dave smiles sweetly. He's got the lead in a movie of his own creation, engaged to the Tantric sex goddess breathing down his neck. He's excited by all the blood, and he's probably forgiven Jain on the basis of entertainment value alone, but he looks thoughtfully at his bodyguard.

"Ask me nicely," he suggests.

"Will you forgive me, Dave?"

"No!" he roars with laughter.

Jain looks crestfallen, but as he turns to walk away, Dave yells.

"No! Wait! Dr. Jain! Ask me again!"

I sink down flat on my back on the lawn. It's a good view looking up at the early evening sky, a blank blue canvas without a single star. The silver crescent moon slices the western horizon with the 'dot' of the evening planet on its heels, like the embellishment of the Omkara. The crescent is the curtain of Maya behind which the dot of infinite truth continually manifests.

I lick the blood on my lips and think of my big empty bed. I've got it back. Everything is perfect just as it is. Brandy leans over to take a look at my bloody smile and kisses me on my split lip.

"Are you okay, Sim?" she whispers.

"No, baby," I growl. "I need a nurse."

EPILOGUE

"The Earth would die if the Sun stopped kissing her."
~ Hafiz

†

BABY

"Pass on that, Roger," I say with a smirk, not taking my eyes off Highway 1. "It used to be a sweet spot but it's a hole now. I haven't got any patience for vicious locals guarding a wimpy little reef point break. Punch outs and murders, guys getting shot and shot up, heroin dealers on the beach. It's not my cup of tea.

"Let's just give it pass and get to Big Sur before dark."

"Oh, come on, Baby," he begs. "Please do it for me. I grew up surfing there. No punks or gangsters are going to hassle me. I'll just run the fuck over all of them. Please, Baby."

I take my eyes off the road just long enough to see how sincere he is about this. He looks like a lost dog begging for a pat on the head. He's got his sweet little pirate patch over his right eye where the board sliced it. He doesn't really need it, but he's so vain about the scar. He likes the way the patch intimidates people and it lets him rest his eye. He's pouting.

"Please, Baby, with sugar on it. Just a quick peek."

I'm a sucker for beggars. But I also know that sometimes stories are blown up fantasies designed to keep the timid away from an over-crowded sweet spot. You never know if you don't go.

I remember the time I swam out to the 'vicious local' break, the Pass, at Byron Bay and a longboarder shot his board to me so I could take a turn. It was September 11th and we were too blessed by swell to know about the horrors on the other side of the planet.

So I turn off on the exit and drive through town to the beach cliff drive just for the hell of it. And really because – just as I expected – as soon as I do Roger starts bouncing up and down on his seat like a little boy on Christmas morning.

"Fucking right!" he sings. "Surfing the Point!"

I can see a nice clean swell when we pass the main beach and a lot of kids are in the water. Just past the city beach, there's a ribbon across the road but Rog says fuck it, road closures never pertain to surfers, so we drive through it. I've done worse criminal perversions in the search for surf.

And then around the bend I see the beautiful point break, empty filthy waves sucking me, drawing me like my mother's breast. And oh my, there is nobody in the water surfing!

But the cliff is lined with police cars, a fire truck, beach rescue jet skis, a news van, and swarming with people. Kids are skateboarding in the middle of the street.

"Sorry," Roger concedes, "Maybe I should listen to you occasionally, Baby."

I stop abruptly next to all the cop cars to avoid running over a tall dark man standing in the road watching the swell. His wetsuit is half off, pulled so gratuitously low that I can see where his hard belly ends and his pubic hair begins.

He turns and grins at me like he wants to bite my head off. Then he puts both hands on the hood of my van so I'll have to run him over or pay whatever toll he's extracting.

"I'll take care of this, Baby," Roger growls but before he can open the door, a blond guy sticks his head in my window and checks out the interior, camping gear and boards.

"Sweet wagon, sister," he whistles. "I bet you'd like what I could do in trade for a ride in this, honey."

I recognize him, Billy Lee, former surf star who was suspended for heroin. Oh, I was so right about giving it a pass, I think. I stare at Roger and shake my head but when I look back, the half-naked guy has pulled Billy by the back of his hair out of my window and now his nose is inches away from mine.

He's fucking beautiful, if not a mad man. His eyes glow like blue gunmetal.

"Nice of you to come," he smirks. "Of course you know the road is closed, but here you are, just in time."

"Look, we'll just be out of here if you don't mind. I think we made a wrong turn," I grovel.

"Oh, no," he laughs "No such thing. You're here aren't you? And just in time for the finals. It's supposed to be an hour final but I can polish it off in 15 minutes if you like and then the waves are all yours, beautiful. You can't leave now. The road is closed."

I'm speechless. I halfway think he's fucking with me, but he continues.

"It's going to be mad, an 8-man final! Really its 7 men and 1 babe but who's counting. It's just a community fundraiser to clean up our neighborhood. If you want to be a sponsor, it's only $20,000. But we'll let you surf here anyway. Pull in."

There's no place to park and I can see a police officer approaching my van.

"Just leave it right there in the road for now," he says with an easy smile. "Be my guest. When it's over you can take one of the spots the police cars are hogging. Premium parking. It's your lucky day."

He puts his arm around the guy's naked shoulders, puts his cop hat on his wet hair and walks back to the cliff.

The mad guy opens my door and with a sweeping bow invites me to step out. "What's your name, baby?" he asks.

"Um, Baby," I say because nobody calls me by my real name whatever that used to be.

"Nice to meet you, Baby," he says. "You can call me S&M."

I shrug and smile at Roger and step into the street. As I follow S&M to the edge of the cliff I'm shocked by the road map of scars and stitches and tortured skin stretched across the beautiful carved muscles of his back.

"You've met Billy," he grins. "This is the rest of my team, Kama Dave Dixon and Nicky Dixon."

Nicky smiles without taking her hands off the younger guy; she's got her arms wrapped around him like she's trying to keep his feet on the earth. He's bouncing off the walls with joy, watching the empty waves.

"We're winning!" he howls. "We cannot lose, Nim!"

They all scramble down the cliff where four other competitors are waiting down on the beach with a beautiful array of boards, long boards, short boards and a couple mini-mals. We watch them paddle out to the peak and, even before the hooter sounds, they're jockeying for position dominating the reef. It looks like a brawl.

One of the surfers takes off wide and scores a lovely perfect peak alone, but I can see the rest of the pack is in trouble. Billy and S&M are blocking any hope of a wave for their opponents as first Kama Dave and then Nicky get set waves.

S&M paddles across the path of the remaining three surfers as Billy takes off, and then finishes up by dropping in deep behind the peak on the last set wave, howling loud enough to raise the dead.

His team just scored four consecutive solid rides – and then I guess it's over because they all paddle in. What the fuck just happened there, I wonder? That was only one set. S&M climbs up the cliff laughing maniacally while the rest of the crew is down on the beach, shaking hands and slapping backs.

He comes up and puts his dripping wet arm around me and purrs. Roger bristles a little, but I don't mind. He smells like seaweed and salt.

"Go for it, Baby!" he grins. "It's all yours!" He kisses me on the cheek with a loud smack.

"What happened there, S&M?" I wonder. "It didn't look like much of a contest at all!"

"Oh, that? That was just the frosting, sugar. The real contest was getting here."

†††

Acknowledgements:

Original cover art by Vincent Stephens **https://www.facebook.com/RamStar**

Hafiz quotations from "The Gift", translations by Daniel Ladinsky

"Can't Get Next to You" lyrics by Norman Whitfield and Barrett Strong

Sanskrit mantra translations by NJ Travis

Botanical blends and medicinal properties are derived from the work of master alchemist and teacher, David Crow of Floracopeia, available at **http://bit.ly/YwBL83**

Much love to David Simon, M.D. co-founder of the Chopra Center for Wellbeing for his Ayurveda and alternative medicine teachings. **http://bit.ly/ZEJLL3**

Thank you to my colleague and friend, Jessica Winston, yoga and meditation teacher and marketing guru, for her thoughtful editing and encouragement.

Thanks to the Bihar School of Yoga and Swami Satyananda Saraswati for warning me not try Tantra at home! I should've known better.